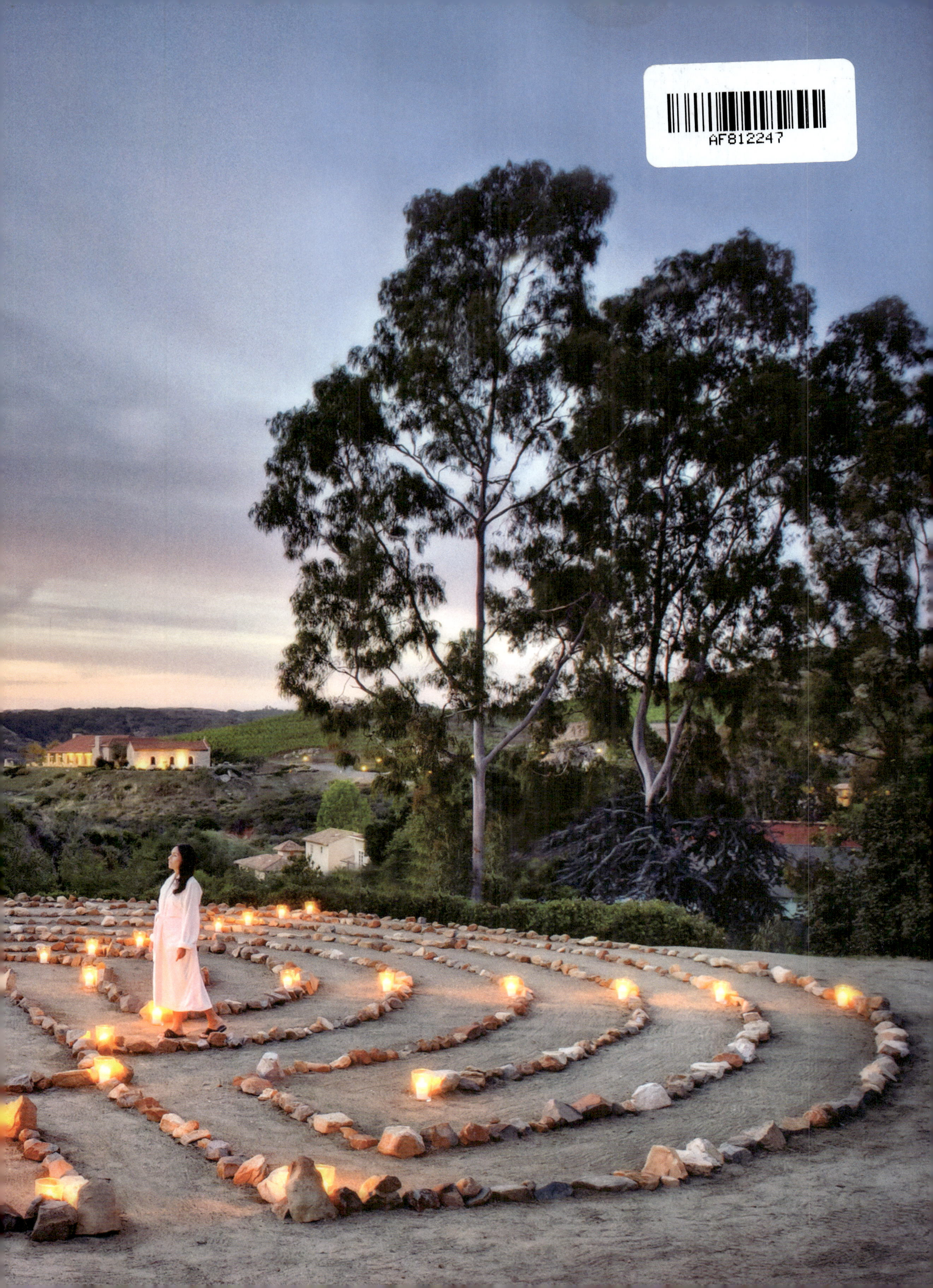

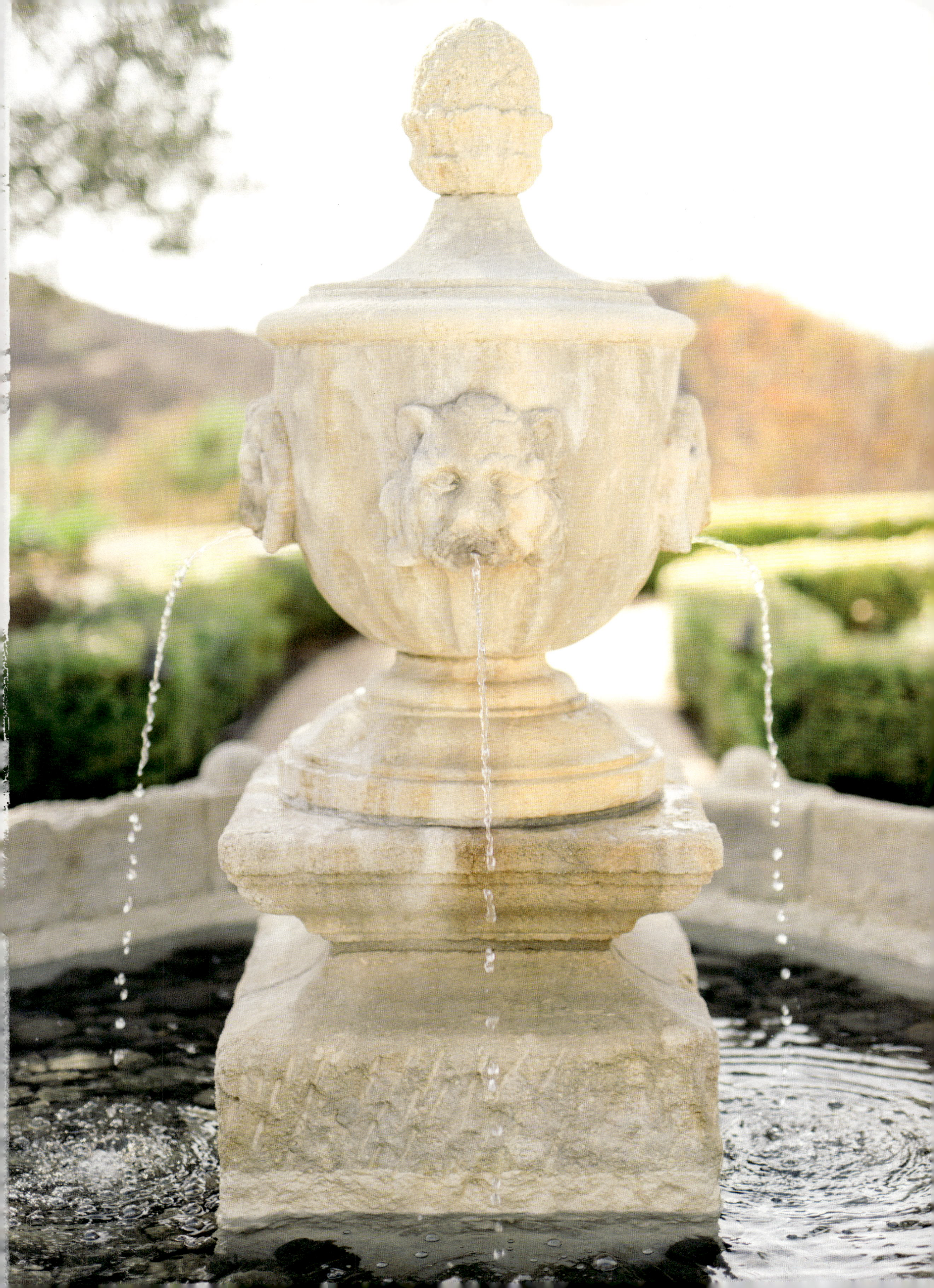

Beautiful Living: Cooking the Cal-a-Vie Health Spa Way

Published by Cal-a-Vie Health Spa
Owners: Terri and John Havens

Website: www.Cal-a-Vie.com
First Printing: November 2019

ISBN: 978-0-9766222-1-5
Library of Congress Number: Pending

Printed in the United States of America by Bayside Printing Company, Inc.

Author: Terri Havens
Book Production Manager, Research and Writing: Roni Atnipp
Cover and Layout Design: Elise DeSilva - Limb Design
Writer: Doug Williams

Photography
Food: Debora Smail
Cover: Anne Watson
Cal-a-Vie location: Max Kim-Bee
Contributors: Brian Leahy, Berra Walsh

Cal-a-Vie Health Spa and Resort
29402 Spa Havens Way
Vista, CA 92084
760-945-2055

In the making of this book, every attempt has been made to verify names and facts. We apologize if any errors have been made.

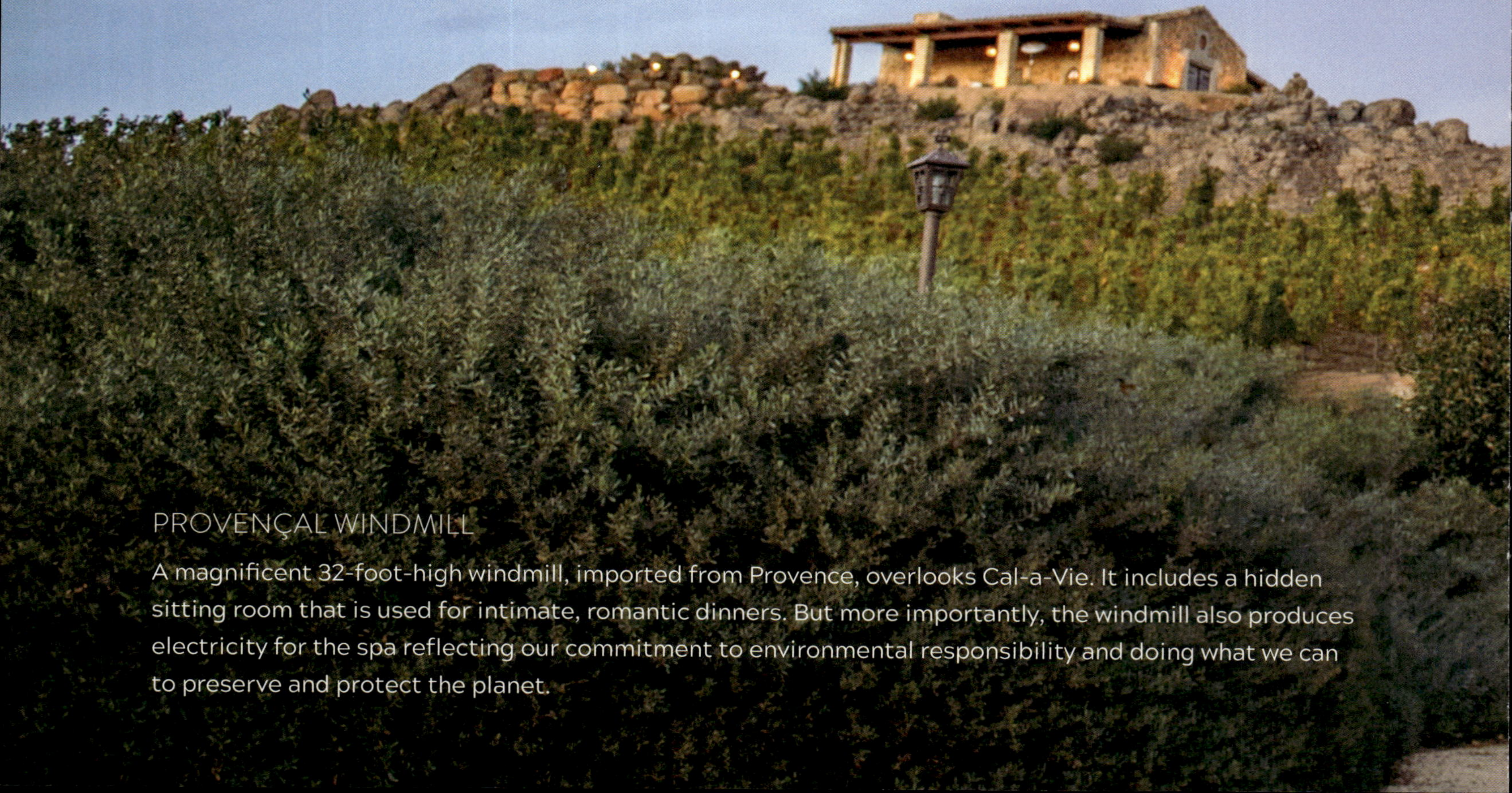

PROVENÇAL WINDMILL

A magnificent 32-foot-high windmill, imported from Provence, overlooks Cal-a-Vie. It includes a hidden sitting room that is used for intimate, romantic dinners. But more importantly, the windmill also produces electricity for the spa reflecting our commitment to environmental responsibility and doing what we can to preserve and protect the planet.

Beautiful Living

COOKING THE CAL-A-VIE HEALTH SPA WAY

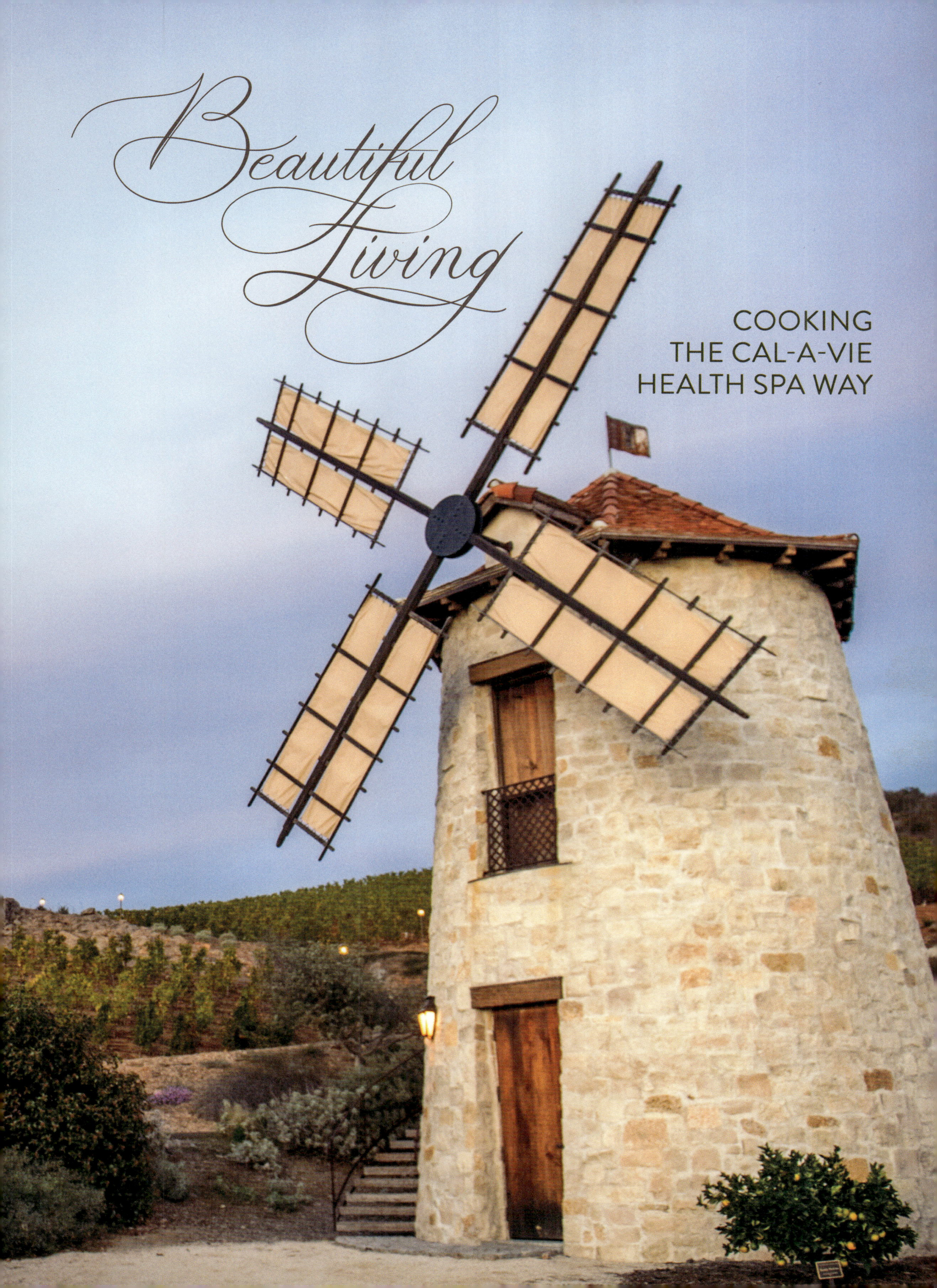

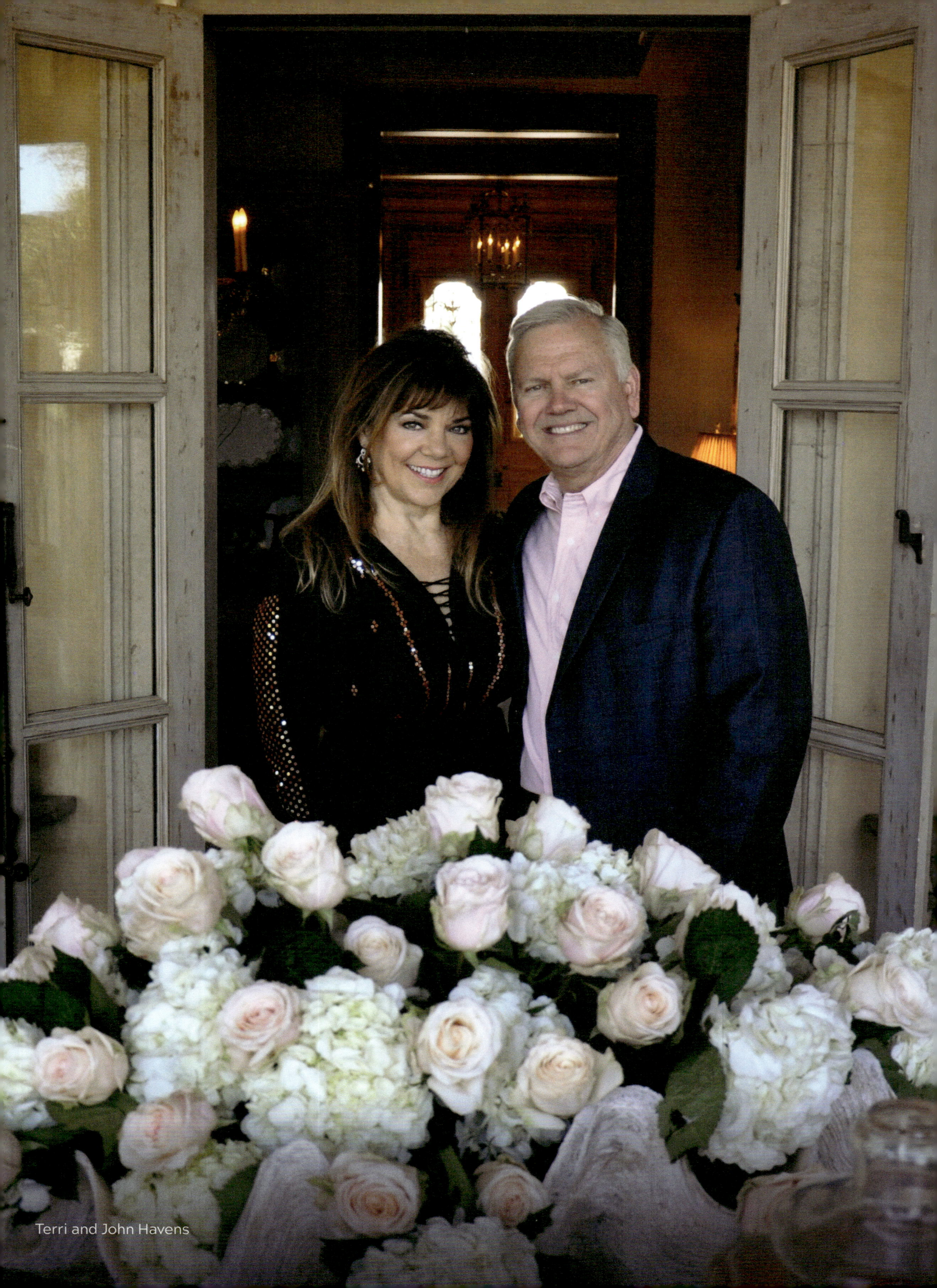
Terri and John Havens

REDEFINING LUXURY

After discovering Cal-a-Vie Health Spa, we had a clear idea of what we wanted the spa to be. We weren't aiming to be best in class. We were aiming to create a destination that produced a new class of its own.

In the years that followed, we feel like we've accomplished that goal, providing our guests with unparalleled opportunities for personal restoration, rejuvenation, and renewal. It's on display everywhere.

You can see it in the 17th-century French-country décor and the world-class, state-of-the-art weight room and exercise pavilion. You can feel it in the customized daily programs, the more than 150 fitness classes, and treatments and therapies that relax the mind and refresh the soul. You can especially taste it in our food, with healthy, savory meals that feature organic fruits and vegetables grown from a farm that is just steps from the kitchen.

That is the Cal-a-Vie Health Spa way: Redefining luxury in every possible way, in every possible detail.

As you look through these pages, we hope that you will experience the same sense of awe, wonder, and pure joy that moved us the first time we saw the retreat. With its European flavor, graceful beauty, romantic ambience, and singular focus on your physical and mental well-being, Cal-a-Vie Health Spa is, truly, a shelter from the rigors and stresses of day-to-day life, and a paradise for the spirit.

Welcome. We hope you enjoy it.

Terri and John Havens

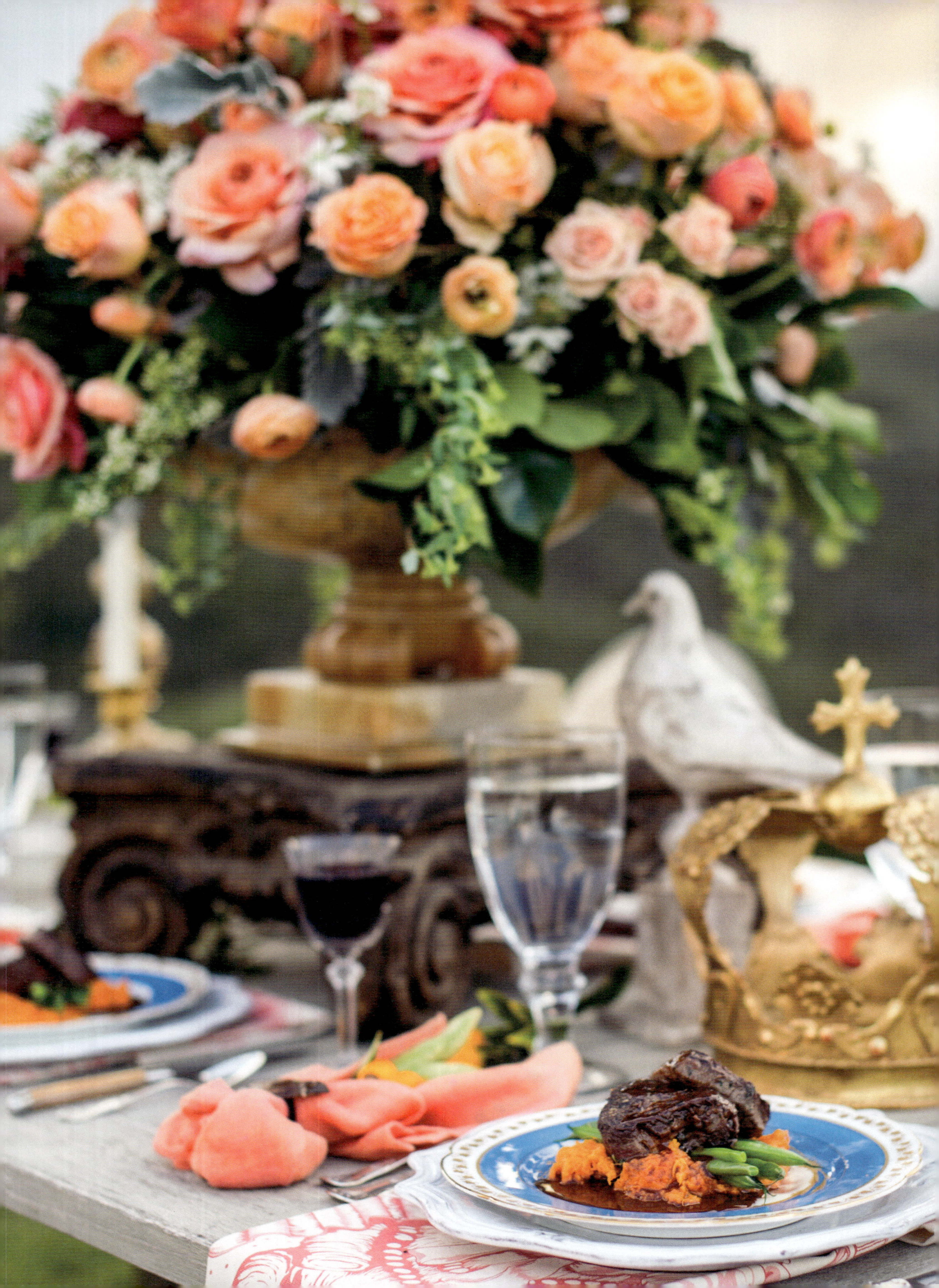

Beautiful Living

TABLE OF CONTENTS

5 FOREWORD LETTER FROM TERRI AND JOHN

8 THE CAL-A-VIE WAY

54 CHAPTER 1 APPETIZERS

78 CHAPTER 2 SOUPS

100 CHAPTER 3 SALADS

126 CHAPTER 4 ENTRÉES

194 CHAPTER 5 SIDES

200 CHAPTER 6 SNACKS AND SMOOTHIES

220 CHAPTER 7 BREAKFASTS

244 CHAPTER 8 DESSERTS

274 NUTRITION RESOURCES

286 ACKNOWLEDGMENTS

293 PHOTOGRAPHY REFERENCE AND INDEX GUIDE

297 INDEX

THE BEGINNING

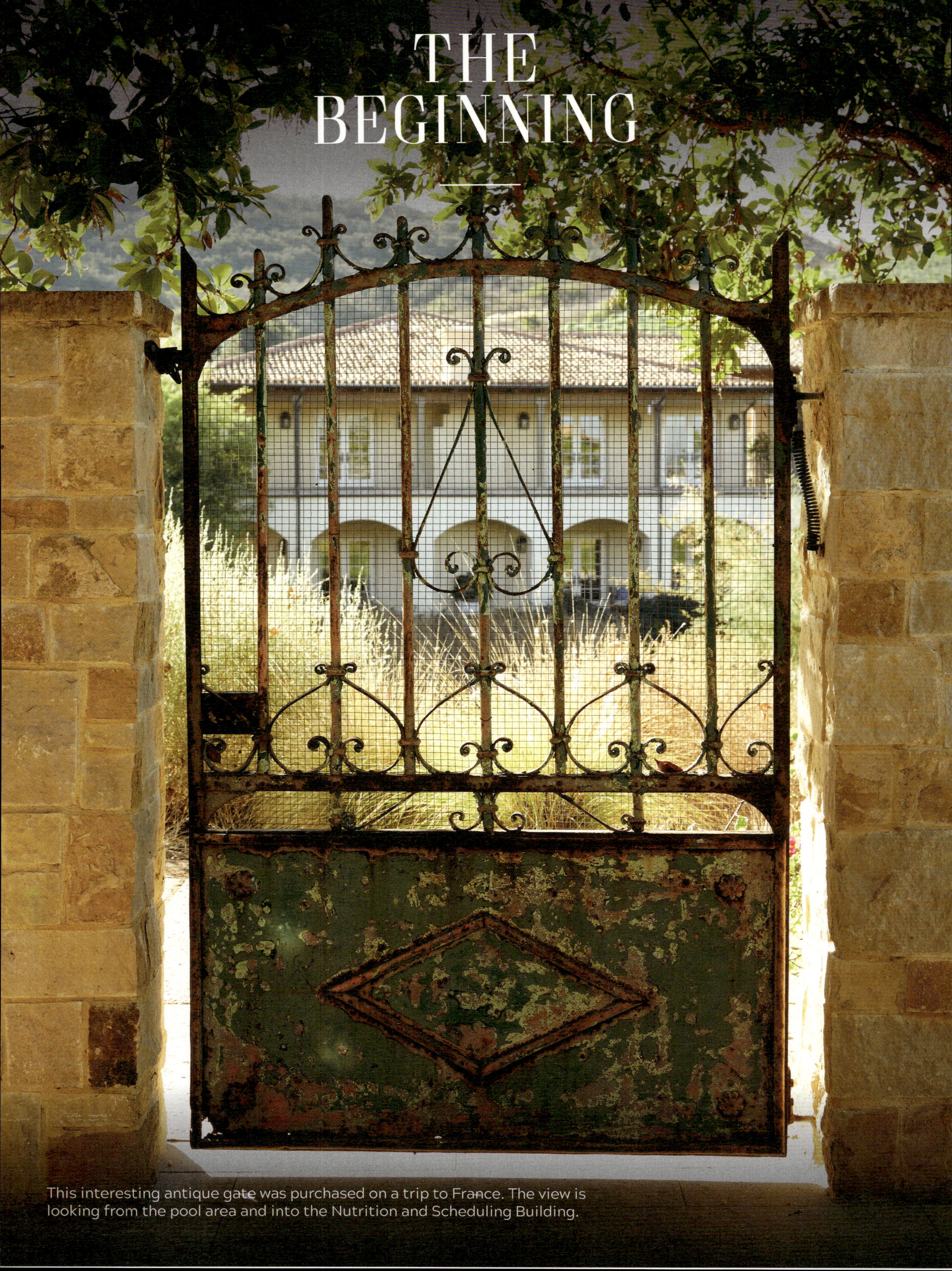

This interesting antique gate was purchased on a trip to France. The view is looking from the pool area and into the Nutrition and Scheduling Building.

OUR LIFE WITH CAL-A-VIE HEALTH SPA STARTED ON THE RUN. LITERALLY.

John was a marathoner, and he was always looking for another city to run in for boredom reasons. It really didn't matter where. If there was a course, and he could fit it into his schedule, he was off to the races. That was fine, but I had kind of a different thought on how we should make the destination decision.

One day, I asked him, "Why don't you run in a city that has a health spa?" I was really into health spas. I read about them constantly and I knew a lot about them, so naturally I wanted to visit the spas that I had studied—and I wanted John to go with me. "Are you kidding me? No way! That's just a bunch of fluff," he exclaimed. That was 35 years ago and men had not quite figured out what spas were all about.

Fine, but I was not going to get brushed off quite that easily. I needed a plan.

After John finished the Houston Marathon in 1994, I surprised him with a gift—a massage set up in our home. I had given him one for Valentine's Day, but he had never used it. This time it would be much more difficult getting out of it if the masseuse came to him. He wasn't thrilled, but being a good guy and a caring husband with a big heart, John humored me and got on the table.

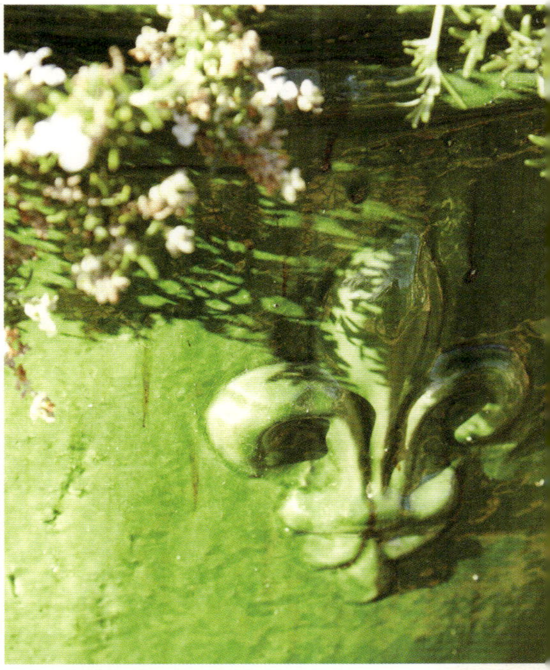

What can I say?

He got the massage, and a whole new world opened up. "What have I been missing all this time?" he asked. We were on our way, his interest totally piqued.

Shortly after that, I sort of conned him into going to a spa in Austin, where he was doing another marathon. Massages were one thing, but spas were something else, and he wasn't exactly wild about the prospect. But he was, after all, a runner, and runners have to be concerned about what they eat, having enough energy, getting enough sleep—just generally taking care of themselves. I didn't think it would be a huge leap for John to go from not being crazy about a spa to loving every second of it.

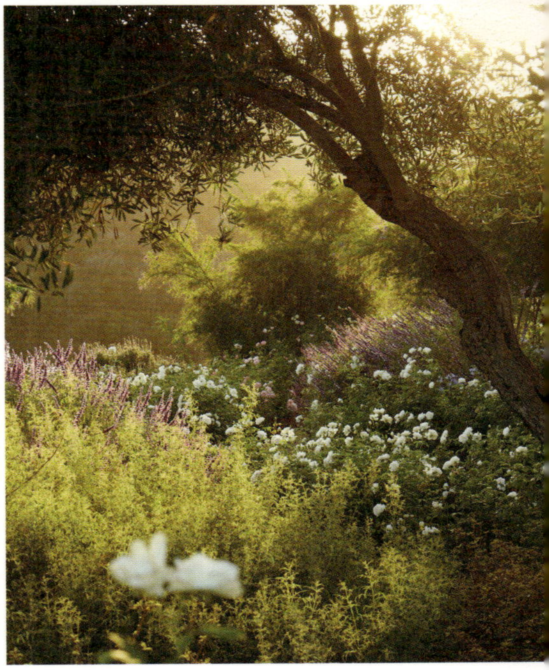

Guess what? I was right. When we walked in the door of that spa, health and wellness was in the air. You could sense it, and John was in awe. At that point, I knew that I had him hooked, and it didn't even bother him that he was the only guy there.

Right after that, we began researching marathons in places that had spas, and we hit as many of them as we could. Eventually, our "tour" headed west, where in 1998, we discovered the inaugural Rock 'N' Roll Marathon in San Diego—but that wasn't all we discovered.

North of the city, on 220 acres of rolling hills in a setting that can only be described as an idyllic haven, was one of the most gorgeous wellness retreats I had ever seen. It was quiet and romantic, far from the stresses of life, tucked into fields of jasmine, oleander, and lavender, kissed by the sun, and looking every bit like a country village in the South of France.

It was called Cal-a-Vie Health Spa.

And all I could think was, Bingo.

"WHAT HAVE I BEEN MISSING ALL THIS TIME?"

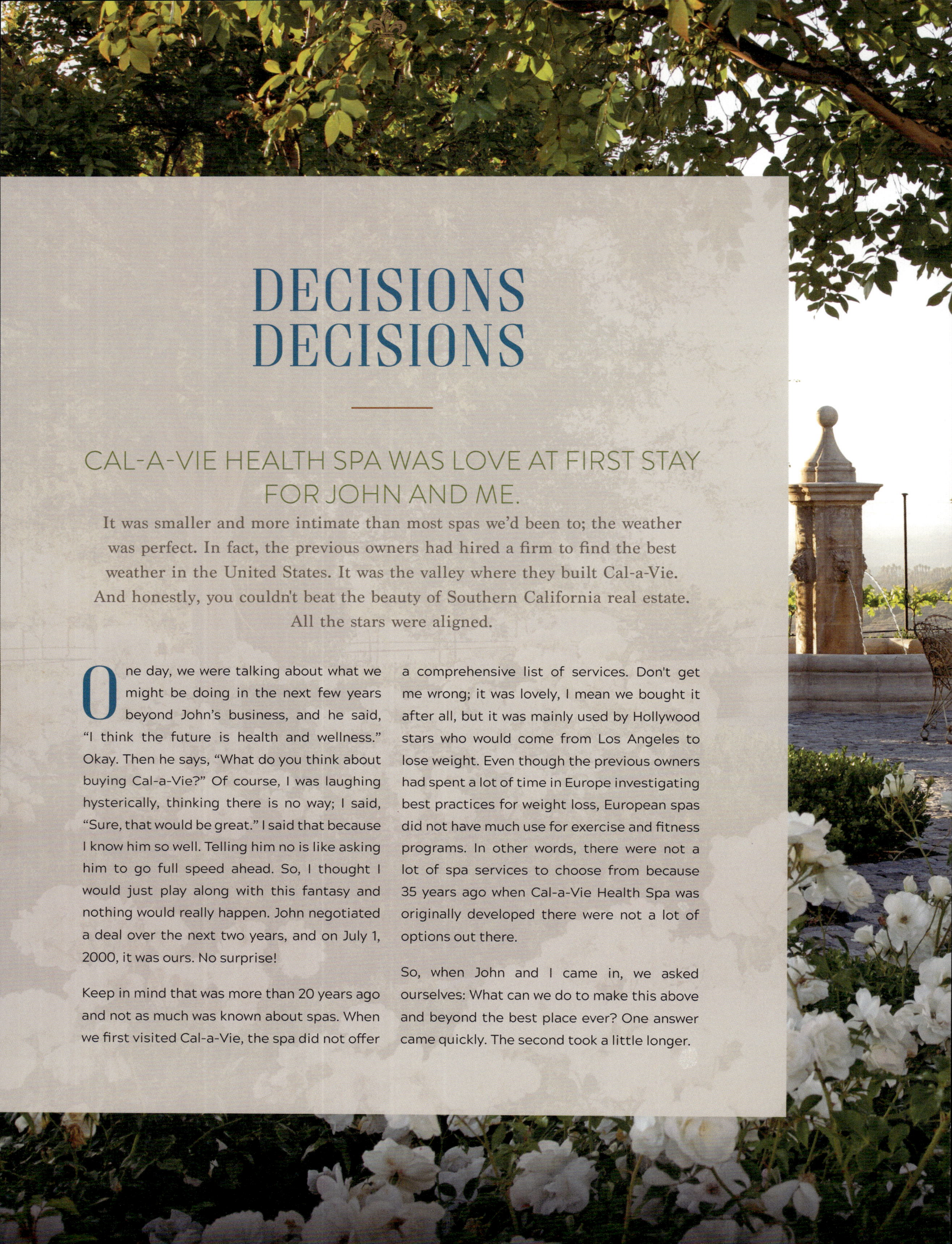

DECISIONS DECISIONS

CAL-A-VIE HEALTH SPA WAS LOVE AT FIRST STAY FOR JOHN AND ME.

It was smaller and more intimate than most spas we'd been to; the weather was perfect. In fact, the previous owners had hired a firm to find the best weather in the United States. It was the valley where they built Cal-a-Vie. And honestly, you couldn't beat the beauty of Southern California real estate. All the stars were aligned.

One day, we were talking about what we might be doing in the next few years beyond John's business, and he said, "I think the future is health and wellness." Okay. Then he says, "What do you think about buying Cal-a-Vie?" Of course, I was laughing hysterically, thinking there is no way; I said, "Sure, that would be great." I said that because I know him so well. Telling him no is like asking him to go full speed ahead. So, I thought I would just play along with this fantasy and nothing would really happen. John negotiated a deal over the next two years, and on July 1, 2000, it was ours. No surprise!

Keep in mind that was more than 20 years ago and not as much was known about spas. When we first visited Cal-a-Vie, the spa did not offer a comprehensive list of services. Don't get me wrong; it was lovely, I mean we bought it after all, but it was mainly used by Hollywood stars who would come from Los Angeles to lose weight. Even though the previous owners had spent a lot of time in Europe investigating best practices for weight loss, European spas did not have much use for exercise and fitness programs. In other words, there were not a lot of spa services to choose from because 35 years ago when Cal-a-Vie Health Spa was originally developed there were not a lot of options out there.

So, when John and I came in, we asked ourselves: What can we do to make this above and beyond the best place ever? One answer came quickly. The second took a little longer.

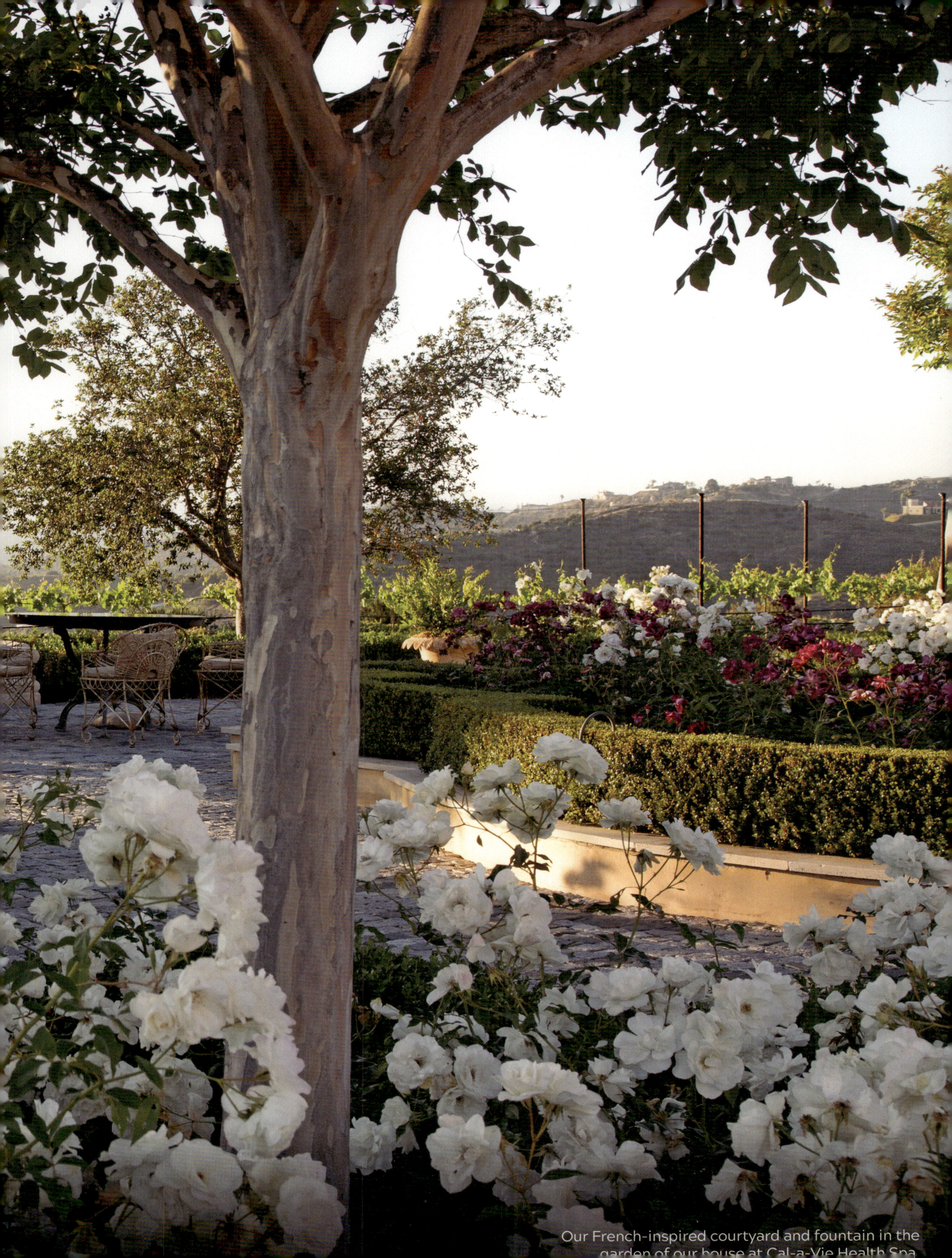

Our French-inspired courtyard and fountain in the garden of our house at Cal-a-Vie Health Spa

RENOVATING FOR

BODY, MIND, SOUL, AND SPIRIT.

WE'RE PROUD AND ADMITTED FRANCOPHILES,

so as we were trying to figure out what direction to take the spa, the first call was a no-brainer: Let's renovate the whole place with the kind of French antiques that we love. We did it slowly, over several years, starting with the rooms.

John and I both agreed that we didn't want Cal-a-Vie Health Spa to look and feel like some big, bland hotel or an institutional spa. I wanted it to be luxurious, an inviting space for the body, mind, soul and spirit. I think in this day and age, when everything is corporate and little is personal, we were looking to create an experience and environment that was not only unique, but also unique to each individual guest.

The rooms reflect that. No two are the same, and every one has at least three antiques. Maybe it's a mirror or a painting, maybe it's a lamp. All the chandeliers are different. We brought the sinks in from Italy and France, and they're really cool. The countertops are marble. The bathrooms are big, with grand tubs surrounded by French Travertine and shower doors with half-inch-thick glass. The walls are Venetian plaster and the king-sized beds have tripled-sheeted Frette linens, memory foam mattresses, and down comforters and pillows. I wanted it to feel like you were in someone's guest bedroom. No expense spared. John didn't quite get that until women kept telling him how they couldn't believe we had Frette sheets on the bed. He had never heard the word Frette before. And 20 years ago mostly women went to spas.

The common areas are just as elegant. You see it the second you walk in. The Pavilion lobby is welcoming—two stories high—with terra cotta flooring from France and a fountain with a nine-foot backsplash with 18th-century tiles from Portugal. Treasures from the 17th and 18th centuries dot the public spaces, including a tapestry that was woven for Louis XIV that hangs in the Great Room.

This was my way of fulfilling my desire for shopping for beautiful things. Once again John went along kicking and screaming. But, once again, he dove in full speed ahead after he saw how many compliments we were receiving. I knew he was hooked.

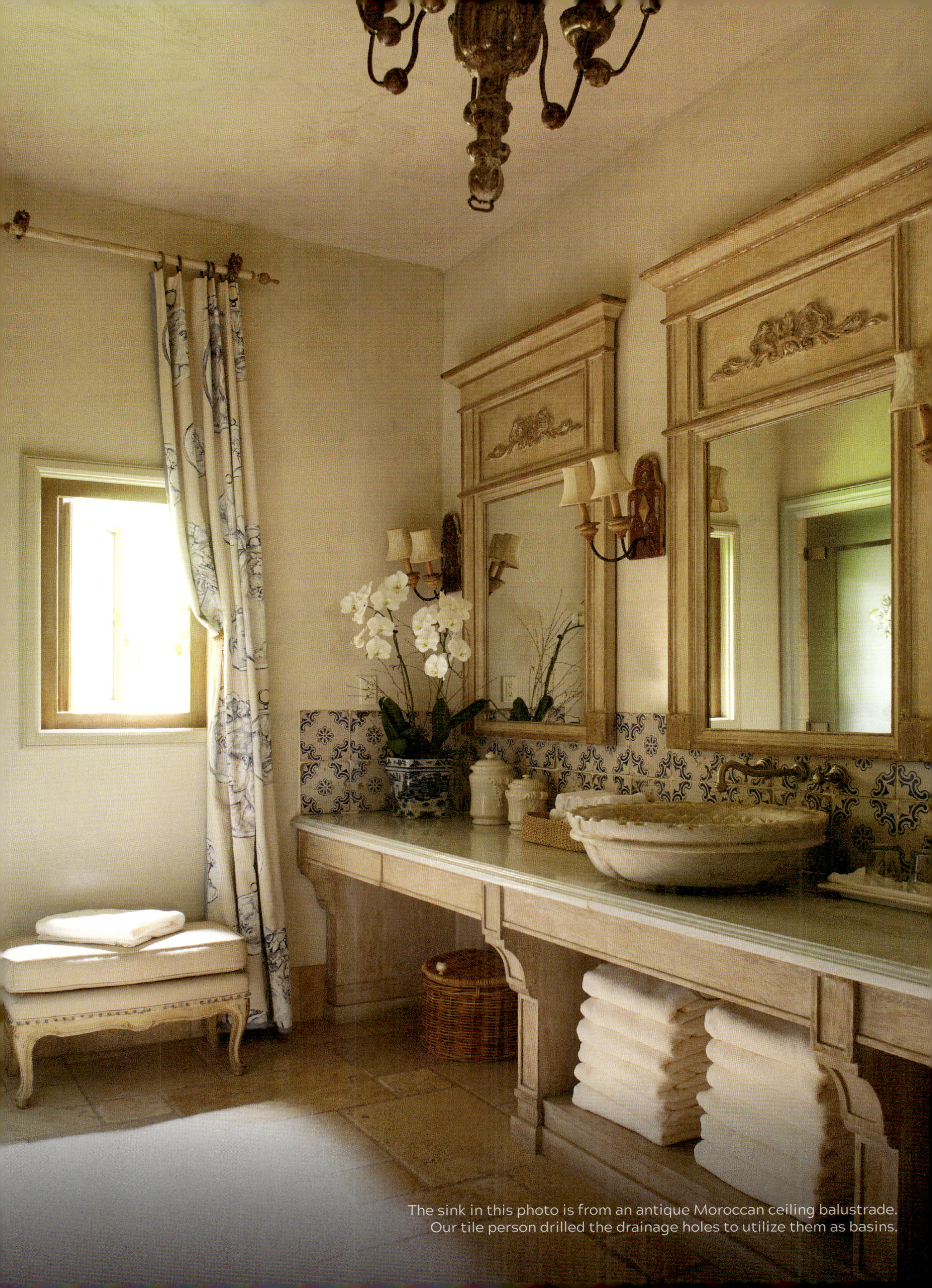

The sink in this photo is from an antique Moroccan ceiling balustrade. Our tile person drilled the drainage holes to utilize them as basins.

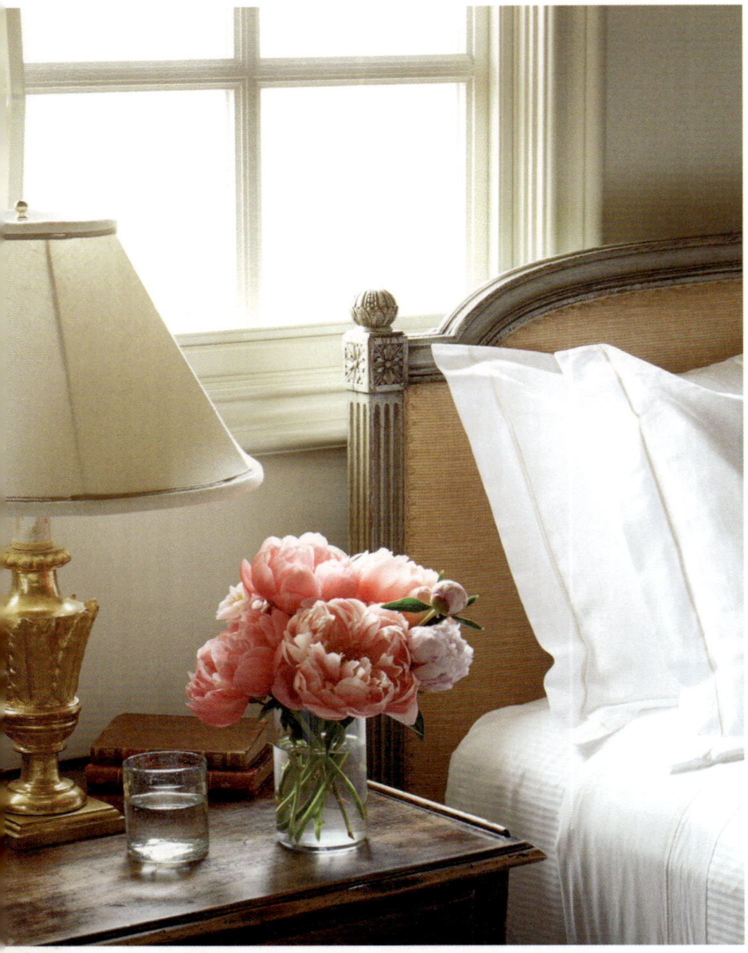

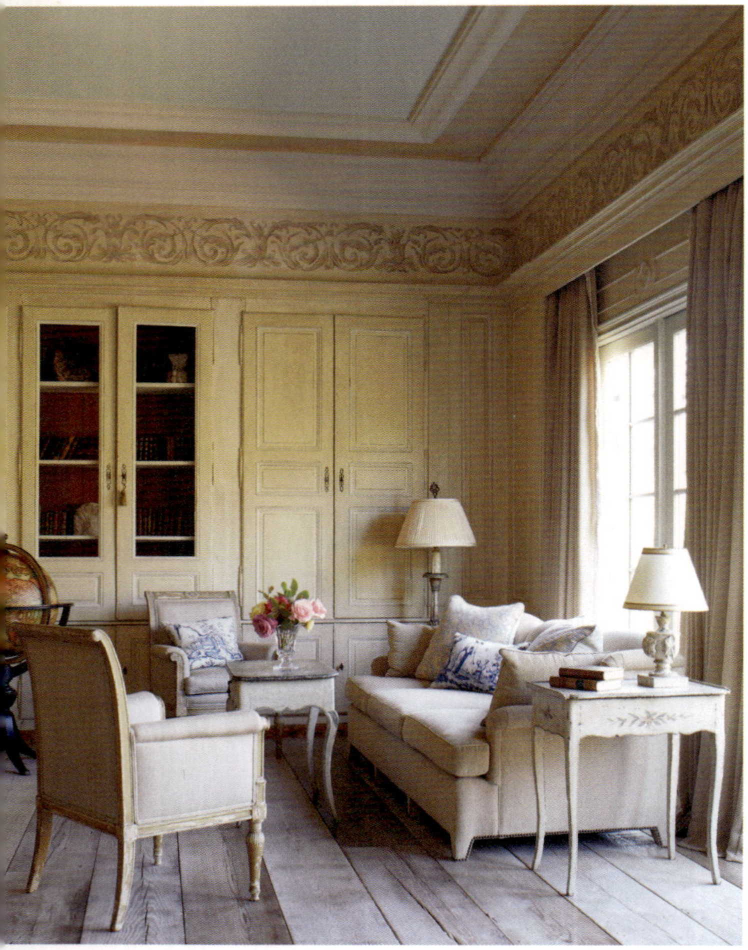

Beyond all that, at the top of the hill overlooking the spa grounds, you'll see a chapel that was originally from Dijon and built in 1615 (a great place for yoga and meditation, and the perfect destination for a wedding). Next to it, also from Dijon and dating back to 1615, is L'Orangerie, which is ideal for classes, receptions, and sampling estate wines from the grapes we grow in our own vineyard.

By now, it is probably obvious that this is not the kind of attention to luxury that one finds in a hotel. I understand that hotels have to be concerned about expenses and the bottom line, but our concern at Cal-a-Vie is about shaping an environment that brings peace, balance and rejuvenation to anyone who enters our front door. No expense was spared in creating this atmosphere and this philosophy remains our passion.

What's interesting is that you might think with all these antiques and magnificent 17th-century structures, guests would feel a little awestruck, like they're in a living museum. But nothing could be further from the truth. Cal-a-Vie Health Spa isn't overly formal. It's comfortable and casual. You can relax and enjoy the surroundings without being intimidated by all this glorious furniture, artwork, and architecture.

In fact, many of our guests actually do see Cal-a-Vie Health Spa as a home away from home. We've had people come here and ask to stay in "their room"—the same one they've always had. They bring their own pillows from home, or their own blankets for the bed, because they feel like it's their personal room.

Our vision became a reality. Located on the most beautiful hillside south of Los Angeles, Cal-a-Vie blossomed into a luxurious French château with lush gardens and vineyards wrapping around the property that provide an inviting space to rest and heal the body, mind, soul, and spirit. We were more than satisfied with our efforts. Now we faced our next goal—how do we solve our "man" problem?

CAL-A-VIE IS ABOUT SHAPING AN ENVIRONMENT THAT BRINGS PEACE, BALANCE, AND REJUVENATION TO ANYONE WHO ENTERS OUR FRONT DOOR.

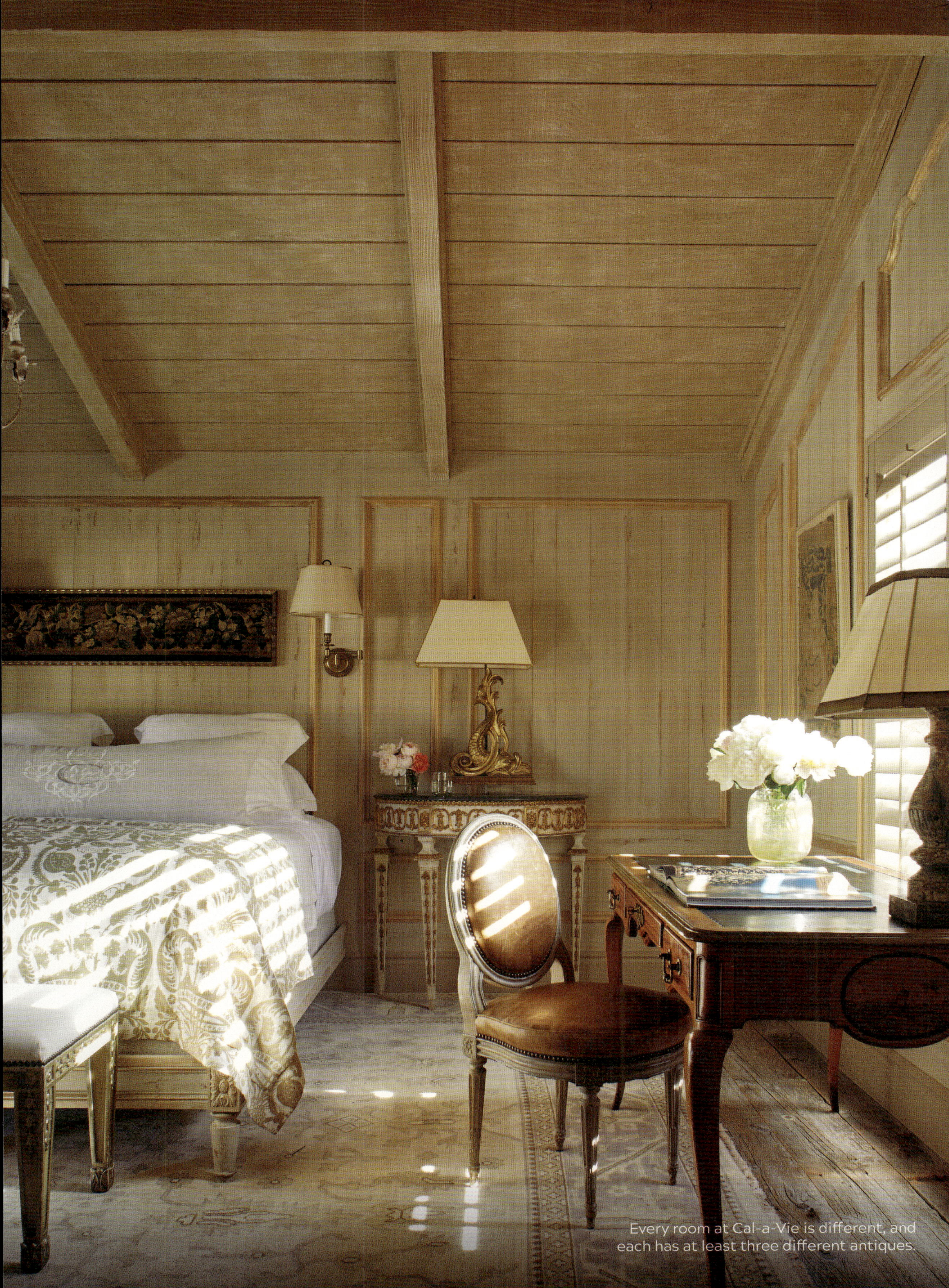

Every room at Cal-a-Vie is different, and each has at least three different antiques.

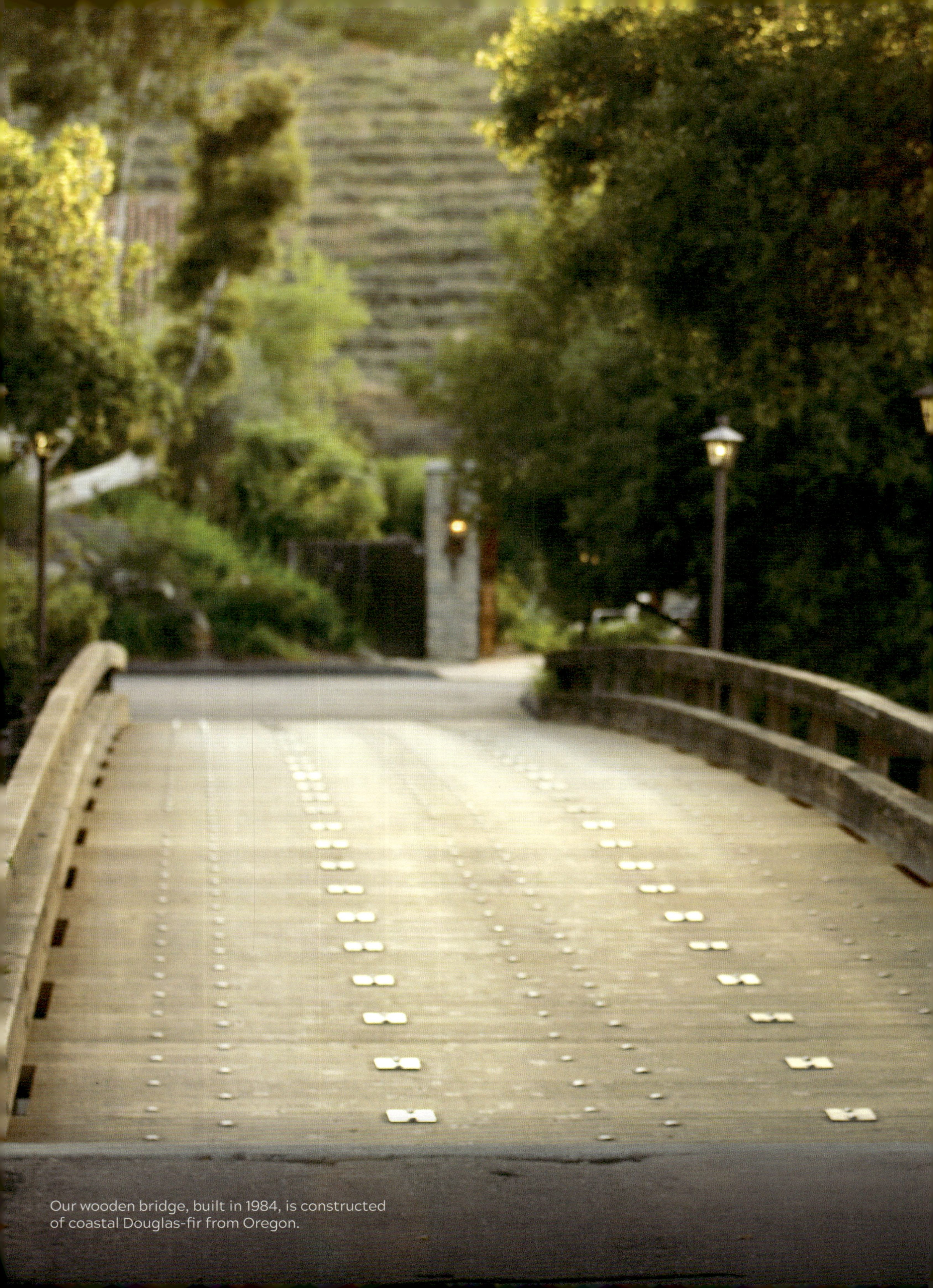

Our wooden bridge, built in 1984, is constructed
of coastal Douglas-fir from Oregon.

IF WE BUILD IT WILL THEY COME?

JOHN KNEW THAT MOST MEN WOULD PROBABLY LOOK AT A SPA AND THINK THE WAY HE DID AT FIRST, BEFORE HE GOT HOOKED: IT'S ALL FLUFF. So he told me, "My mantra is to get men in here." I said, "Great. But just how can we do that?" His easy answer: "Build a massive weight room, and they will come."

Good idea, except we did not have any place to build it. Cal-a-Vie only had two exercise rooms at the time with no ideal space to expand.

When you arrive at Cal-a-Vie, you get to the spa by crossing a large wooden bridge over a peaceful running stream. Most of the land for building was on the entrance side of the bridge not on the Cal-a-Vie side. We spent about a year trying to decide if our guests would walk from the lush comforts of the spa, back over the bridge to workout. We were afraid the bridge might be a psychological separation. Finally, it hit us! Why wouldn't they? After all, they came here to get healthy, right?

Now we had a site so the building began. We didn't just build a big weight room. Oh no; we built a 17,000-square-foot exercise pavilion with top-of-the-line fitness equipment, a full Pilates studio, and a spinning room, and just like the rest of Cal-a-Vie, we made it super luxurious in every single respect. For example, the boxing gloves are done in custom Ralph Lauren-rich leather—not exactly what you would find in your basic gym. We ordered for our weight equipment a specially dyed leather made for us and monogrammed with our logo.

Thanks to John's vision, we went from having just two exercise rooms to five—as well as that humongous weight room—and now offer pretty much everything a man (or woman) could possibly want. We've also increased the number of fitness classes from eight to about 150, everything from yoga and stretching, to cardio and kickboxing, to TRX, aqua jogging, and ab shredding. It is our goal to always have the latest fitness classes and equipment. Cal-a-Vie Health Spa provides the perfect atmosphere to try something new that you might not try at home.

We built a place that helped our guests get stronger, fitter, and more toned, and that delivered a whole lot of benefits to their body and brain.

So, back to the question: Did men come? This past summer during one week we had more men than women at the spa!

Also, when New Orleans Saints' quarterback Drew Brees celebrated signing a contract extension, he did it at Cal-a-Vie. I think that pretty much answers the question.

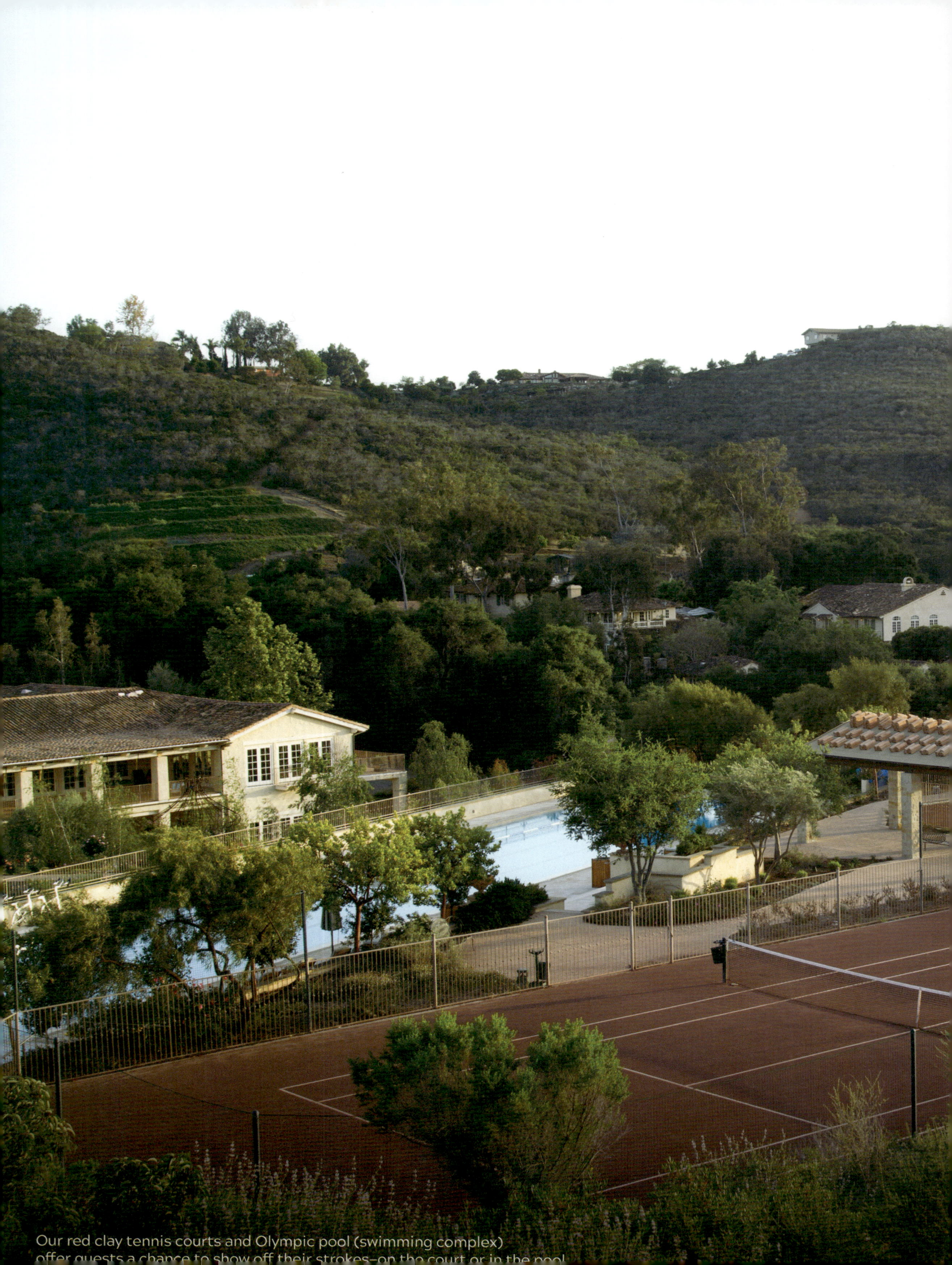

Our red clay tennis courts and Olympic pool (swimming complex)
offer guests a chance to show off their strokes–on the court or in the pool.

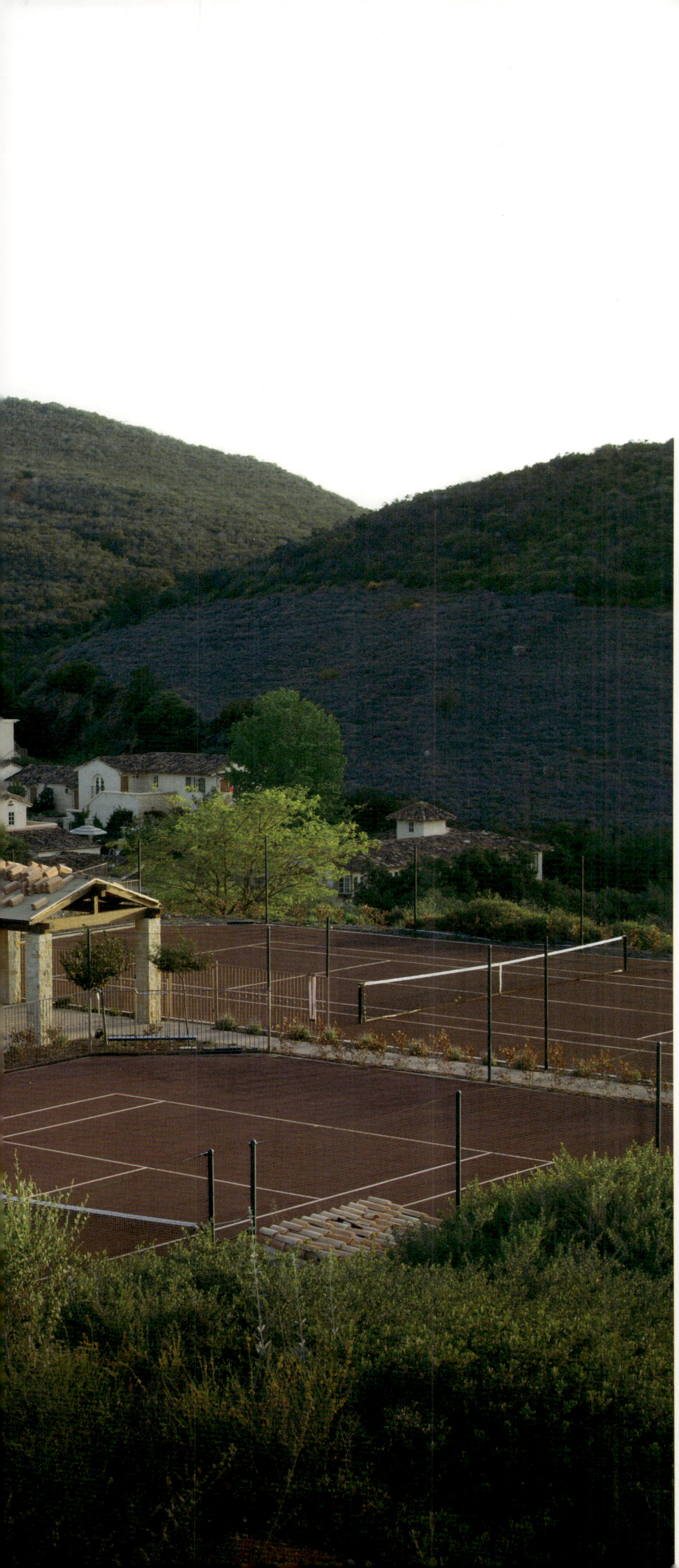
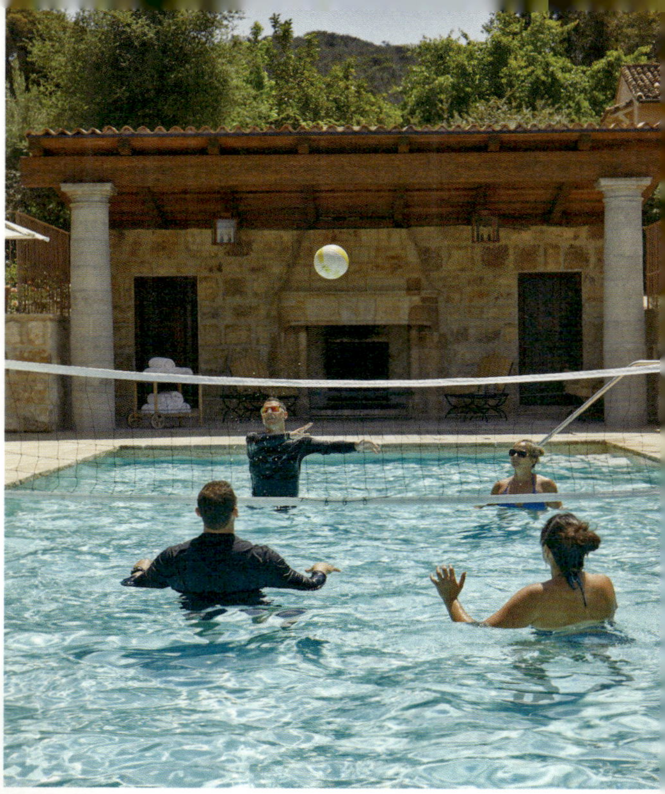
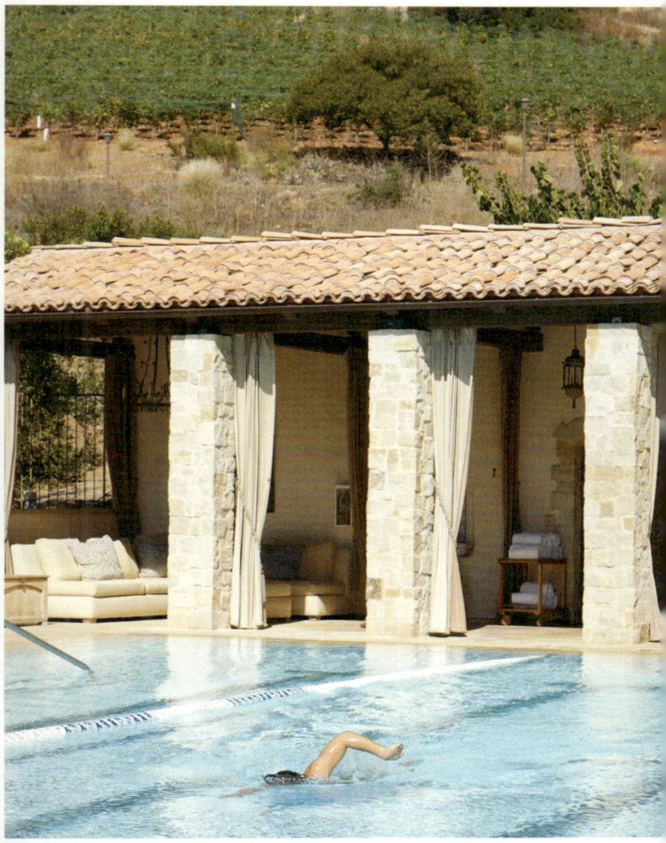
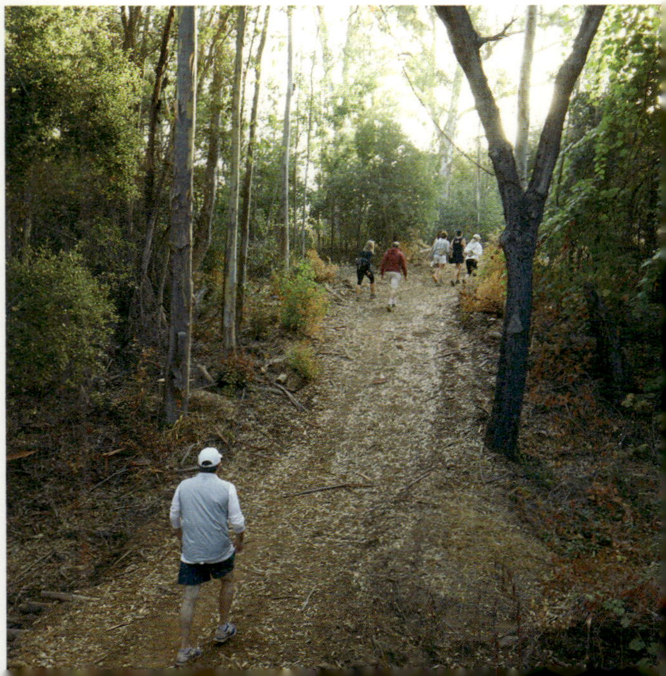

OUR COOKING PHILOSOPHY:

RESPECT MOTHER NATURE.

I ONCE ASKED CURTIS COOKE, OUR CLASSICALLY TRAINED EXECUTIVE CHEF AT CAL-A-VIE, TO SUM UP HIS PHILOSOPHY ON FOOD PREPARATION.

His answer was unexpected—and unexpectedly simple.

"I think we should respect what Mother Nature gives us," he replied. "I want our guests to taste what nature gives. And I don't want to mess up nature's work."

It's tough to argue with that. At Cal-a-Vie Health Spa, Curtis has put that kind of thinking into practice, creating meals that are as flavorful and energizing as they are fresh and natural.

He and his culinary team respect farmers and where food comes from. We even have a farmer on staff, and she shares an office with Curtis, who by the way, has been growing food for 20 years. They talk every day, and for good reason: growing food is hard to get right, as Curtis has often said, especially when you are not using chemicals (which we aren't).

We get it right. Most of the fruits, vegetables, and herbs we use are grown on our own organic farm, which is literally 100 steps from the kitchen. So when we say "farm to table," it's not an exercise in trendy branding. It really describes what we do and how we do it. And it's the reason the food tastes so great.

Curtis has described his cooking technique as "mindful" and being "present in the moment" rather than "robotic." That's an important distinction. He'll be the first to tell you that, many chefs are programmed: they get an order, they throw the food onto the stove, cook it fast, and the order goes out. Then do it all over again, like rinse and repeat, except in the kitchen.

But Curtis wants his team to be engaged.

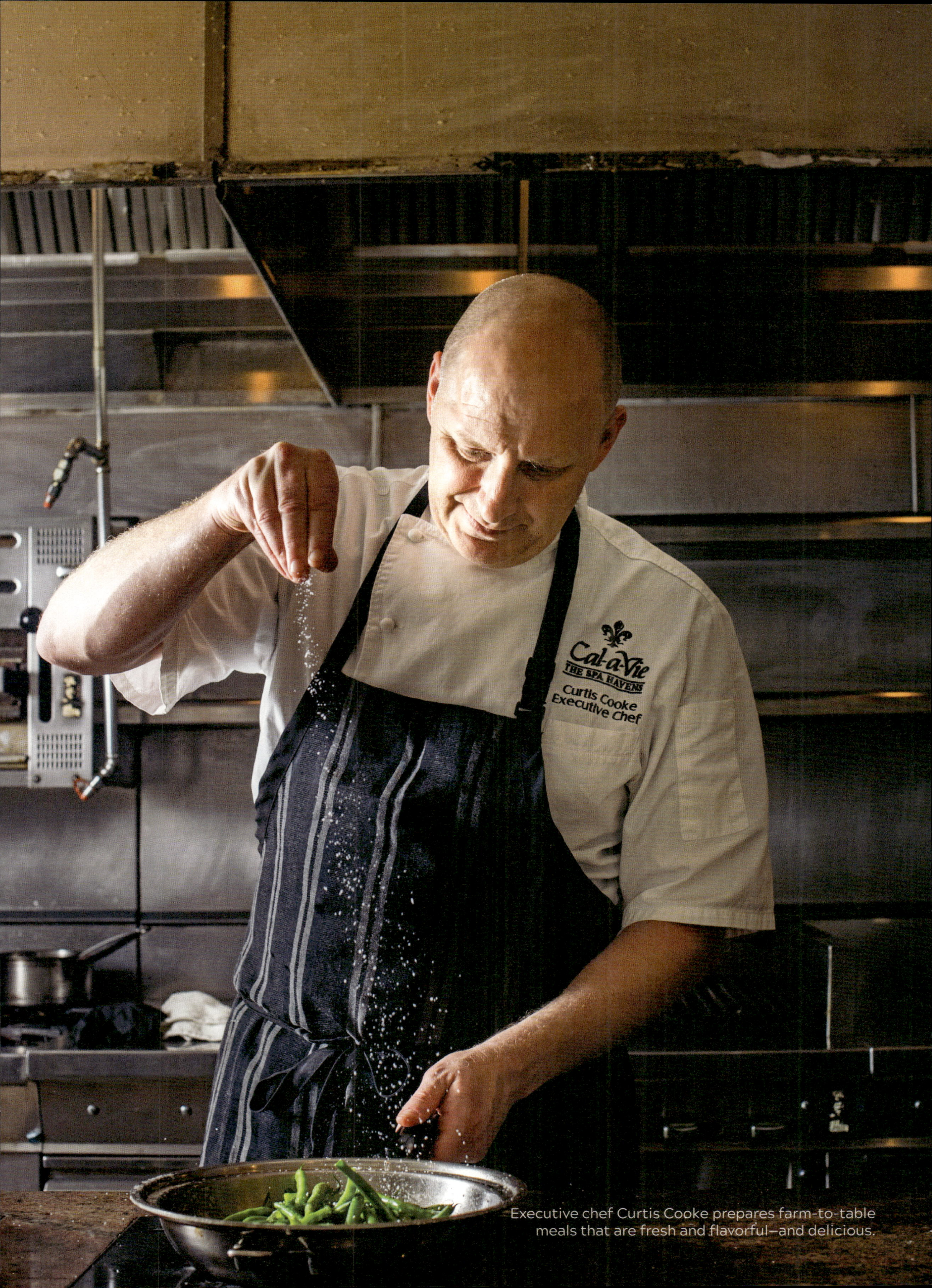

Executive chef Curtis Cooke prepares farm-to-table meals that are fresh and flavorful—and delicious.

He has mastered the art of slow cooking. He spends more time and attention in the preparation stage, making sure everything is done just right before he ever turns the burners on. In the classes he offers at Cal-a-Vie Health Spa, I've heard him describe what seems like the most basic task in almost cosmic terms.

"Think about slicing an onion," he said. "You do it so many times, it becomes a habit. Mechanical. But if you look down at the onion, how thick or thin the slice is, you are right there with it, right there in the moment. You are on the right path when you respect the food and the technique."

I realize this may sound like chef speak, and maybe even a little mystical, but that's fine with me, because Curtis is passionate about what he does and he channels that passion to his team. Our guests are the winners, and, he is right. We need to slow down and be present when we are eating our food.

Besides, at the end of the day, the proof is in the taste, right? And the taste of Curtis' creations is super fantastic. Try any one of the recipes in this cookbook, and you'll be hard-pressed not to agree. That is why all our guests were begging us for a cookbook!

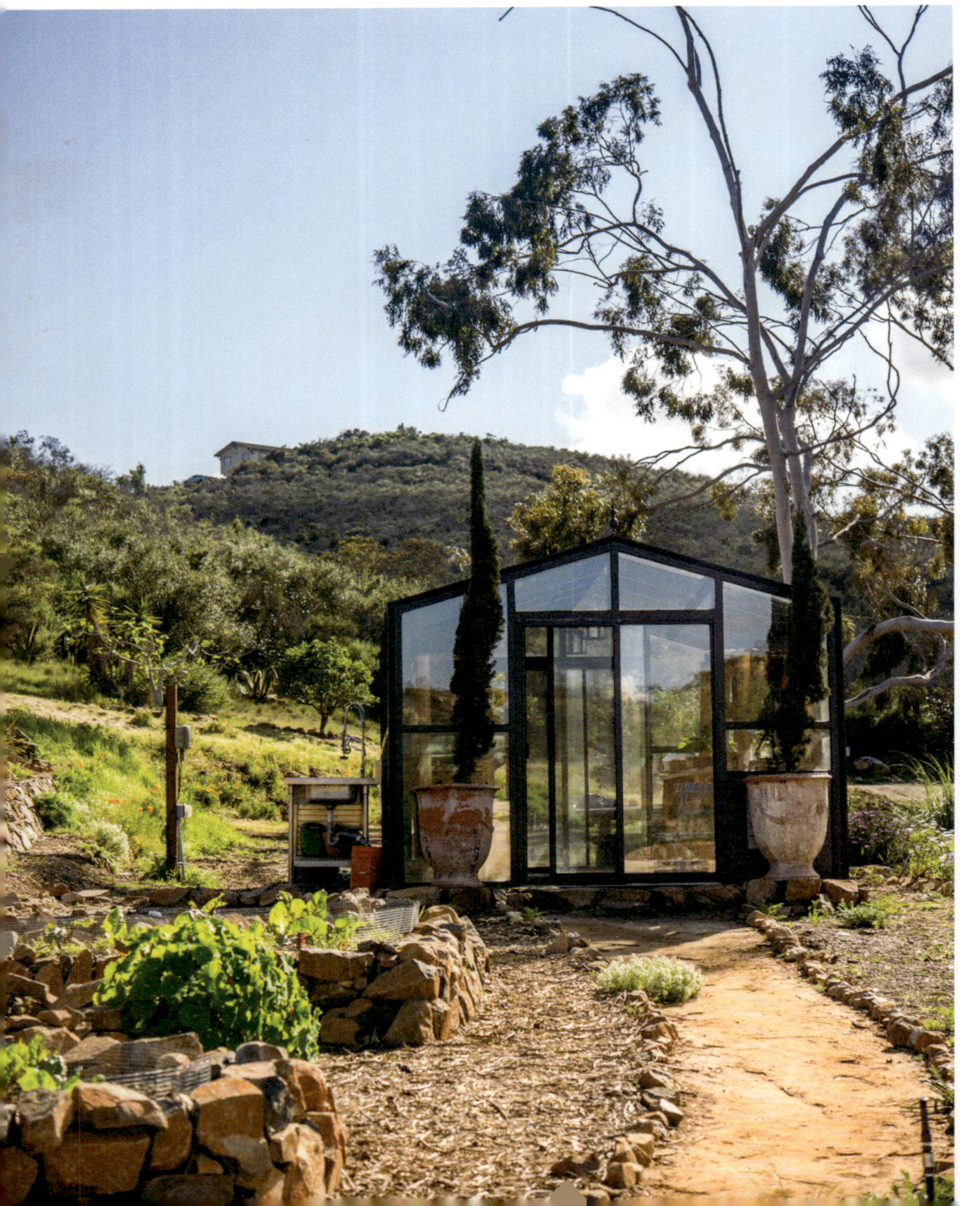

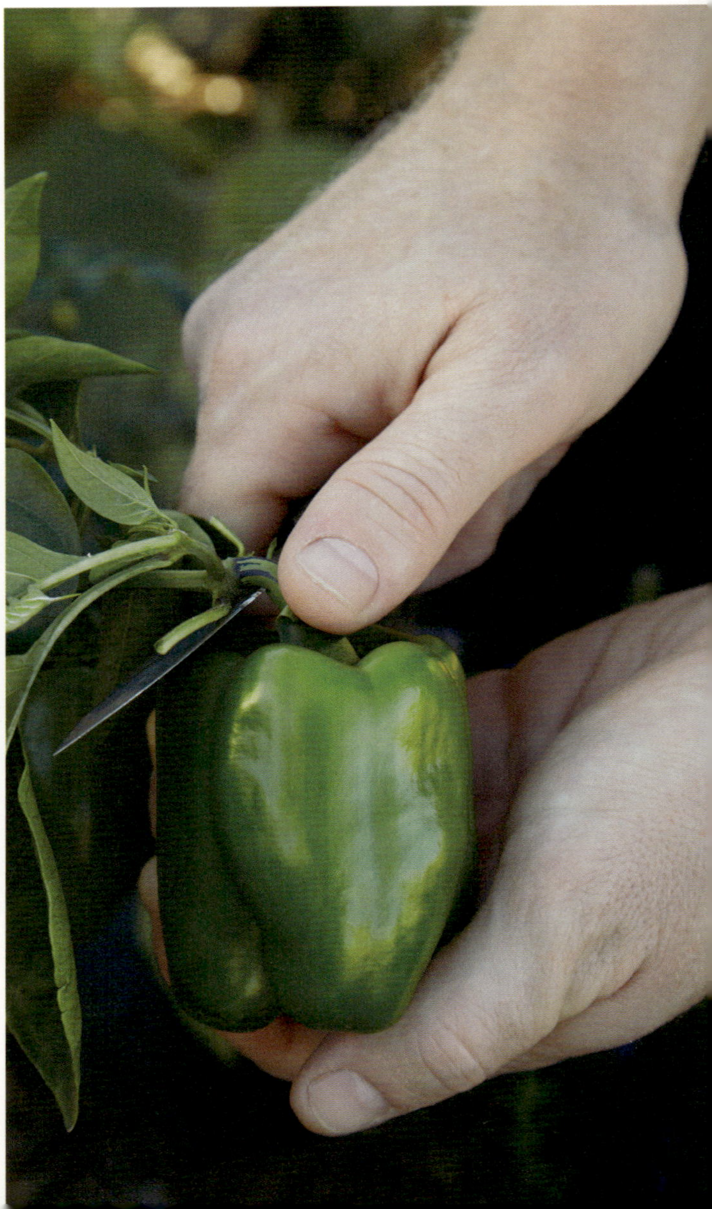

"THE BEE IS MORE HONORED THAN ANIMALS NOT BECAUSE SHE LABORS BUT BECAUSE SHE LABORS FOR OTHERS."

– Saint John Chrysostom

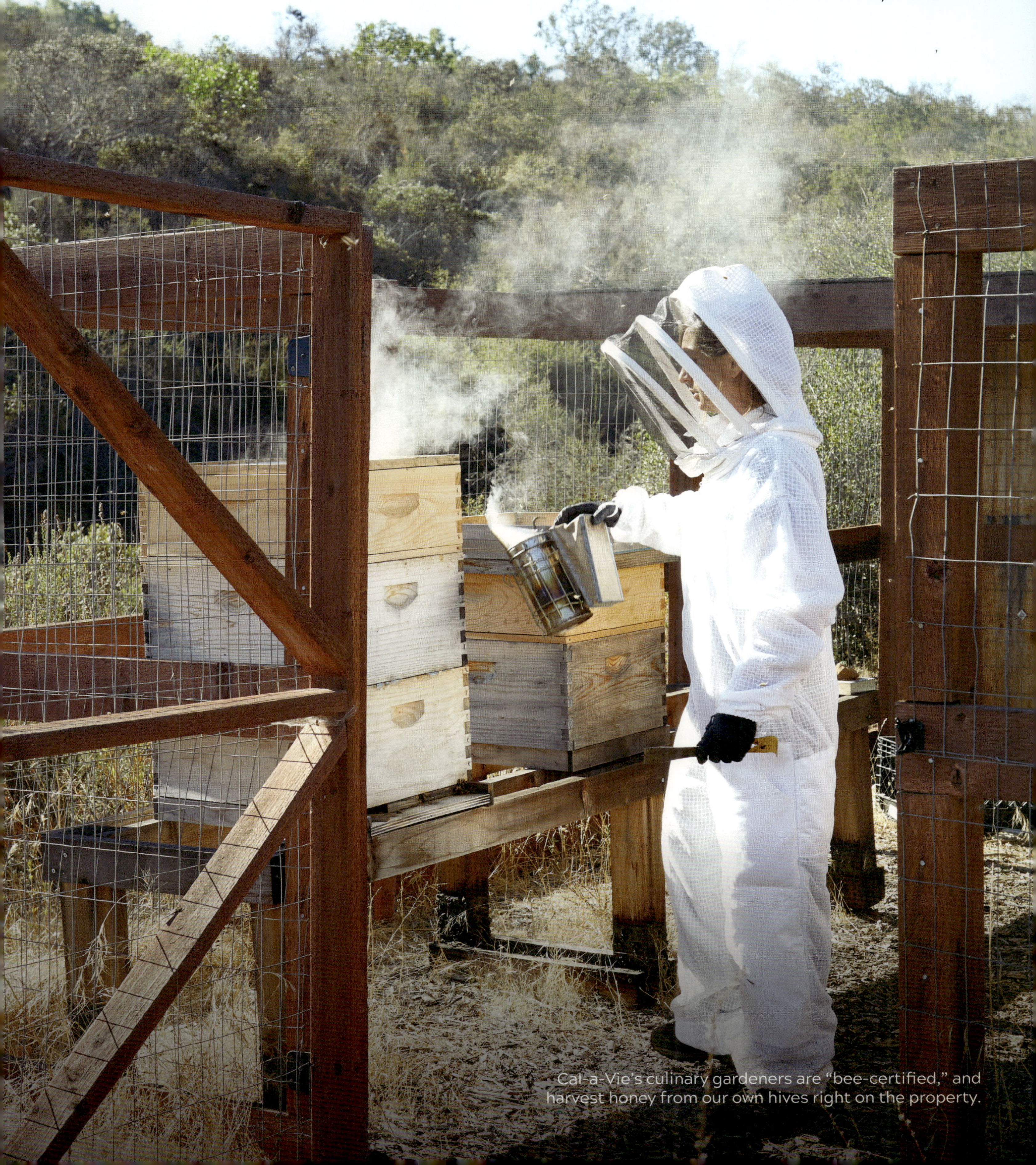

Cal-a-Vie's culinary gardeners are "bee-certified," and harvest honey from our own hives right on the property.

NUTRITION DONE RIGHT

WE HAVE TWO NUTRITIONISTS AT CAL-A-VIE HEALTH SPA,

and their job in many respects is to apply the magic Curtis creates in the kitchen to the quality of life of our guests.

May Tom and Gina Worful are both registered dieticians with master's degrees and share our commitment to taking a functional, customized approach to health and well-being—without sacrificing the flavor and enjoyment that is central to the Cal-a-Vie Health Spa way.

I've talked a lot about how we tailor every experience to every individual guest. The same is true for nutrition. We believe that when it comes to diet, one size does not fit all. We don't all have the same genes, diet or health concerns. So it doesn't make much sense to give generic nutrition advice. Like everything else, personalization is the key. Let's take calories, for example. Conventional wisdom would have you believe that cutting calories leads to weight loss and a healthier lifestyle. I suppose that's true to some degree, but Curtis, May, and Gina all believe that you shouldn't be fixated on the number of calories you consume, but on the quality of those calories.

Their focus is on eating real food that is properly prepared and mindfully enjoyed. Our cuisine is nutrient-dense, balanced, and plant-based. As Curtis has said, our goal is to make the vegetables the star of the plate, and the meat the garnish. Our guests discover pretty quickly that if they eat the right foods, in the right amounts, and don't rush, they'll be satisfied perfectly.

With their extensive training in functional medicine, May and Gina are not your typical dieticians. Functional medicine is a systems-biology approach to identifying and addressing the root cause of common

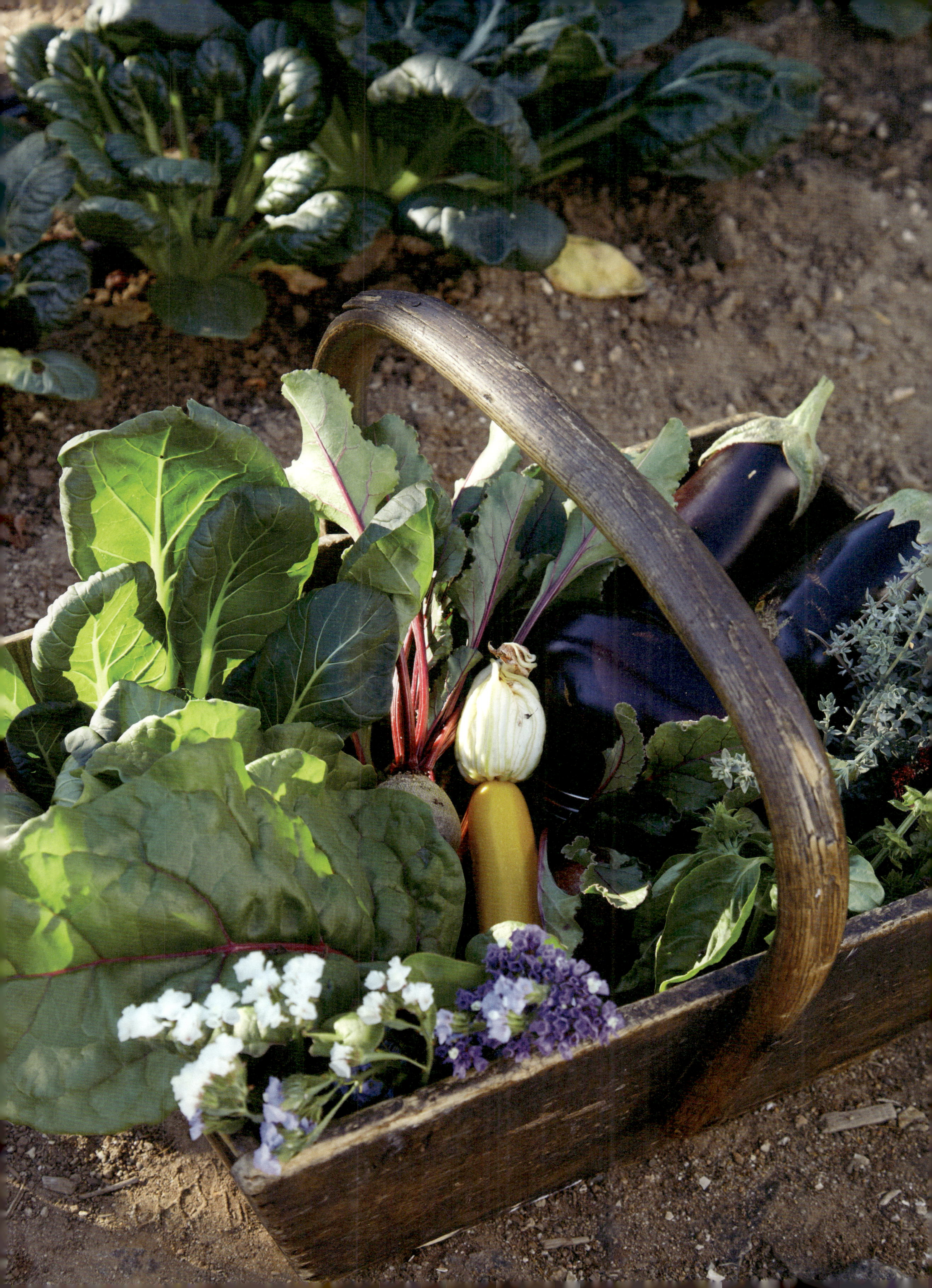

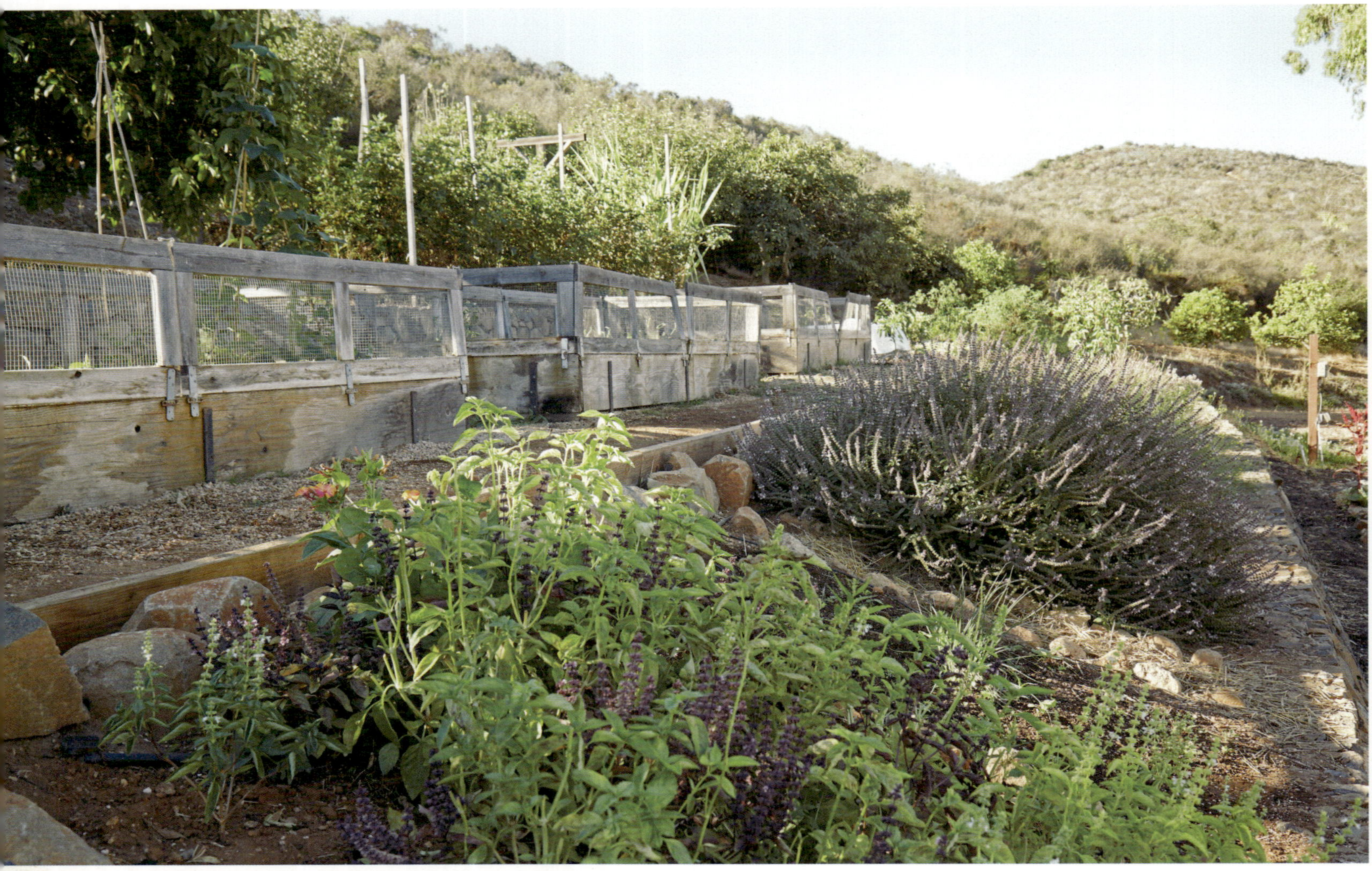

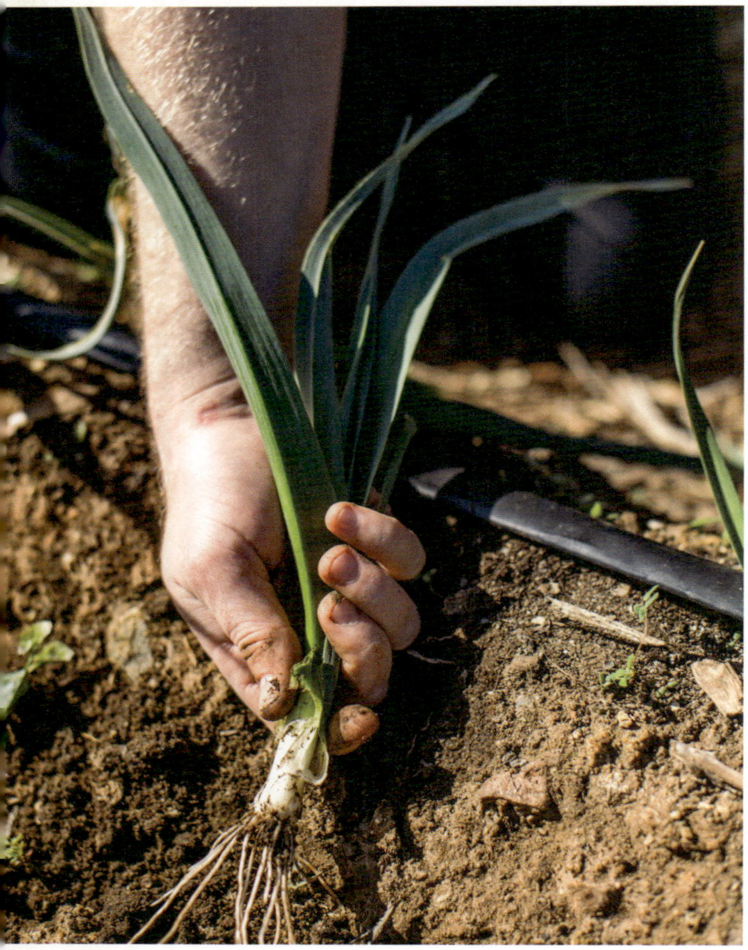

health concerns, such as gut issues, hormone imbalances, slow metabolism, and poor sleep. Our dieticians utilize testing and comprehensive consultations to help guests come up with a detailed game plan to take their health to the next level. This includes tailored diet, lifestyle, and supplement recommendations.

We offer lab tests to help you see which foods are best for you to eat and which ones are causing inflammation. We have IV Vitamin Therapy, and B-12 shots, all in an effort to get you tuned up to face the world again.

THEY ARE PASSIONATE ABOUT HELPING OUR GUESTS INTEGRATE THEIR PERSONAL HEALTH PLAN ONCE THEY RETURN HOME.

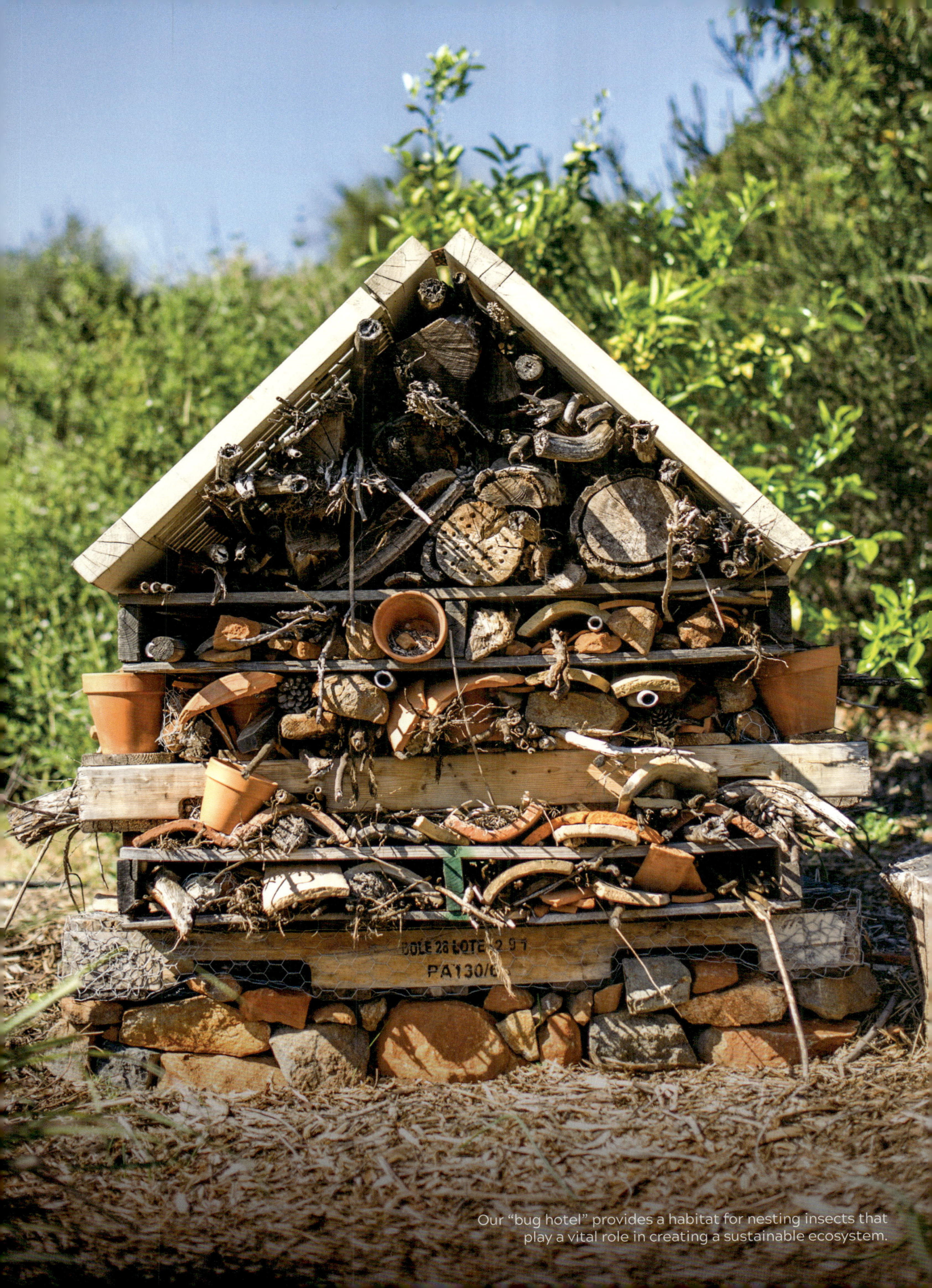

Our "bug hotel" provides a habitat for nesting insects that play a vital role in creating a sustainable ecosystem.

NEVER SATISFIED

ALWAYS GOING FOR THE BEST.

CAL-A-VIE HEALTH SPA'S GENERAL PHILOSOPHY CAN BE DEFINED BY A LOT OF THINGS IN A LOT OF WAYS.

But I think one of the qualities that guides us most is that we are never satisfied. We just do not sit still or rest on our laurels.

We are always on the lookout for the next new thing, and we are always thinking about what we don't have. Once a year, we meet with the managers and ask them; "What do you want?" "What would be amazing?" They get it almost every time.

I remember once I read about a Zumba class. At the time, no one really knew Zumba from zebra, but I thought, "Hey let's try it." So I researched to find the world's best Zumba teacher. As it happened, she lived in Barcelona, so we flew her in. Yes, she was the best, and you cannot begin to imagine how she danced, and what fun and excitement she brought to our guests. At the same time, she taught our instructors advanced-level Zumba. I always want to make sure our instructors are having fun along with the guests . . . and it shows. Everyone is always happy.

Another time, I was watching "Dancing With The Stars," and there was this one guy I really, really liked, so I just called him up, told him what I needed, and said, "Will you come and teach some classes?" You know what? He did, and now he comes all the time. Guests love him and they come back each year just to see him.

I have a teenage daughter, so I decided it would be great to do a Teen Week at the spa. I sent out a notice to mothers saying, "Bring your daughters and let them learn about nutrition before it's too late. What mom wouldn't want their little girl to know the value of eating healthy and getting exercise at an early age, right?" Then I started thinking, "Okay, what can I do to make the experience a little more special? Oh, I know, I'll get a teenage movie star to come in," which I did, and it was huge. Now, the week is so popular we don't even need the star.

These are all just examples of my belief that if you want or need something, you should get the absolute very best you can. We never stop going for it at Cal-a-Vie. Ever.

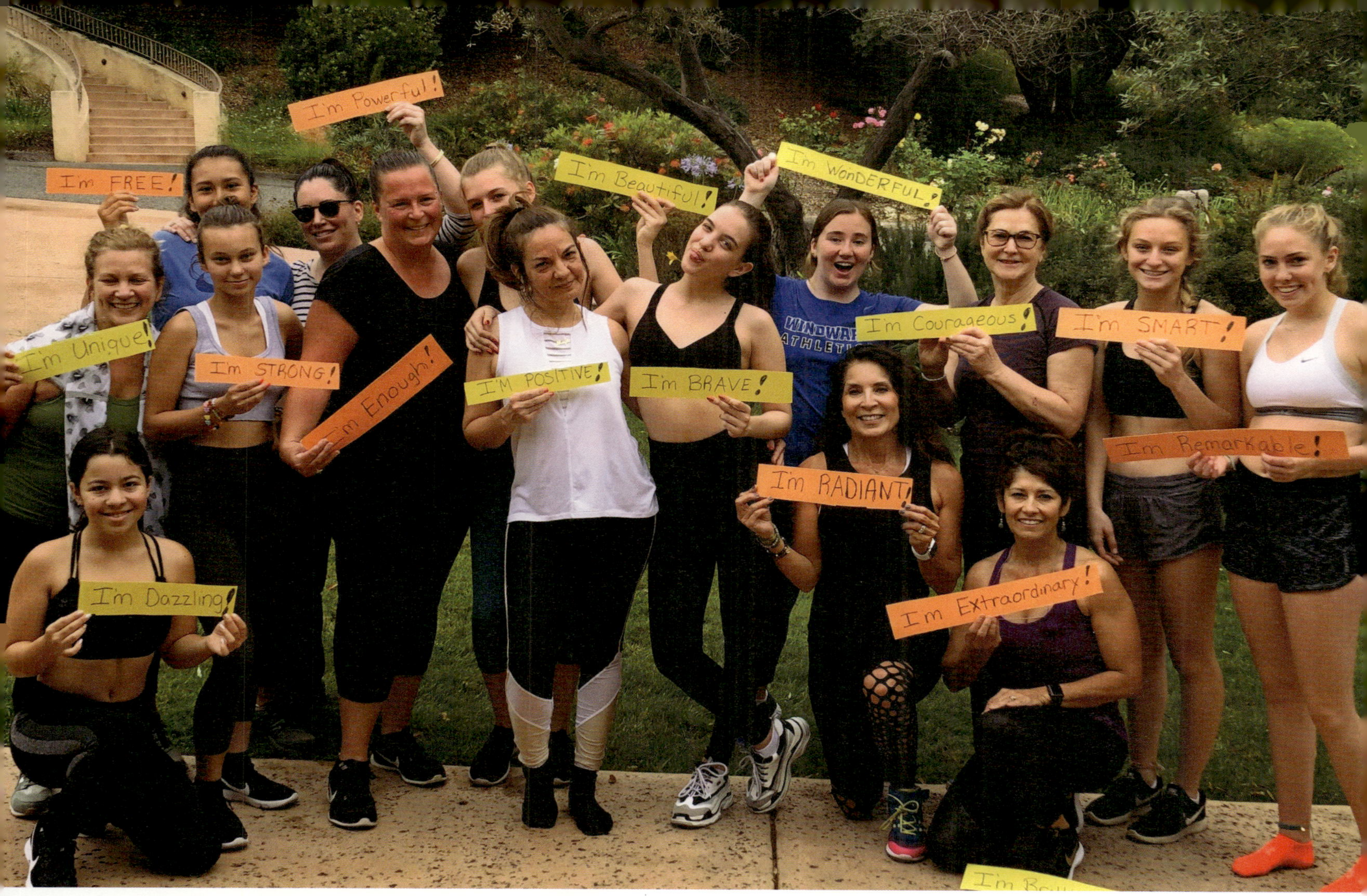
I'm Powerful!
I'm FREE!
I'm Beautiful!
I'm WONDERFUL
I'm Unique
I'm STRONG!
I'm Enough!
I'm POSITIVE!
I'm BRAVE!
I'm Courageous!
I'm SMART!
I'm Remarkable!
I'm RADIANT
I'm Dazzling!
I'm Extraordinary!

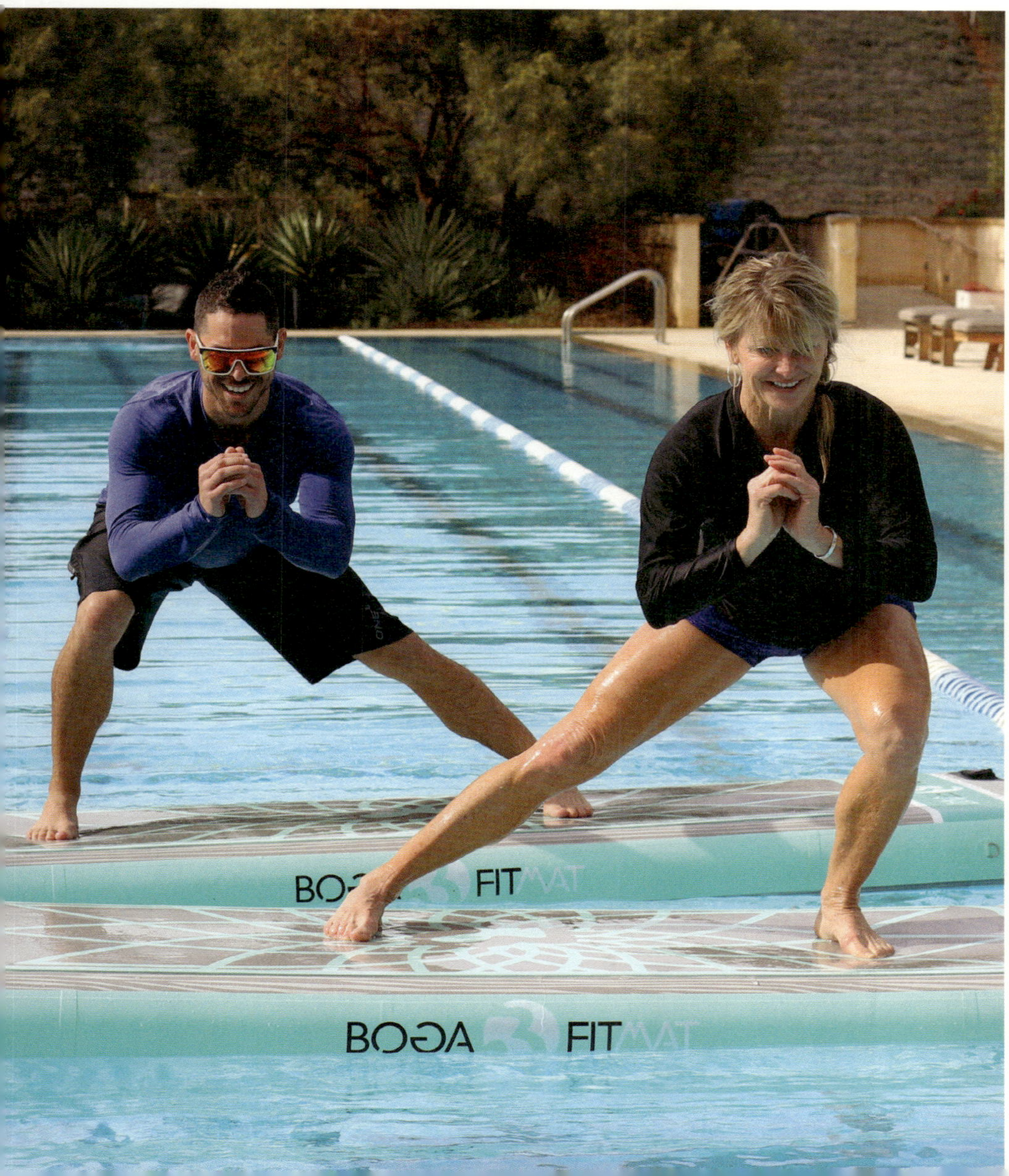
BOGA FIT MAT

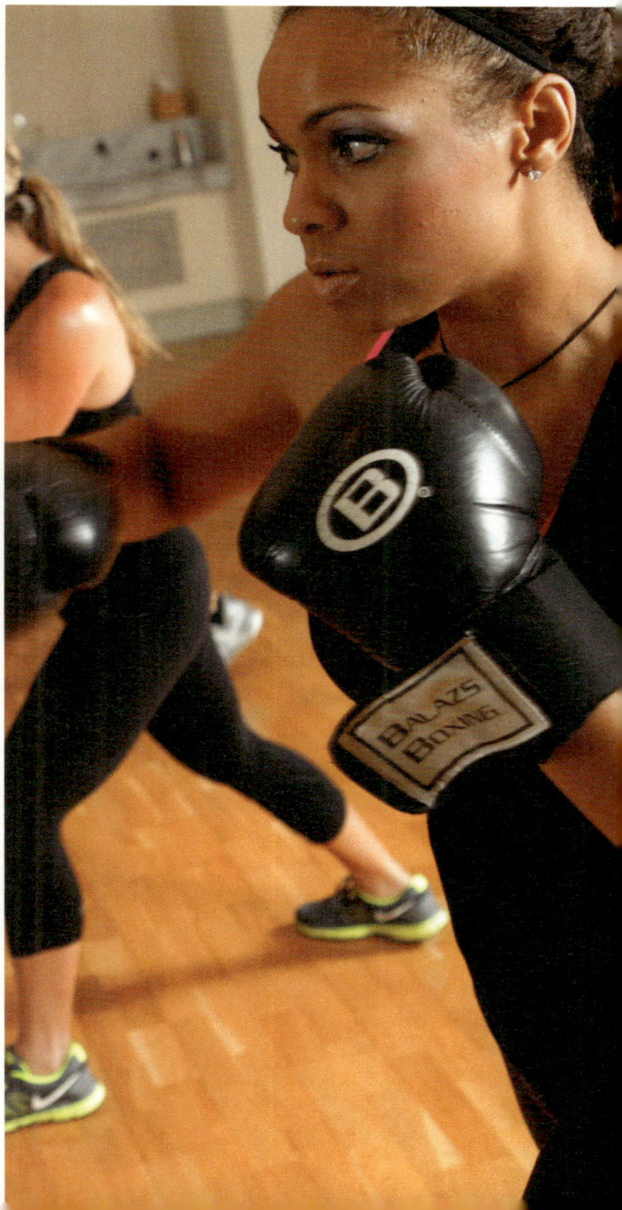
BALAZS BOXING

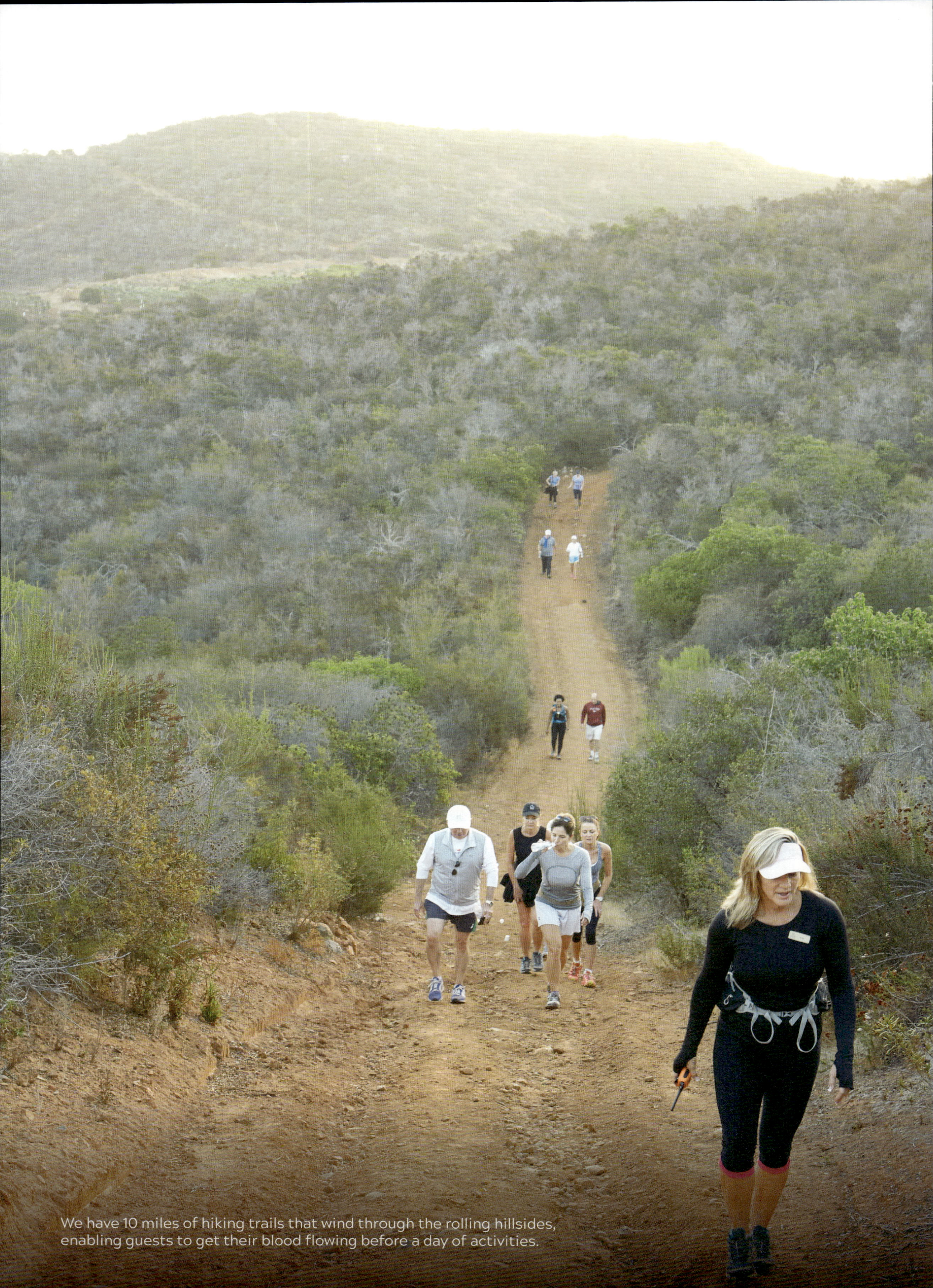

We have 10 miles of hiking trails that wind through the rolling hillsides, enabling guests to get their blood flowing before a day of activities.

GIVING BACK

SOMETHING SPECIAL AND MEANINGFUL.

I GET ASKED A LOT ABOUT HOW I MAINTAIN MY PASSION FOR WHAT WE DO AT CAL-A-VIE.

I am always trying to teach my children that it is important to give back to this world, and whenever they have a chance to do something positive for something or someone, they should seize the moment. In a different way, I think that is what John and I are trying to do at Cal-a-Vie. We are providing a new way of life for our guests and we receive so much satisfaction in seeing the change in their lives—right before our eyes. It matters.

When we realize how many lives Cal-A-Vie has touched through the years and we hear our guests say, "Wow, this is amazing," it makes us feel good to know that we are providing positive life-changing results for our guests who visit our spa. Then it becomes an on-going cycle—guests tell their friends about this beautiful environment and these great programs and more people come and on and on—while we just keep providing this golden opportunity for self-improvement.

Our guests come from all over the world, even places like Russia and Australia. We never advertise; it is all word of mouth, and we have a return rate of almost 70 percent which is unheard of in this business. That says a lot about a lot of things, but to John and me, it says we must be doing something right.

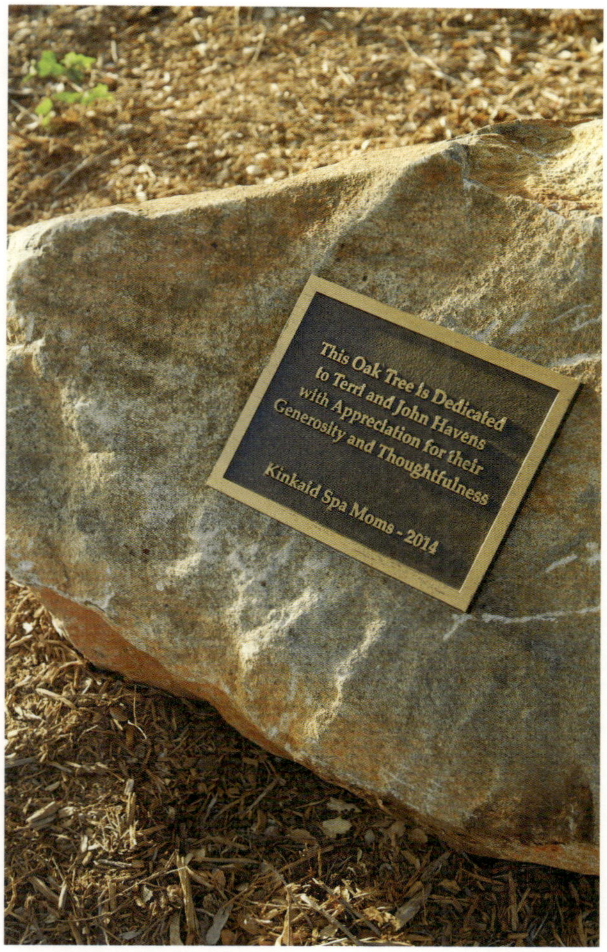

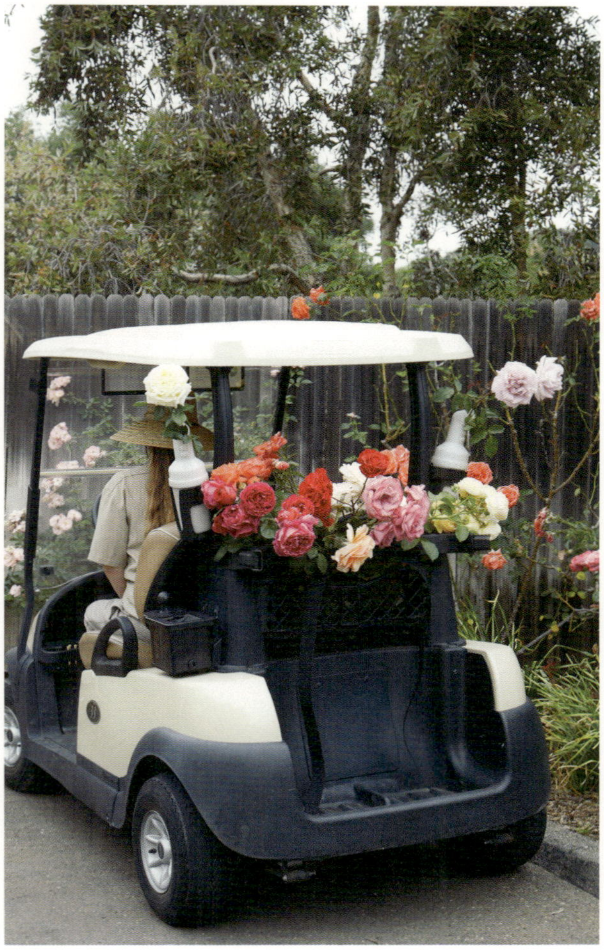

THE CAL-A-VIE HEALTH SPA WAY

IN THE END, CAL-A-VIE HEALTH SPA IS WORLDS AWAY FROM THE WORLD AS YOU KNOW IT.

For everything I've been talking about—recharging, relaxing, reinvigorating—one word that keeps coming to mind is not one you'd typically associate with a spa:

FREEDOM.

We have 32 Mediterranean-styled villas, and only our suites have televisions. Cell service is not good, so you get your news from the person sitting next to you at lunch or dinner, not from the paper or the talk show. It's good news, delivered with goodwill and grace, from newfound friends. In other words, you are free from the chaos and stress that all too often has thrown our day-to-day existence out of balance.

At Cal-a-Vie Health Spa, you are also free to do what you want to do. You can skip an exercise class, eat more (or less), have a private session with a personal trainer, or enjoy popcorn delivered to your room. You can even come to dinner in the Frette bathrobes we provide. It's all up to you.

What this adds up to is that, for however long you stay with us, you are free to be who you are and who you want to be. You can find yourself and think about yourself, and do it in a place that was created specifically for those purposes.

LIFE SHOULDN'T HAVE TO BE HARD. AT CAL-A-VIE HEALTH SPA, WE DO EVERYTHING WE CAN TO MAKE SURE IT'S NOT. THAT'S JUST OUR WAY.

You can rely on us to have done all the research on food, nutrition, fitness, treatments, and even keynote speakers. Our goal at CAV is for you to enjoy your stay, have fun, and start on a new road to fitness and health.

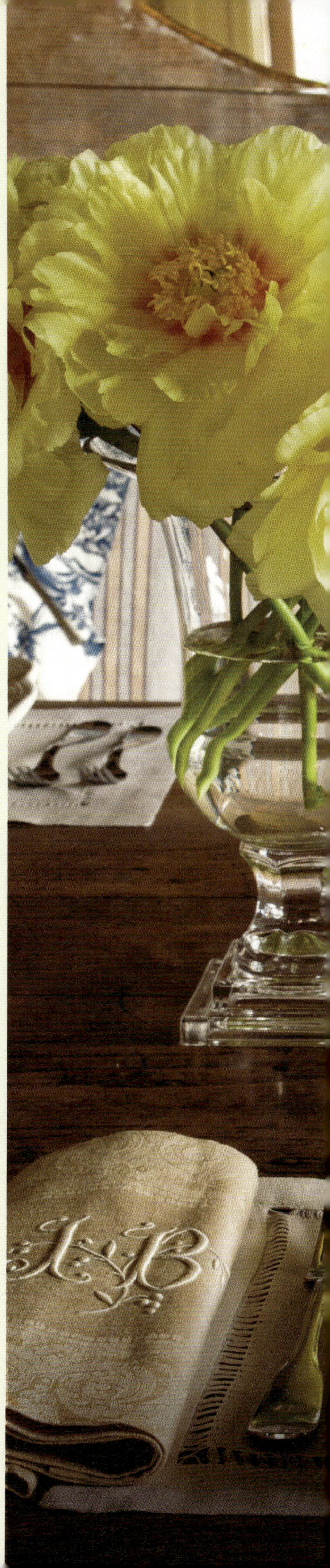

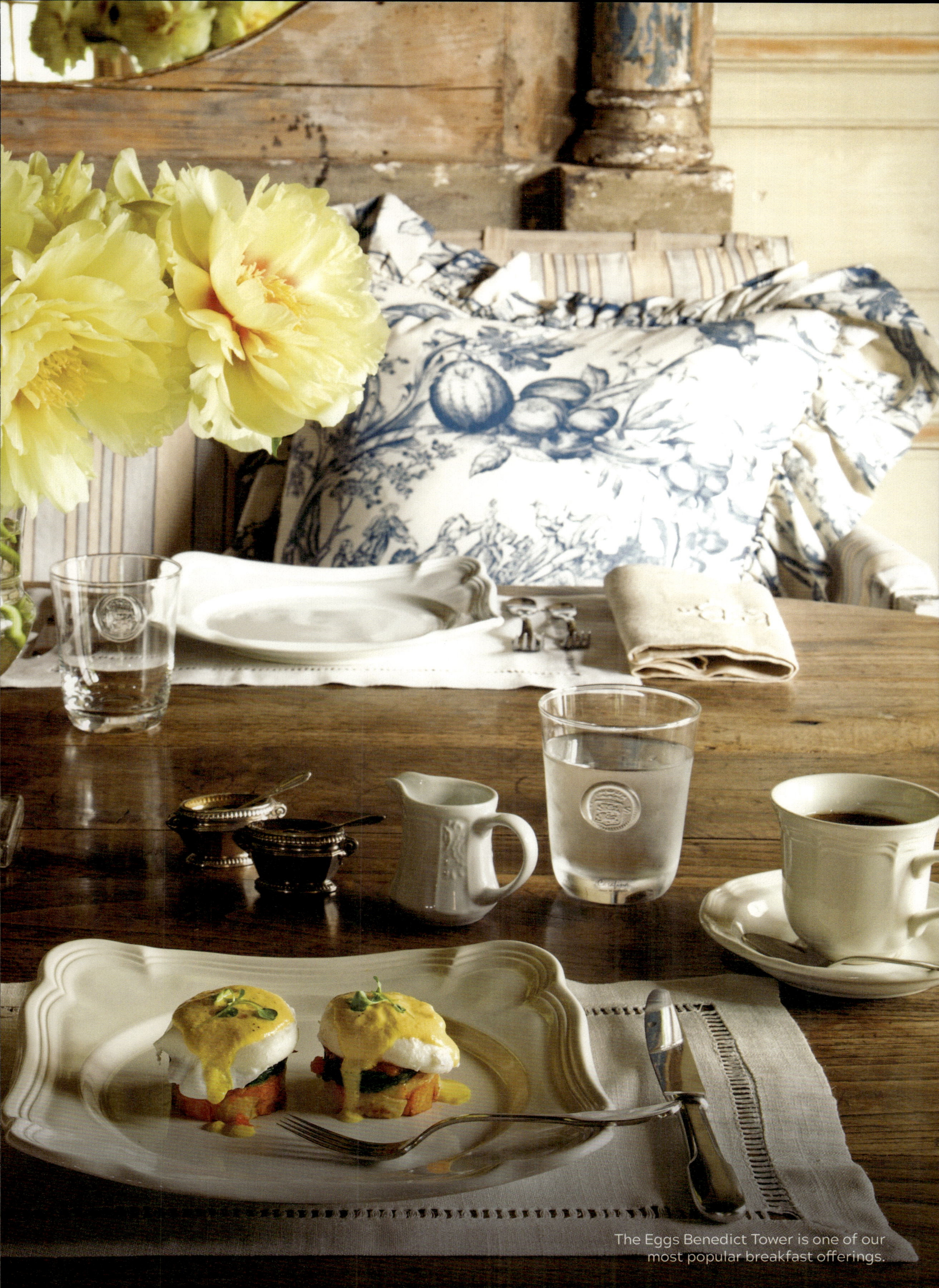

The Eggs Benedict Tower is one of our most popular breakfast offerings.

FRENCH CHAPEL

Our 400-year-old chapel was brought to Cal-a-Vie piece by piece from Dijon, and an architect reassembled it right here on the grounds. Virtually everything is original, and it was even rebuilt to be earthquake-proof. The acoustics are perfect, so our guests can experience the joy of music at its purest, and the rustic-but-romantic vibe provides for a perfect wedding destination.

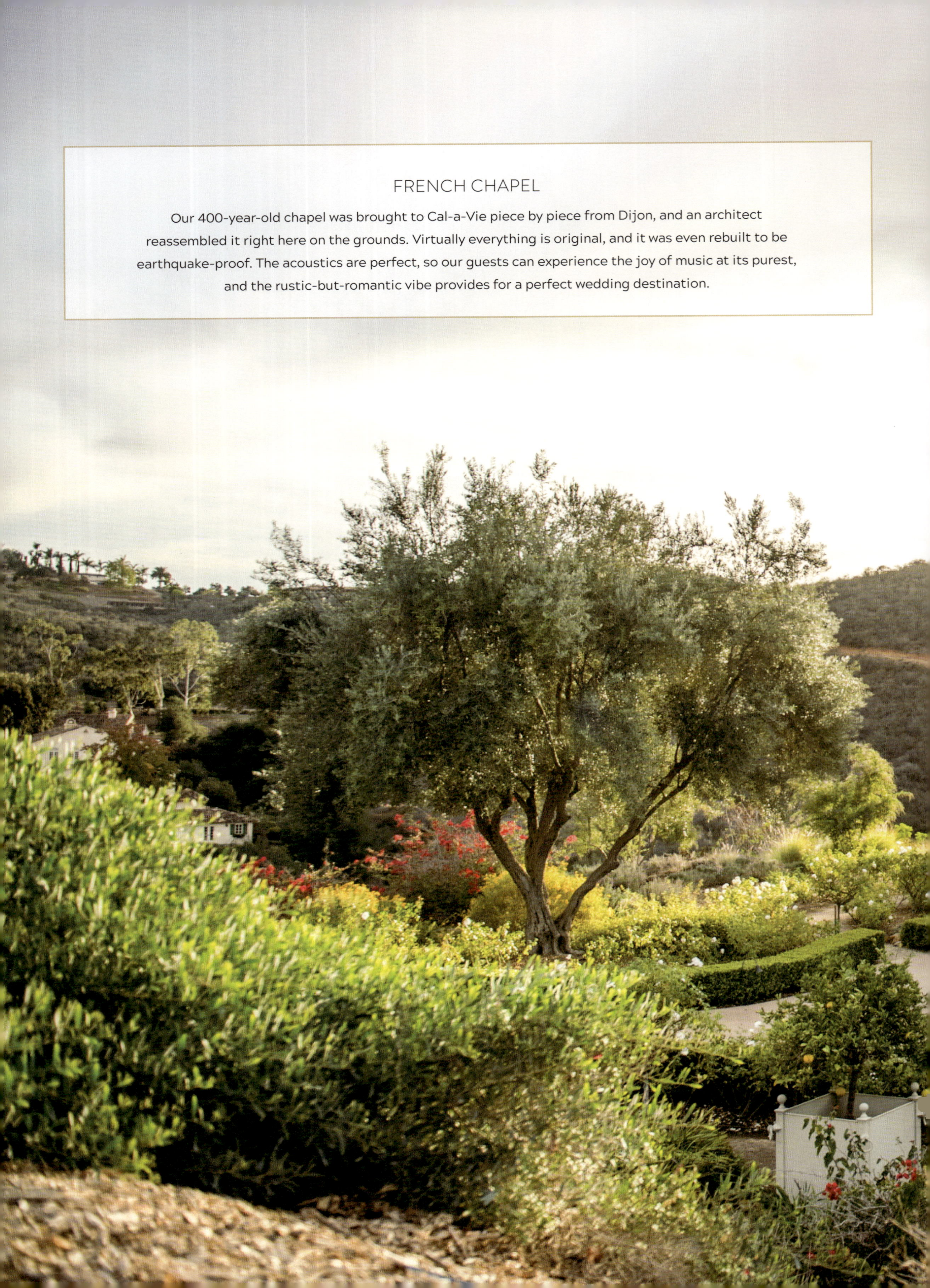

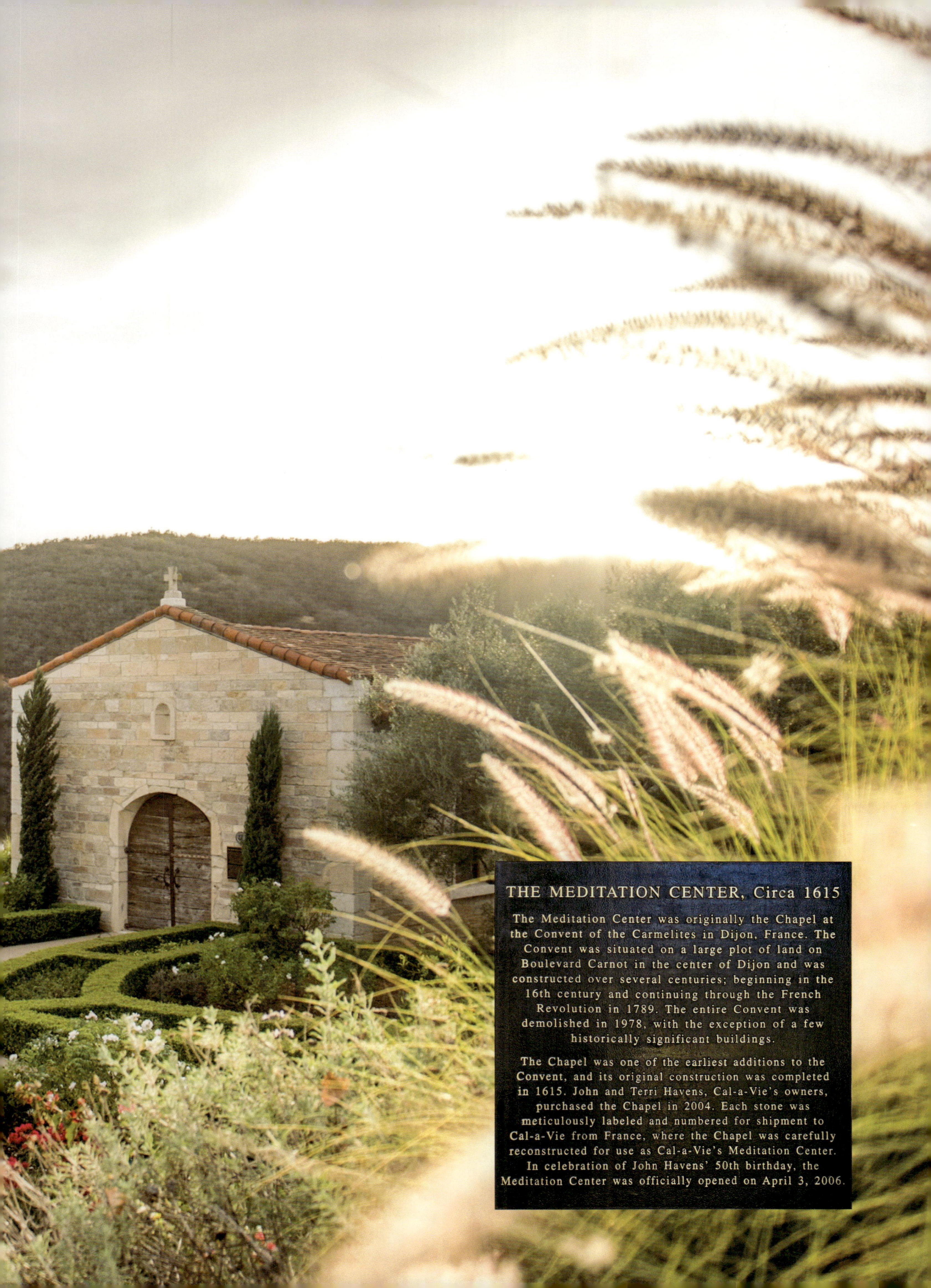
THE MEDITATION CENTER, Circa 1615
The Meditation Center was originally the Chapel at the Convent of the Carmelites in Dijon, France. The Convent was situated on a large plot of land on Boulevard Carnot in the center of Dijon and was constructed over several centuries; beginning in the 16th century and continuing through the French Revolution in 1789. The entire Convent was demolished in 1978, with the exception of a few historically significant buildings.
The Chapel was one of the earliest additions to the Convent, and its original construction was completed in 1615. John and Terri Havens, Cal-a-Vie's owners, purchased the Chapel in 2004. Each stone was meticulously labeled and numbered for shipment to Cal-a-Vie from France, where the Chapel was carefully reconstructed for use as Cal-a-Vie's Meditation Center. In celebration of John Havens' 50th birthday, the Meditation Center was officially opened on April 3, 2006.

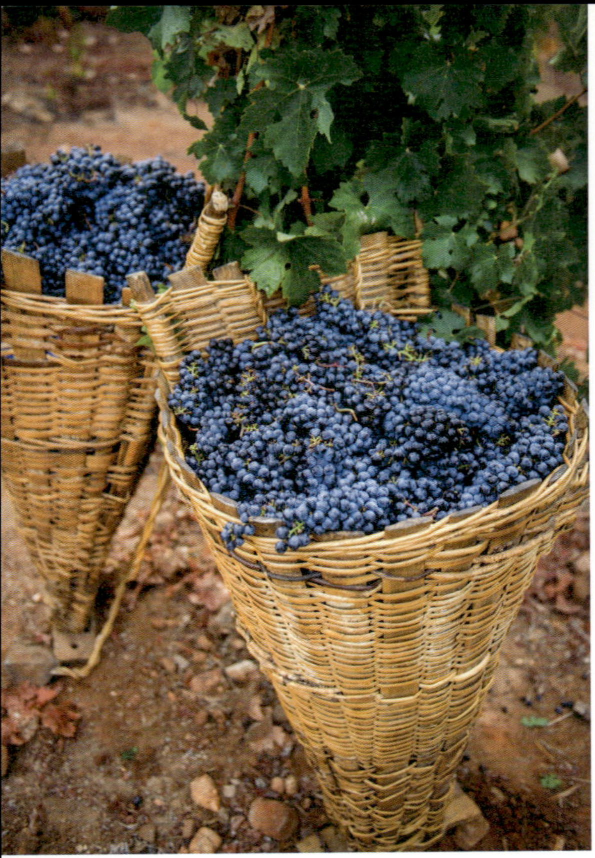

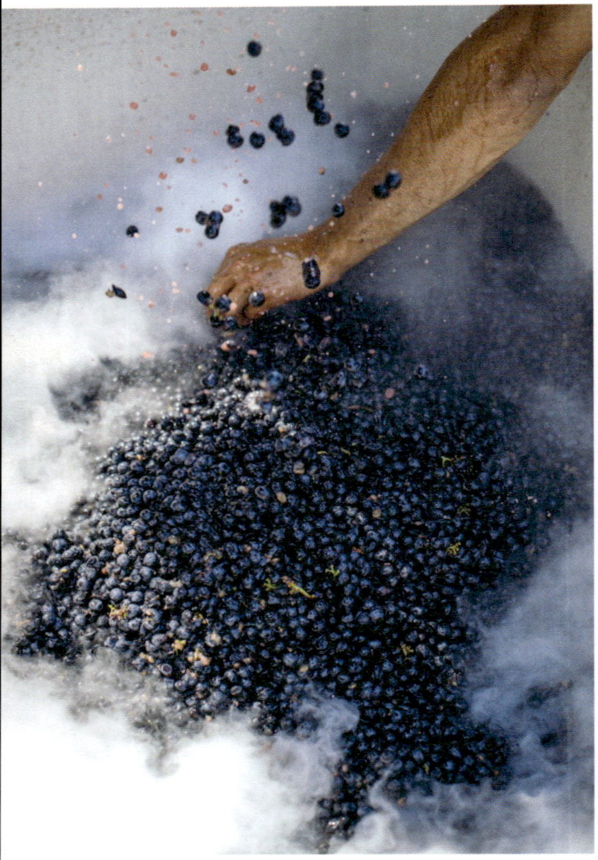

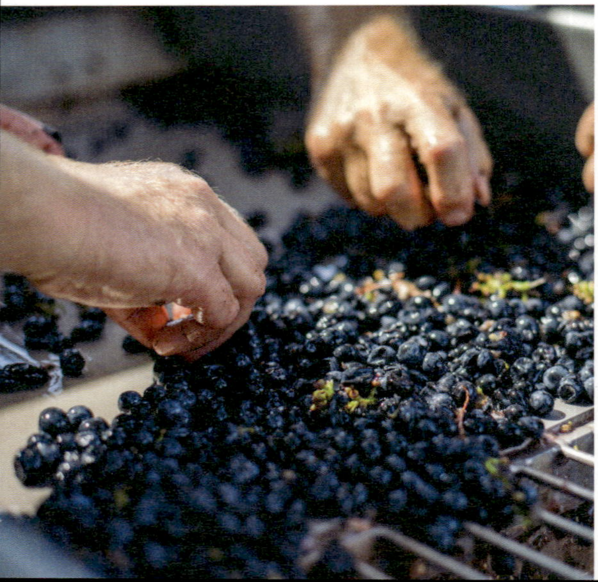

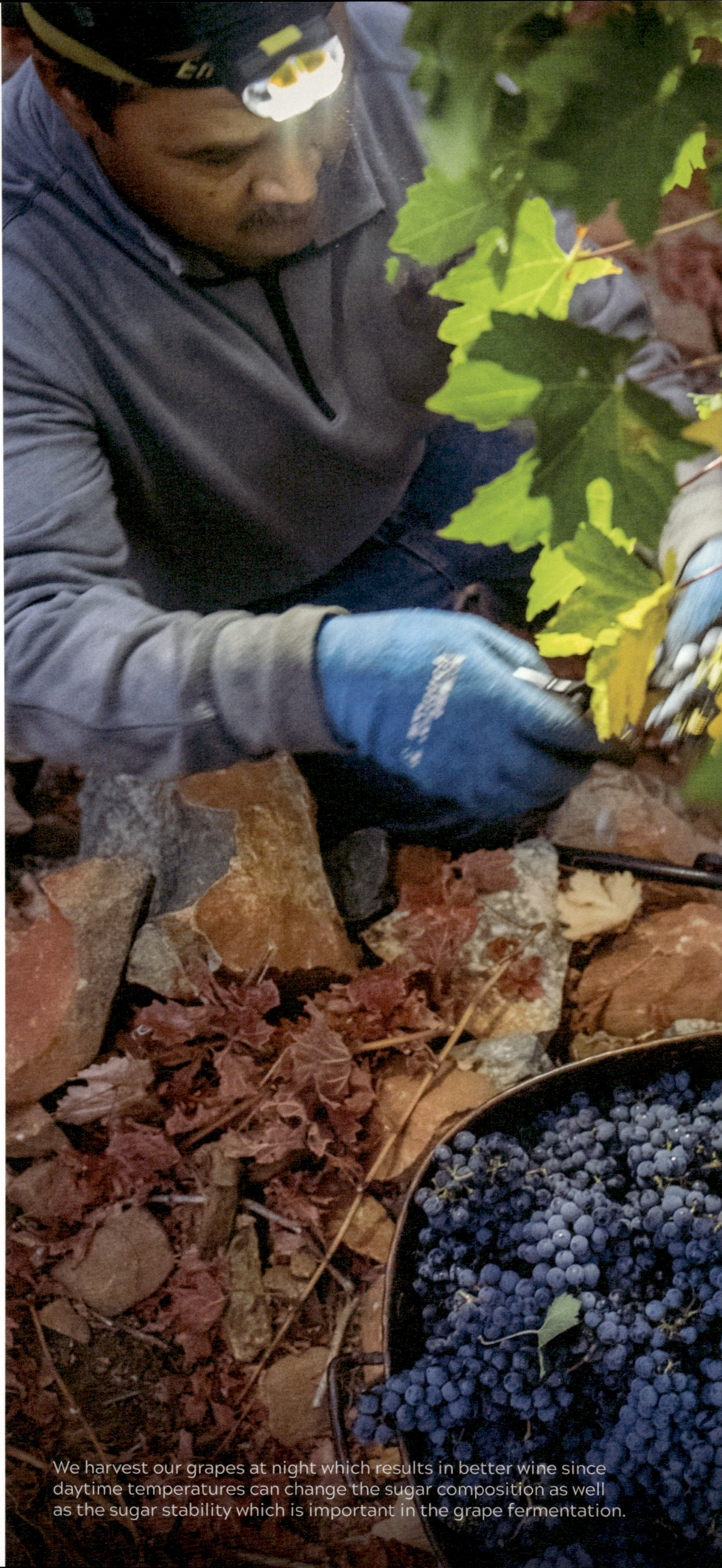

We harvest our grapes at night which results in better wine since daytime temperatures can change the sugar composition as well as the sugar stability which is important in the grape fermentation.

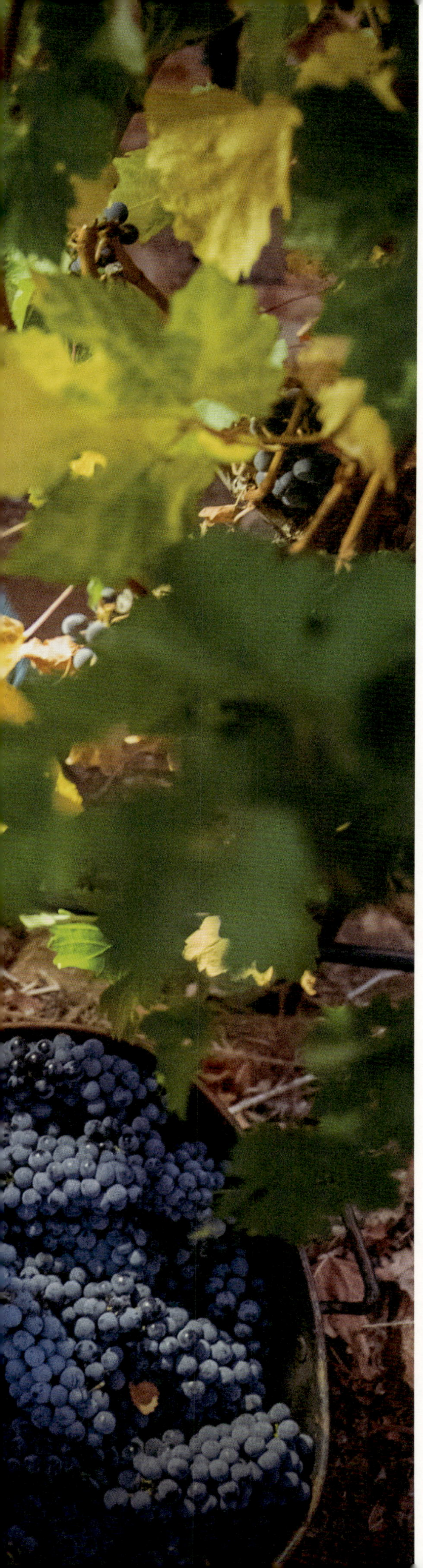

HOW DID WE MAKE CAL-A-VIE EVEN MORE FRENCH?

WINE, OF COURSE!

Since we renovated the retreat with a distinctive Provençal flavor, we were always thinking of different ways to further capture the history and ambiance of France—to make Cal-a-Vie more French. What's more French than wine, right?

It actually made sense. The rolling countryside, pristine soil, ideal California climate, and gentle Pacific breezes are perfect for growing grapes. So we dedicated 15 acres on the site for the Havens Family Estate, a vineyard whose grapes we use in our signature label, Chateau Cal-A-Vie.

We offer a range of wines to satisfy even the most discriminating palette. Our crisp Merlot Rosé has hints of papaya, citrus, and melon, with a touch of lavender. The Sauvignon Blanc is aged to perfection, helping to bring out the nuanced flavors of white peach and gooseberry, with just a suggestion of jalapeño. Dramatic and rich, our Merlot is known for its cherry aromas and classic Bordeaux-style bouquet and finish. And we've blended Cabernet Sauvignon, Cabernet Franc, and Merlot grapes to create a perfectly balanced Grand Vin Rouge.

Often, we're asked if alcohol is served at the spa. It's not, but you can have a bottle of our estate wine sent to your room to enjoy a private glass before or after dinner. We do offer wine-tastings at the Presbitaire, a 17th-century priest's residence that was located 30 miles from Dijon, in the heart of French Burgundy country. We had it carefully disassembled there and then reassembled here, and it offers an exquisite setting for guests to sample our Chateau Cal-a-Vie wine.

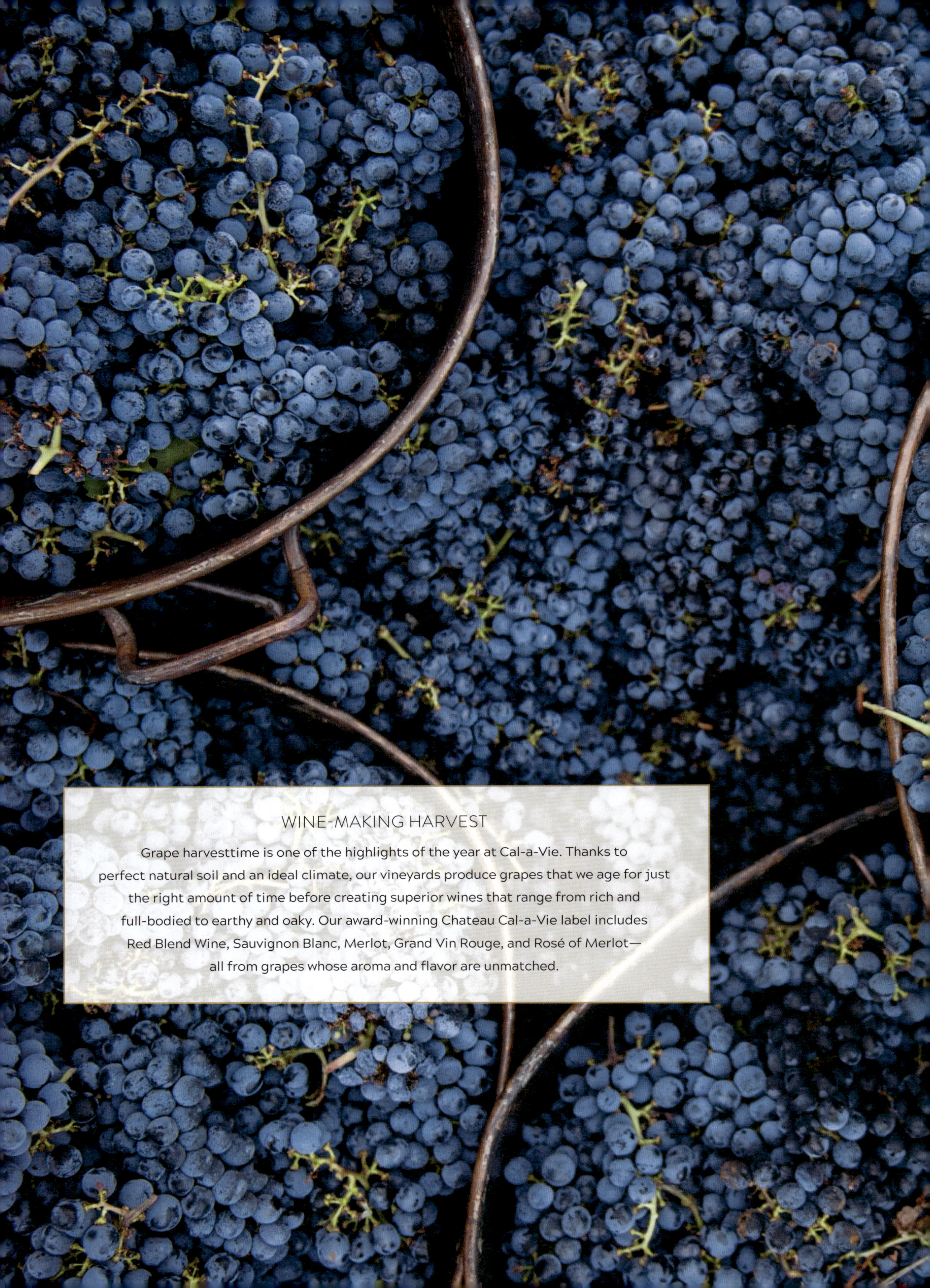

WINE-MAKING HARVEST

Grape harvesttime is one of the highlights of the year at Cal-a-Vie. Thanks to perfect natural soil and an ideal climate, our vineyards produce grapes that we age for just the right amount of time before creating superior wines that range from rich and full-bodied to earthy and oaky. Our award-winning Chateau Cal-a-Vie label includes Red Blend Wine, Sauvignon Blanc, Merlot, Grand Vin Rouge, and Rosé of Merlot—all from grapes whose aroma and flavor are unmatched.

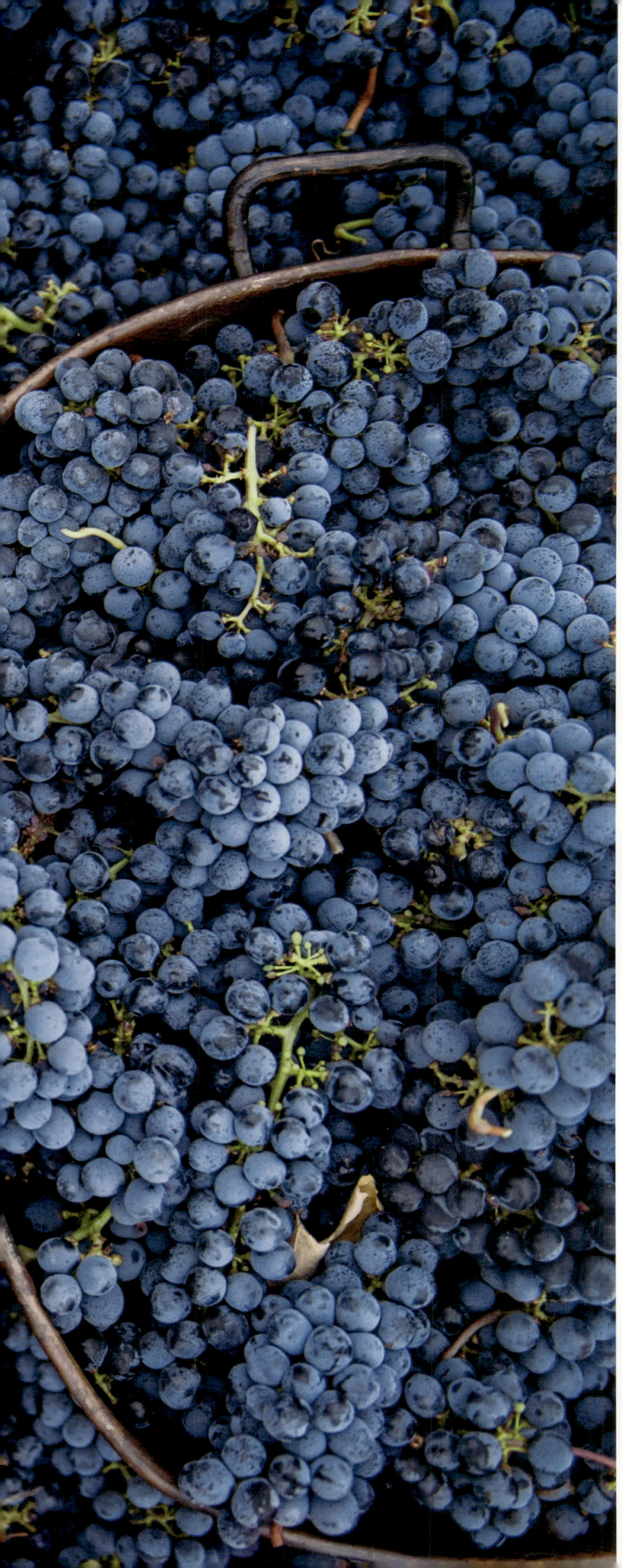
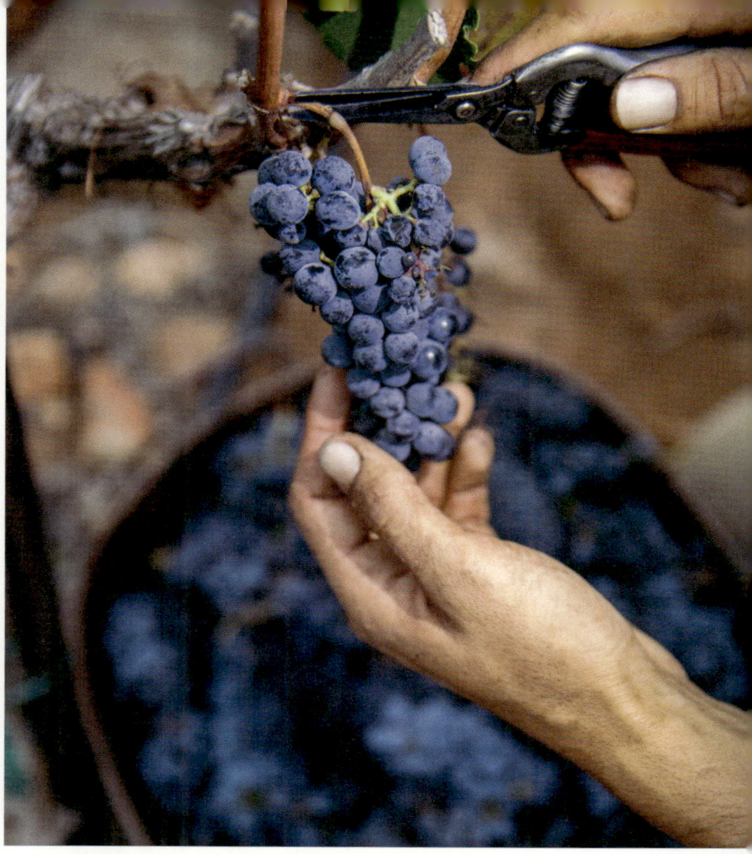
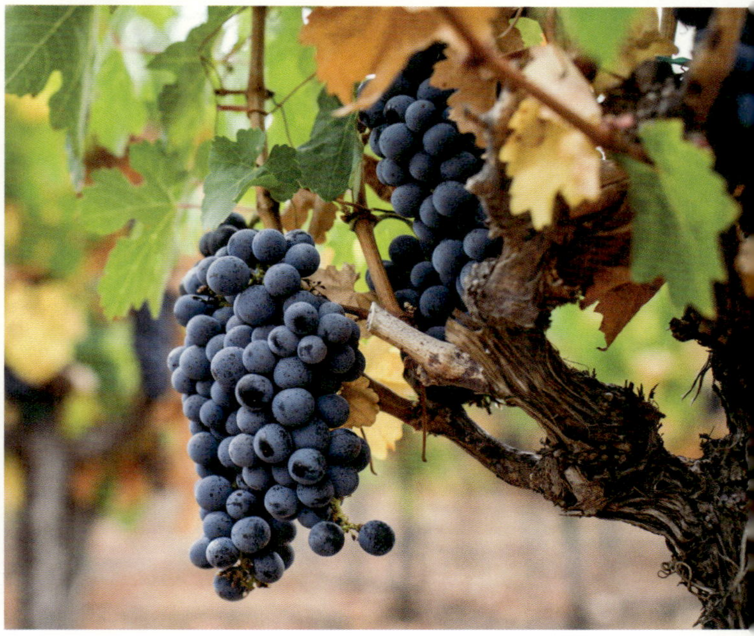
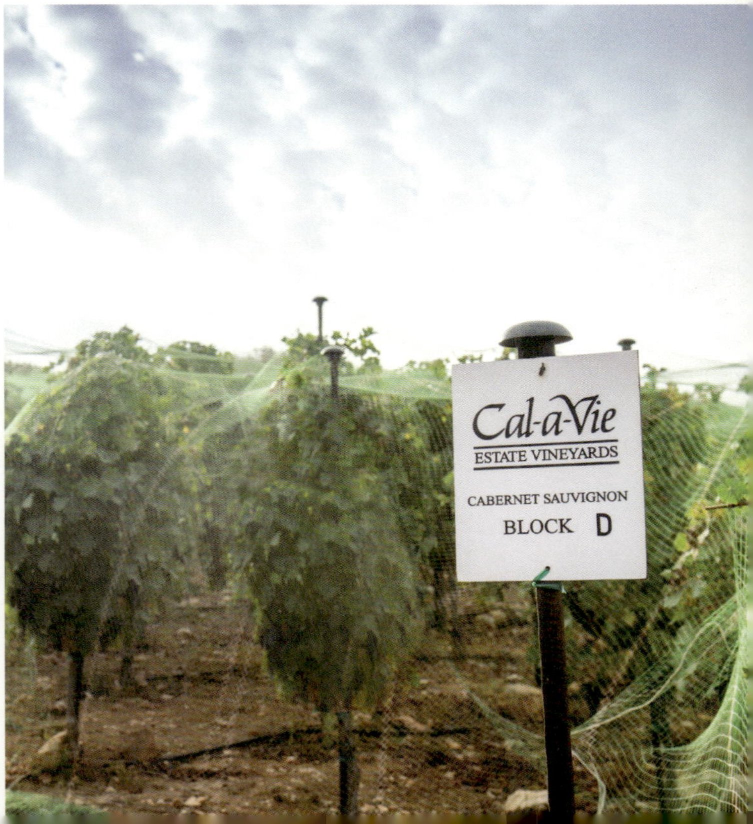
Cal-a-Vie
ESTATE VINEYARDS
CABERNET SAUVIGNON
BLOCK D

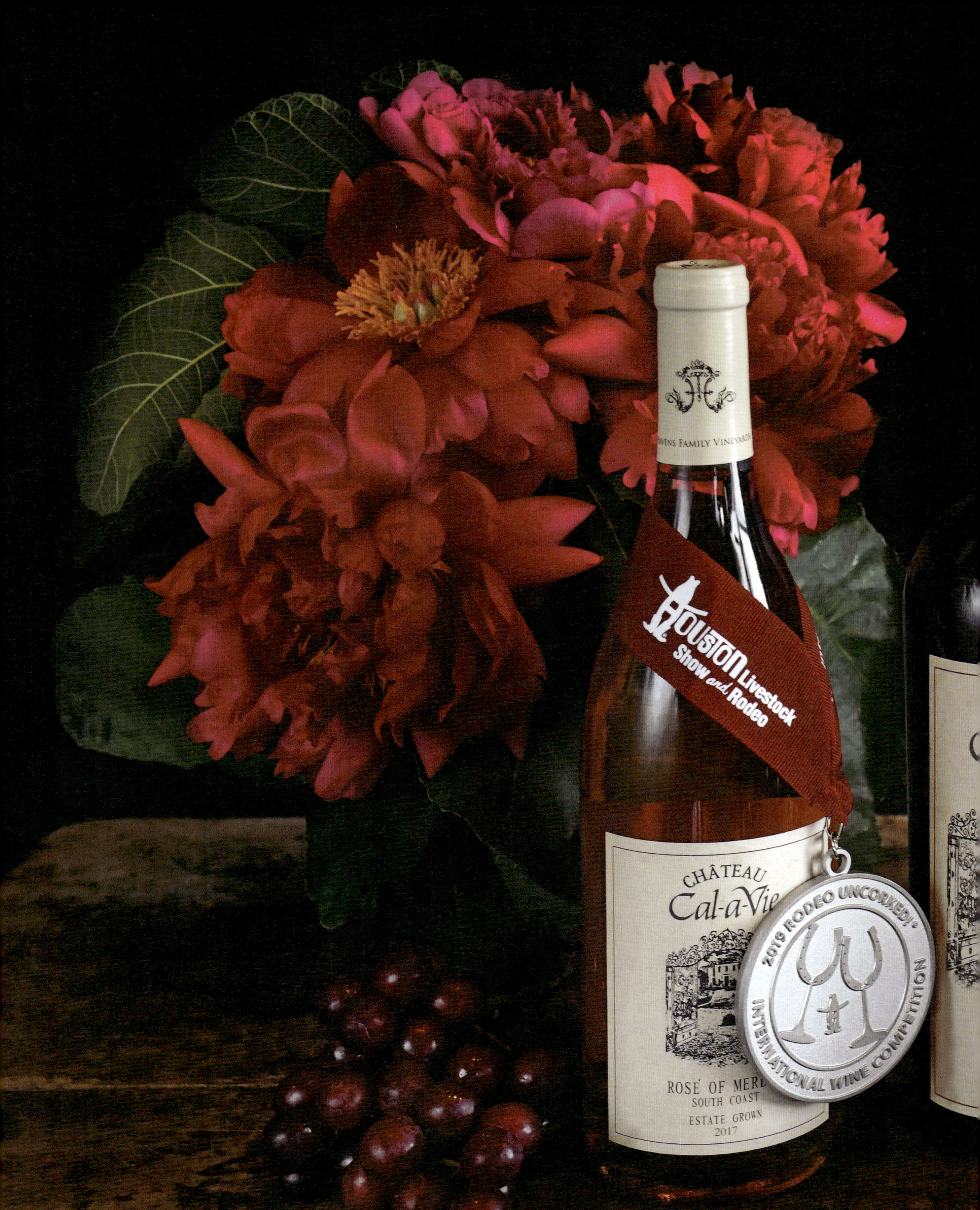

Our Rosé of Merlot earned a silver medal in the 2019 Rodeo Uncorked International Wine Competition from the Houston Livestock Show and Rodeo.

Cal-a-Vie's Sauvignon Blanc was a gold medal winner at the 2019 Rodeo Uncorked International Wine Competition, while our Grand Vin Rouge received a silver.

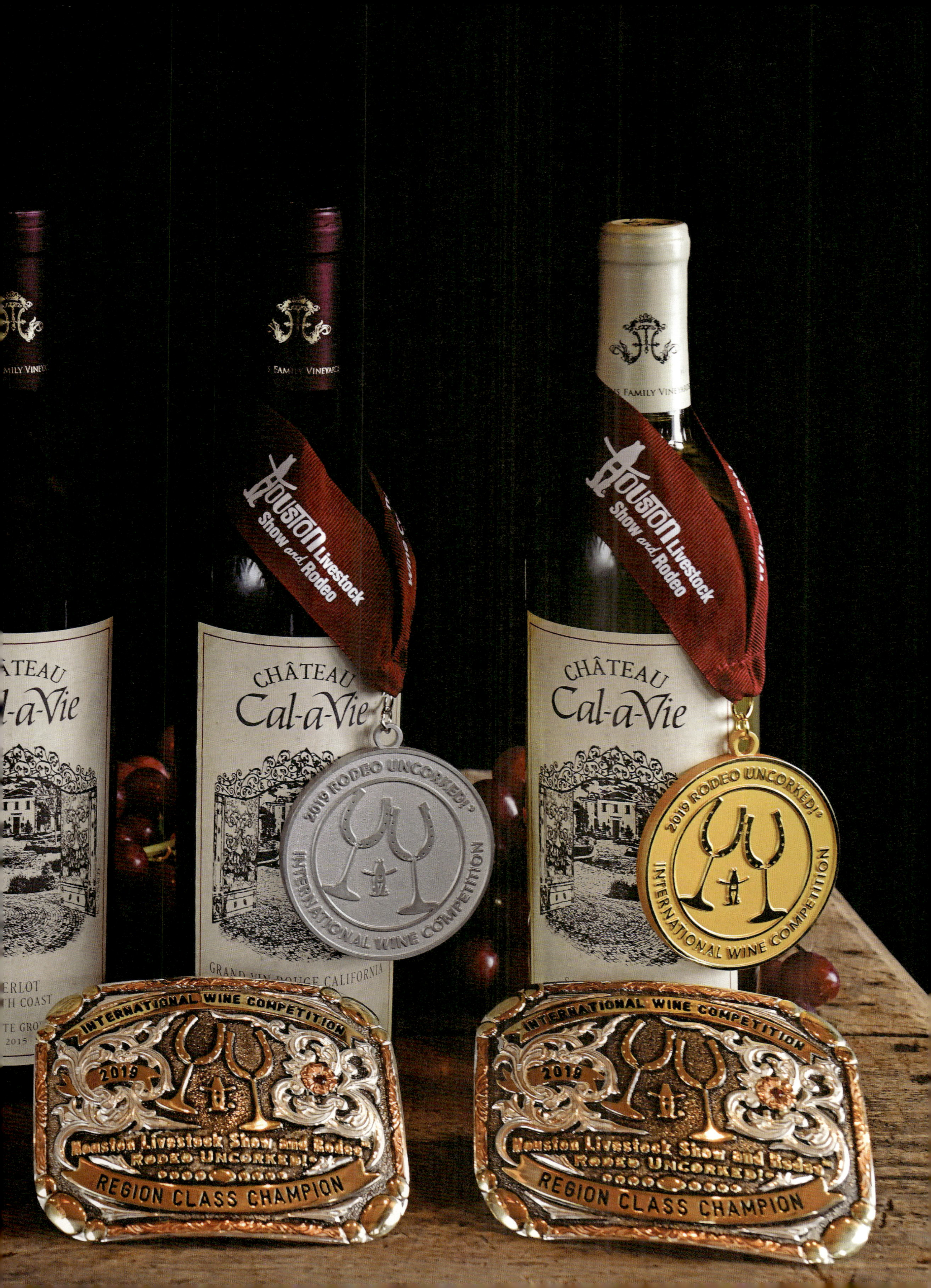
CHÂTEAU
Cal-a-Vie
Houston Livestock Show and Rodeo
2019 RODEO UNCORKED!®
INTERNATIONAL WINE COMPETITION
GRAND VIN ROUGE CALIFORNIA
INTERNATIONAL WINE COMPETITION
2019
Houston Livestock Show and Rodeo
RODEO UNCORKED!
REGION CLASS CHAMPION

A BETTER YOU

FITNESS IS A CENTERPIECE OF CAL-A-VIE, AS MUCH A PART OF THE RETREAT AS THE GORGEOUS DÉCOR AND NUTRITIOUS MEALS.

It just reflects our belief that mind, body, and spirit are all equal parts of the whole person, and that each must be treated with the same respect and focus.

We make it easy, and we do provide a lot of options—and I do mean a lot—to give you just about anything you need to boost your energy, reduce your stress, and condition your body.

We have more than 150 classes. There are eight of them on the schedule at any given hour after the morning hike and before lunch, and they're all overseen by professional trainers and instructors. Like everything else at Cal-a-Vie Health Spa, we wanted to be sure that our offerings went above and beyond those at any other spa, any place in the world. They do.

If you're into heavy-duty workouts, we have programs with names like Muscles on Fire, No Guts No Glory, and R.I.P.P.E.D. (that would be resistance, interval, power, plyometric, and endurance). If you're looking to mix it up a little, there's Piloxing, a blend of Pilates, boxing, and dancing. If fun mixed with fitness is your preference, hit one of our Zumba classes. All that is in addition to classes like circuit training, aerobics, cardio, kickboxing, spinning, and Tai Chi. Of course, some people like sitting by the pool as their activity; that's great, too.

There's something else that's unique. Some people just aren't into the whole group exercise thing. We get that, and it's not a problem. We can arrange for personal, one-on-one sessions that deliver all the fitness benefits you want in a private setting. It's the perfect way to try something you haven't wanted to do in front of everyone at home.

Bottom line, this is a program with one major goal: To make you feel better, be better, and maybe even look better than when you arrived. You can go as hard and fast as you want. But I promise that whatever your pace, you'll be heading in the direction of your absolute best.

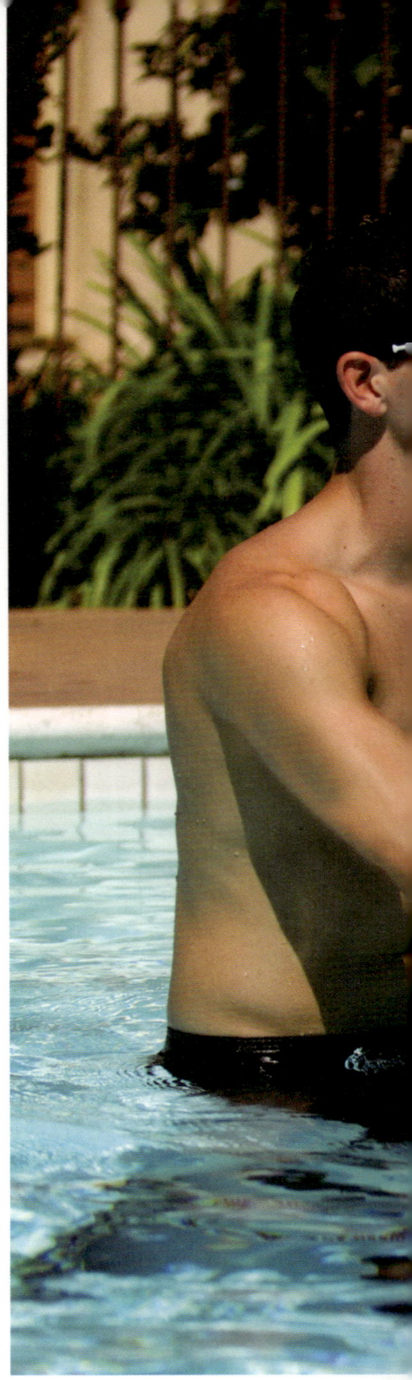

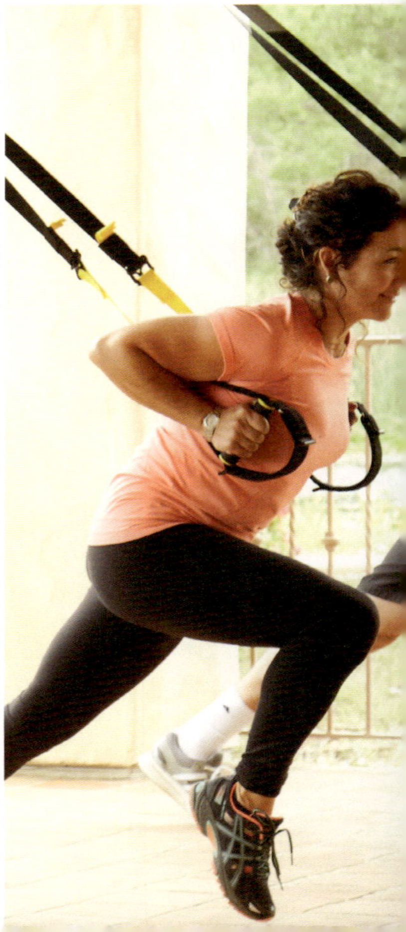

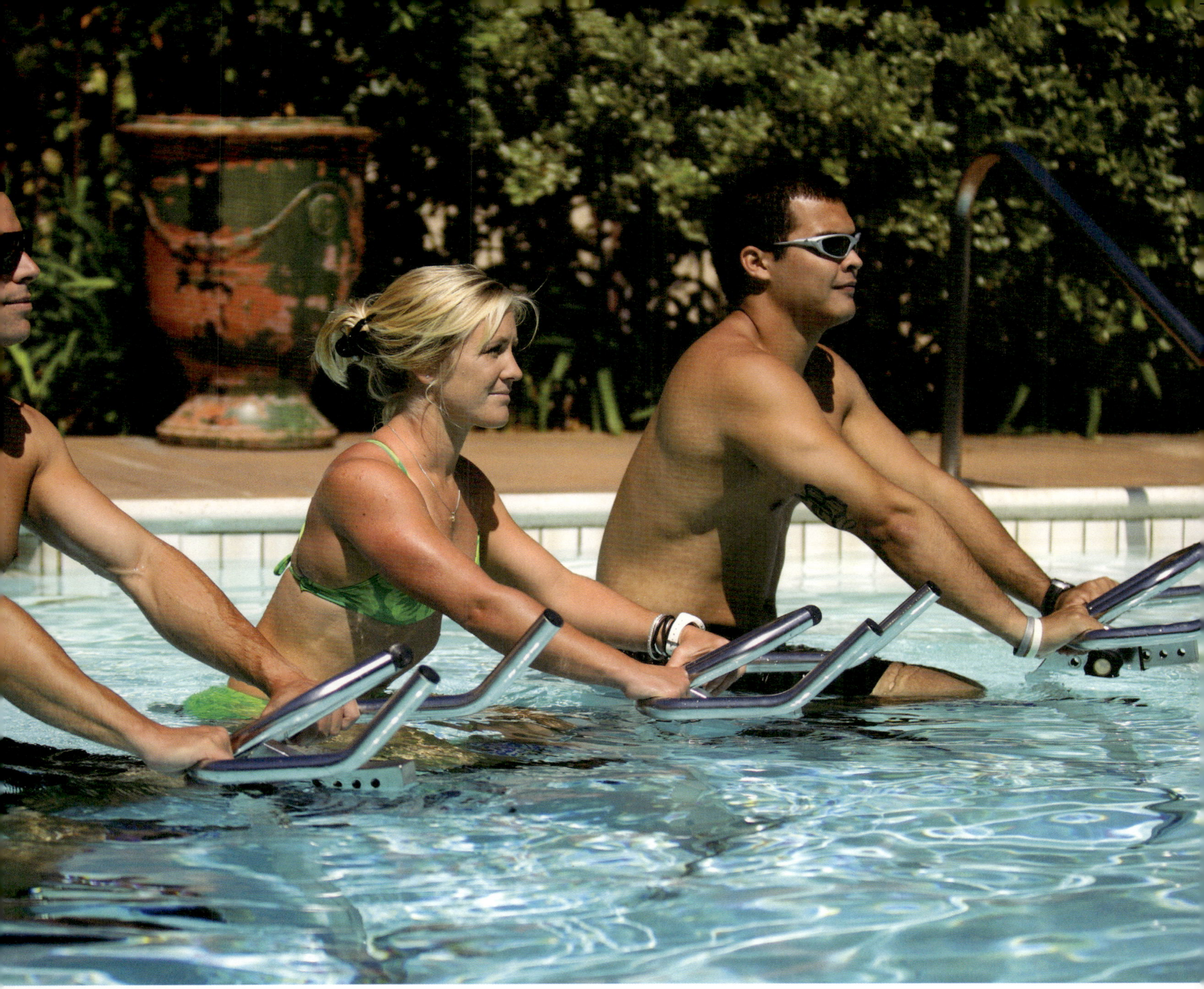
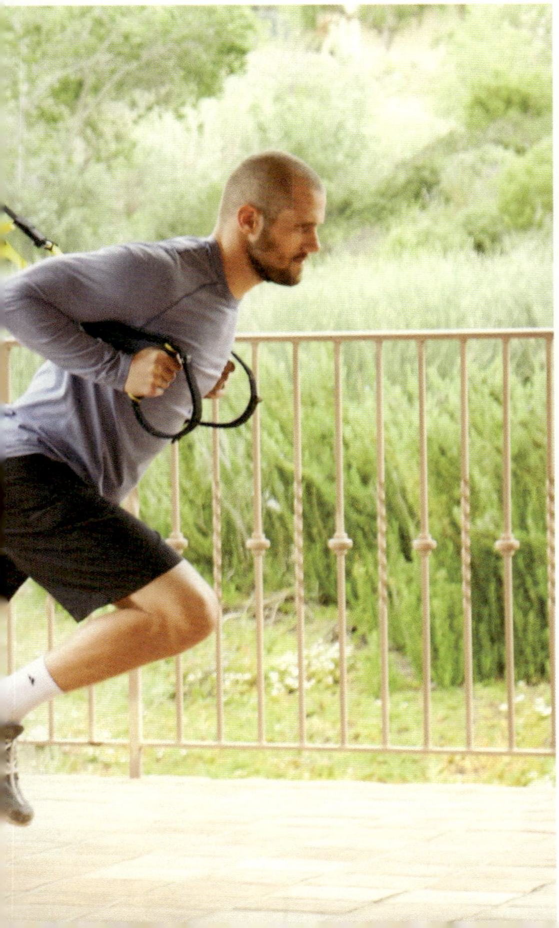
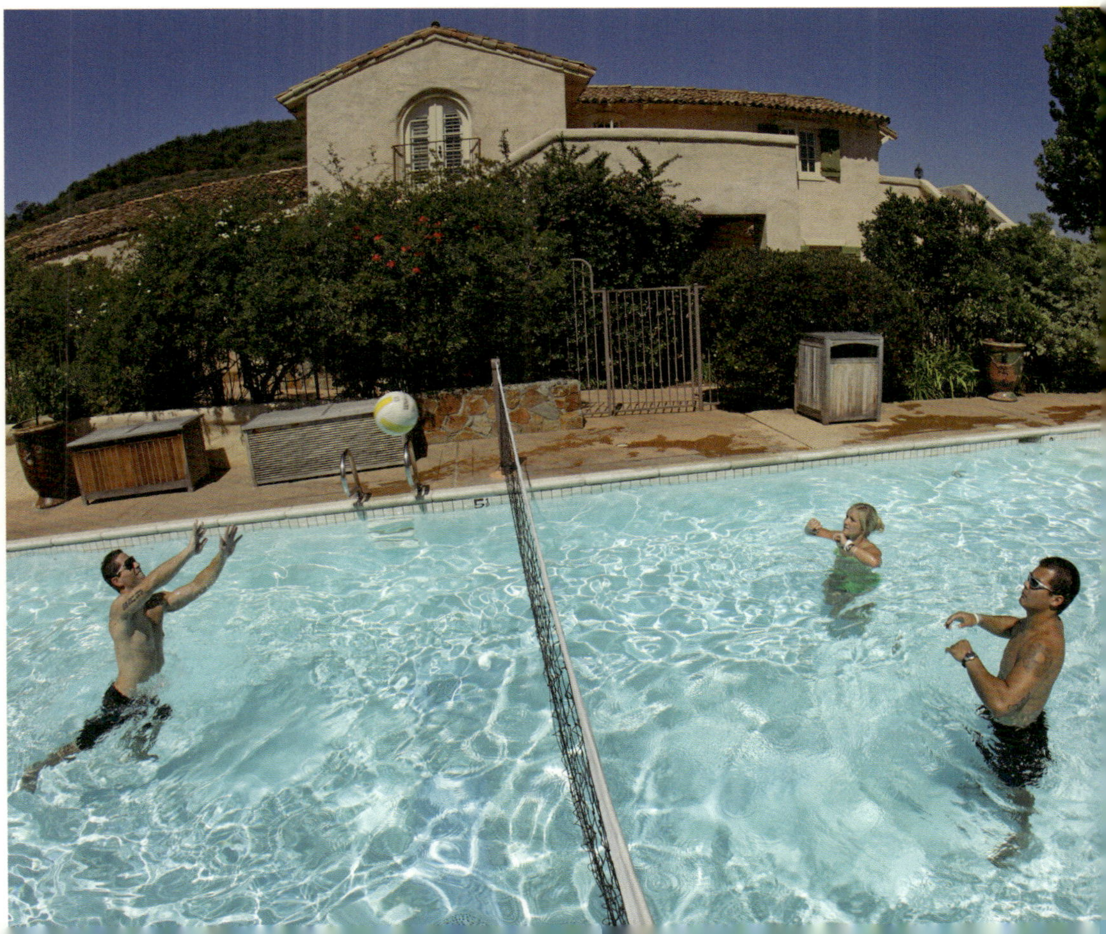

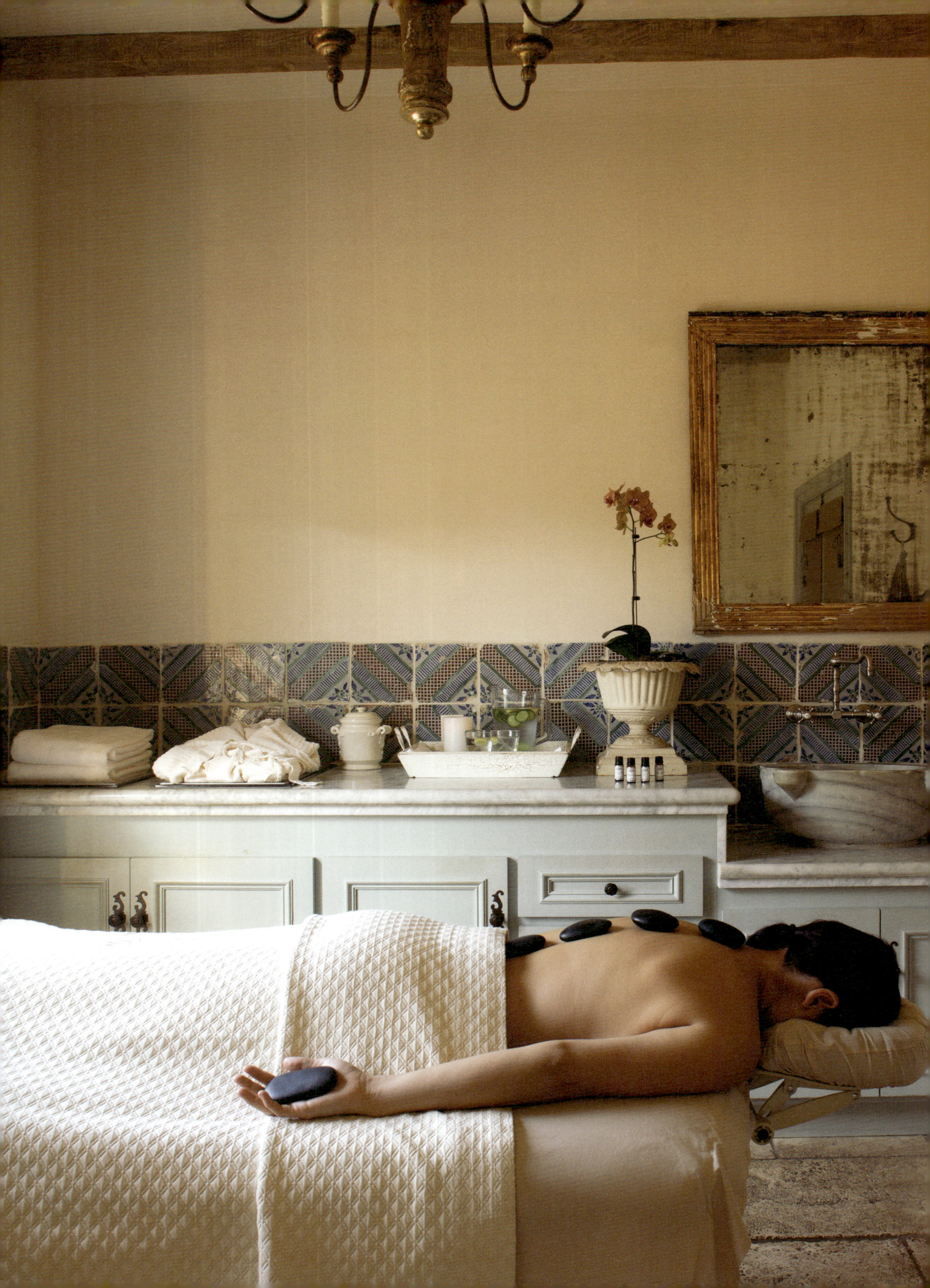

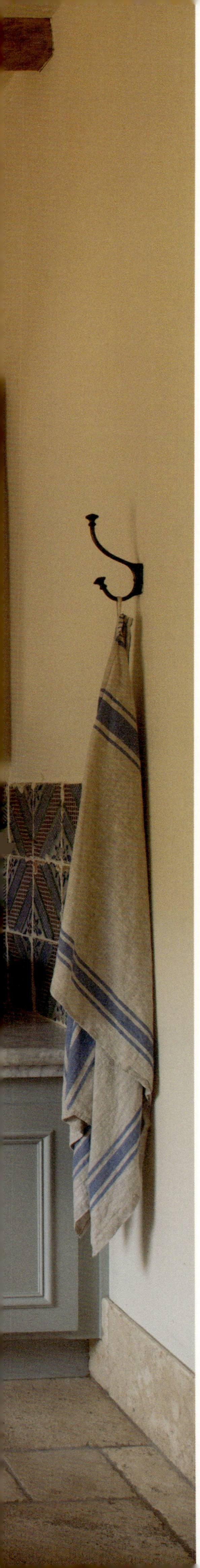

BEAUTY TREATMENTS AND SPA THERAPIES

PAMPER YOURSELF.

SO MUCH OF THE CAL-A-VIE HEALTH SPA EXPERIENCE IS ABOUT SELF-CARE. **While our visitors come here from many places, for many reasons, what we hear as much as anything is that they need some degree of personal recharging. Our spa services and beauty treatments aim to please.**

Of course, these services were the foundation of Cal-a-Vie, and were a big reason John and I were first attracted to the retreat. Because we believe that beauty treatments and wellness therapies are critical to good mental and physical health, we wanted to be sure that what we were offering lifted and nourished the spirits of our guests.

It doesn't matter if you come here like me—a lover of all things spa-related—or like John, who didn't initially have much time for this kind of thing (until he did). Whatever your level of experience might be, Cal-a-Vie Health Spa has what it takes to relax your mind and your body: soothing facials and facial enhancements, like alpha-hydroxy fruit peel and microdermabrasion; hand and foot rejuvenation; traditional and Thai massage; and a full range of salon extras.

We developed them all with the input of international health and beauty experts, too, and we use only the best, natural, plant and sea extracts and fragrant, restorative oils.

But as luxurious and appealing as all that may sound, it doesn't stop there. You could also say we've turned the spa experience into a science. Seriously.

We are the first retreat in America to use what's called MUSE, a wearable brain-sensing headband that measures brain waves to give instant feedback on things like heart rate, breathing, and body movements, and helps our guests stay more relaxed and better focused when they meditate. It promotes calm, reduces stress, controls anxiety, increases joy and happiness, and elevates a sense of self.

Which, now that I think about it, pretty much captures the essence of Cal-a-Vie Health Spa. If our fitness programs help you to become your absolute best, our treatments and therapies help you become the purest version of yourself.

THE DREAM DESTINATION

FOR A DREAM WEDDING.

I'LL BE THE FIRST TO ADMIT I'M AN INCURABLE ROMANTIC.

One of the things that captured me most when John and I first discovered Cal-a-Vie was the way it made me feel.

I'd look out over lavender fields tucked into the lush rolling foothills—all of it drenched in the soft, warm sunshine—and it just took my breath away. I know what love feels like. Cal-a-Vie is what it looks like.

That makes it the dream destination for a wedding. As one bride said, "From our first visit, Cal-a-Vie felt like a fairytale."

You feel the pull and ambiance of the French provincial countryside instantly. The setting is magical—intimate and elegant at once. The wedding ceremonies, lit by hundreds of candles, are held in a 400-year-old chapel we imported from Dijon, France, and you have a choice for a gala reception: The 300-year-old L'Orangerie (also from Dijon), with its antique French chandeliers and three 16th-century fireplaces, or outside on the manicured, 8,000-square-foot L'Orangerie lawn, which overlooks tranquil Vista Valley. You can't lose. They're both stunning.

But a wedding at Cal-a-Vie is not simply about an astonishing venue. We also go the extra mile to make sure that every detail of your event delivers the kind of memories and joy that brides, grooms, families, and friends deserve.

Guests and members of the party can enjoy all the spa's benefits, from fitness classes to nutritional lectures to spa and beauty treatments. Cal-a-Vie's executive chef and his staff prepare gourmet dinners highlighted by natural, organic foods fresh from our on-site garden. We have our own planner who will oversee and guide you through every step of the wedding, including pictures, flowers, rehearsals, color palettes, and entertainment. And we offer all the perfect accessories and amenities that will make your happiest day even happier than you could imagine.

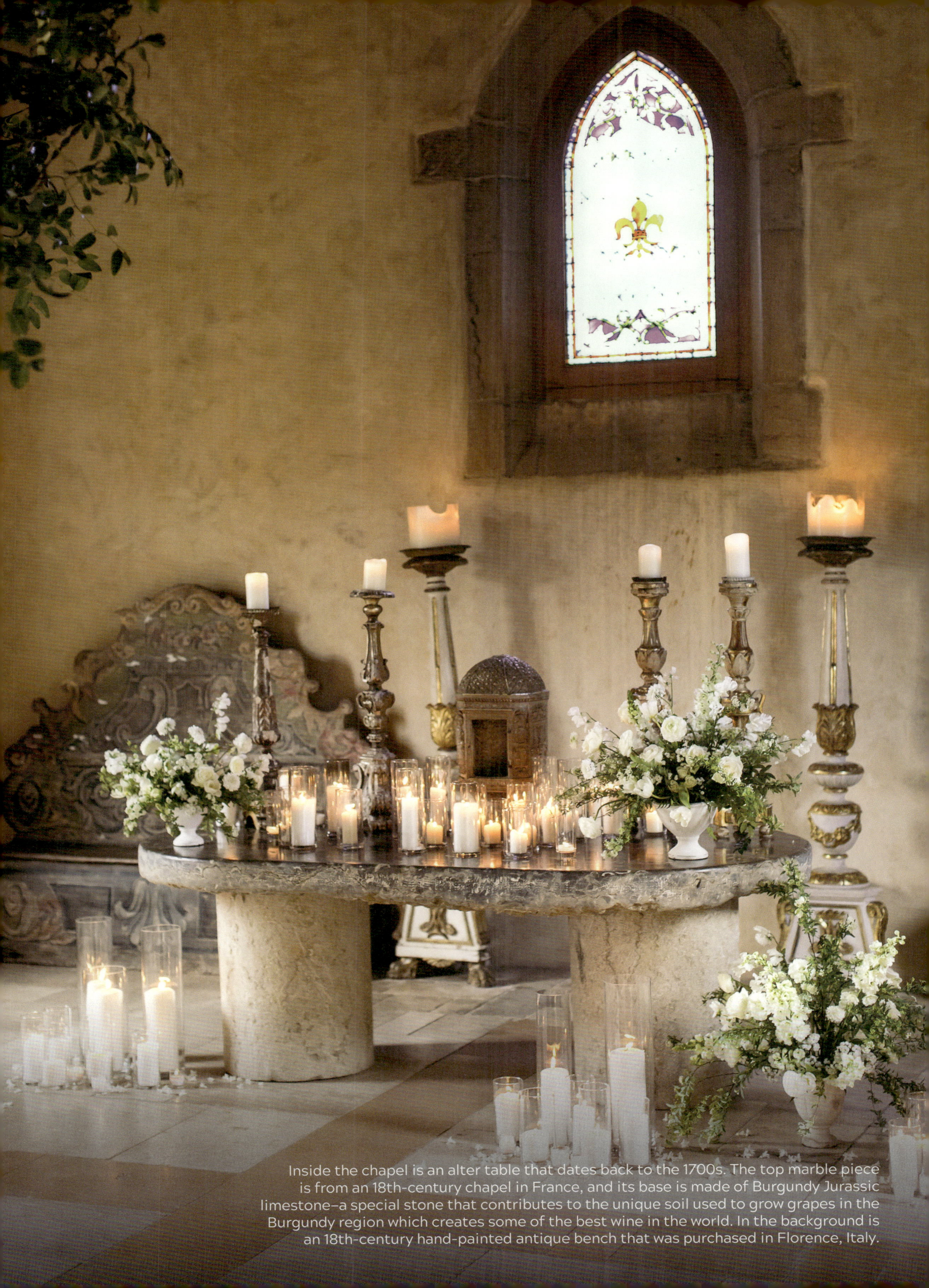

Inside the chapel is an alter table that dates back to the 1700s. The top marble piece is from an 18th-century chapel in France, and its base is made of Burgundy Jurassic limestone–a special stone that contributes to the unique soil used to grow grapes in the Burgundy region which creates some of the best wine in the world. In the background is an 18th-century hand-painted antique bench that was purchased in Florence, Italy.

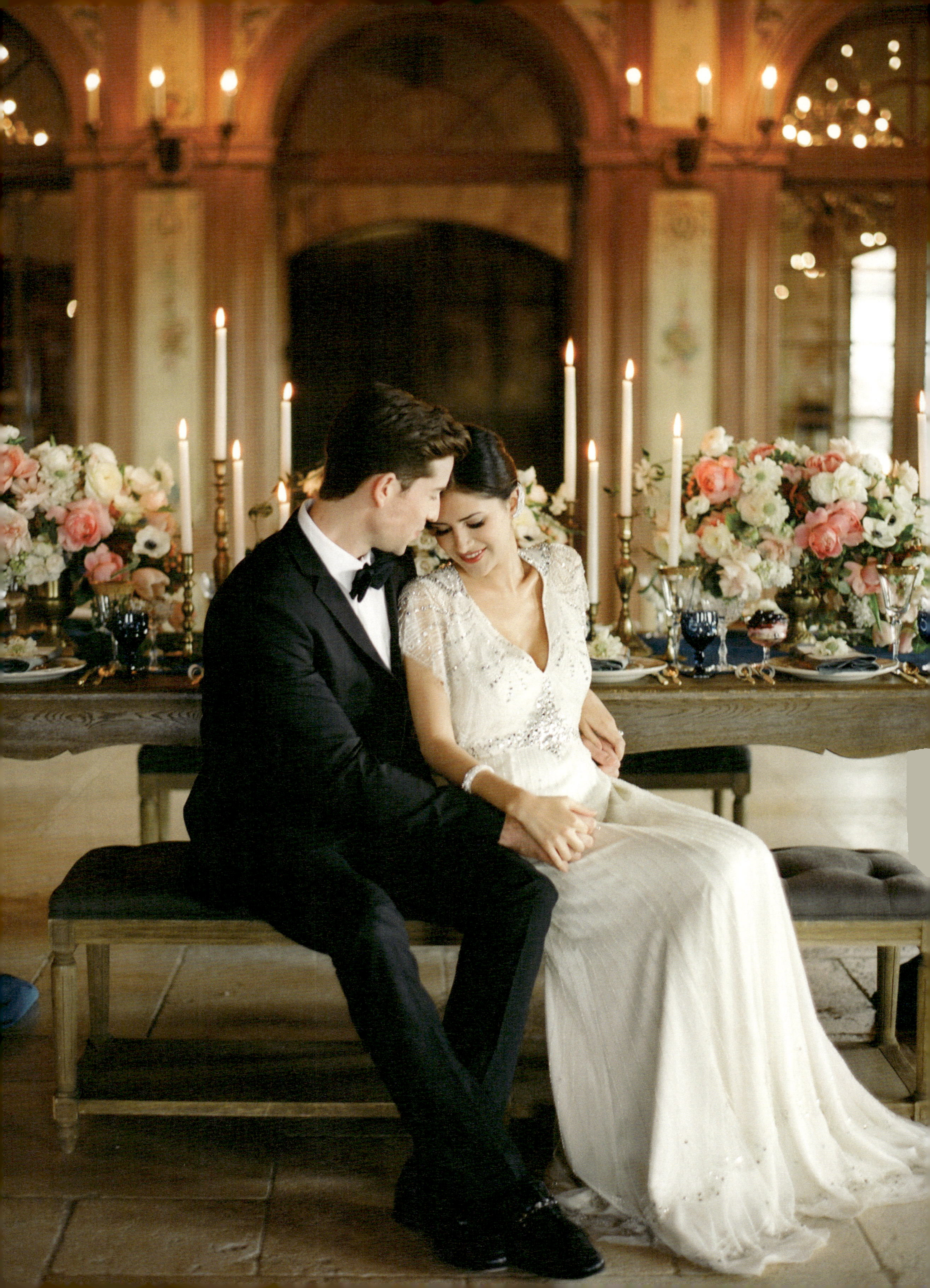

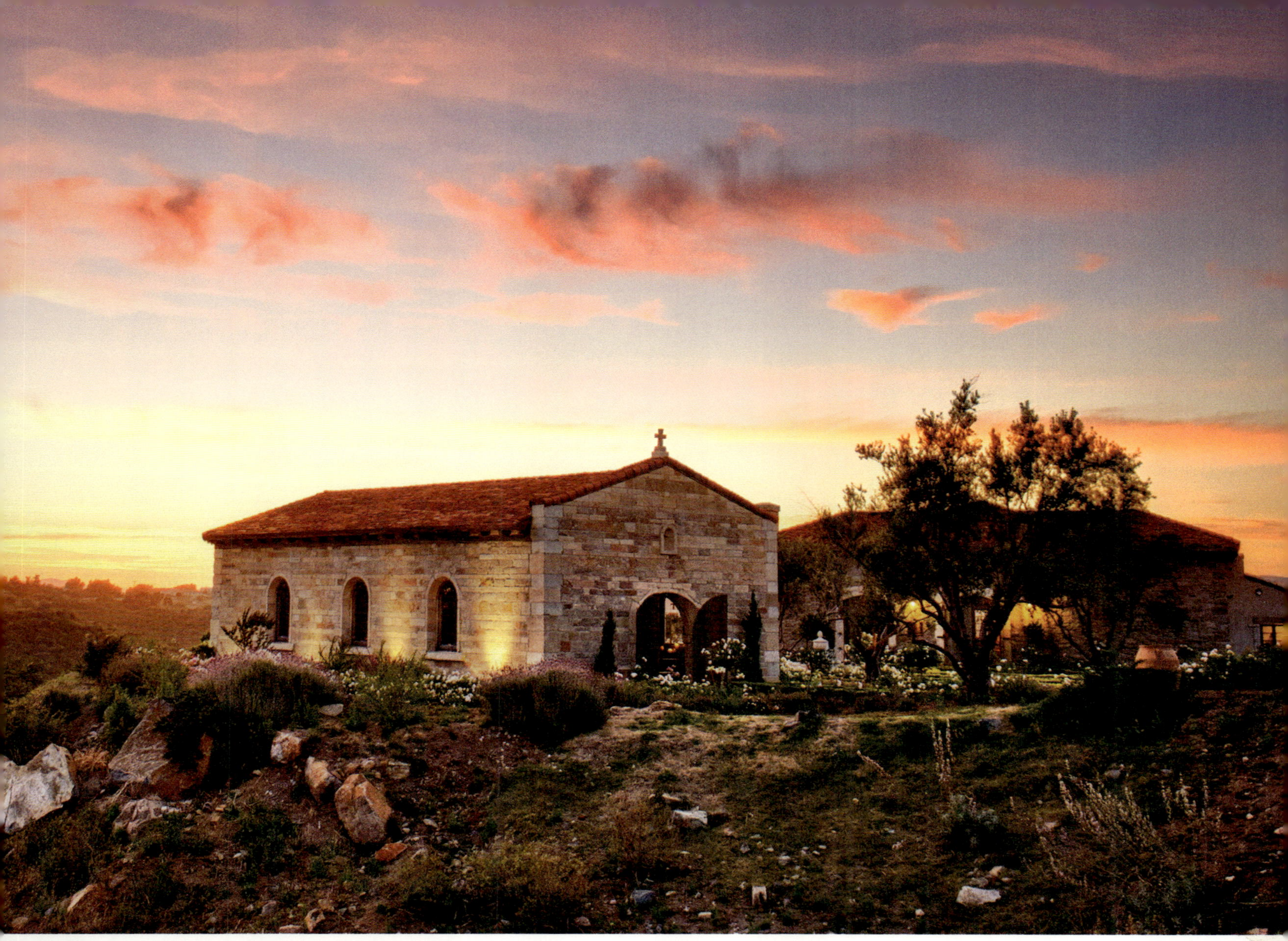
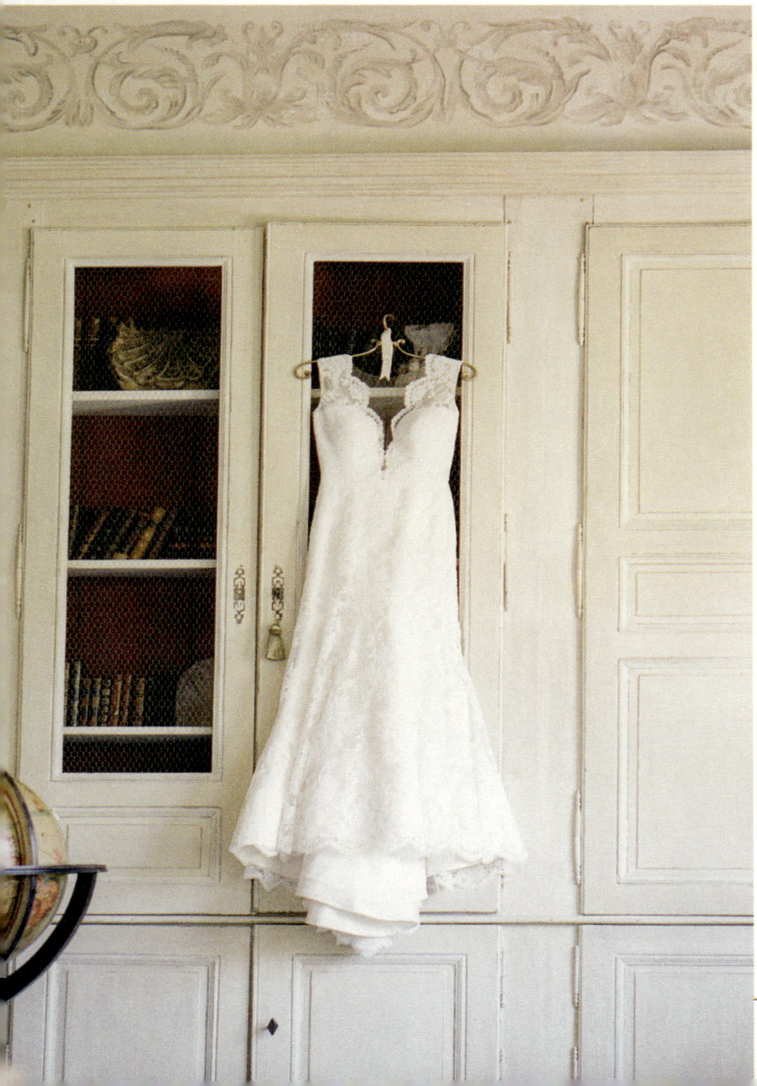
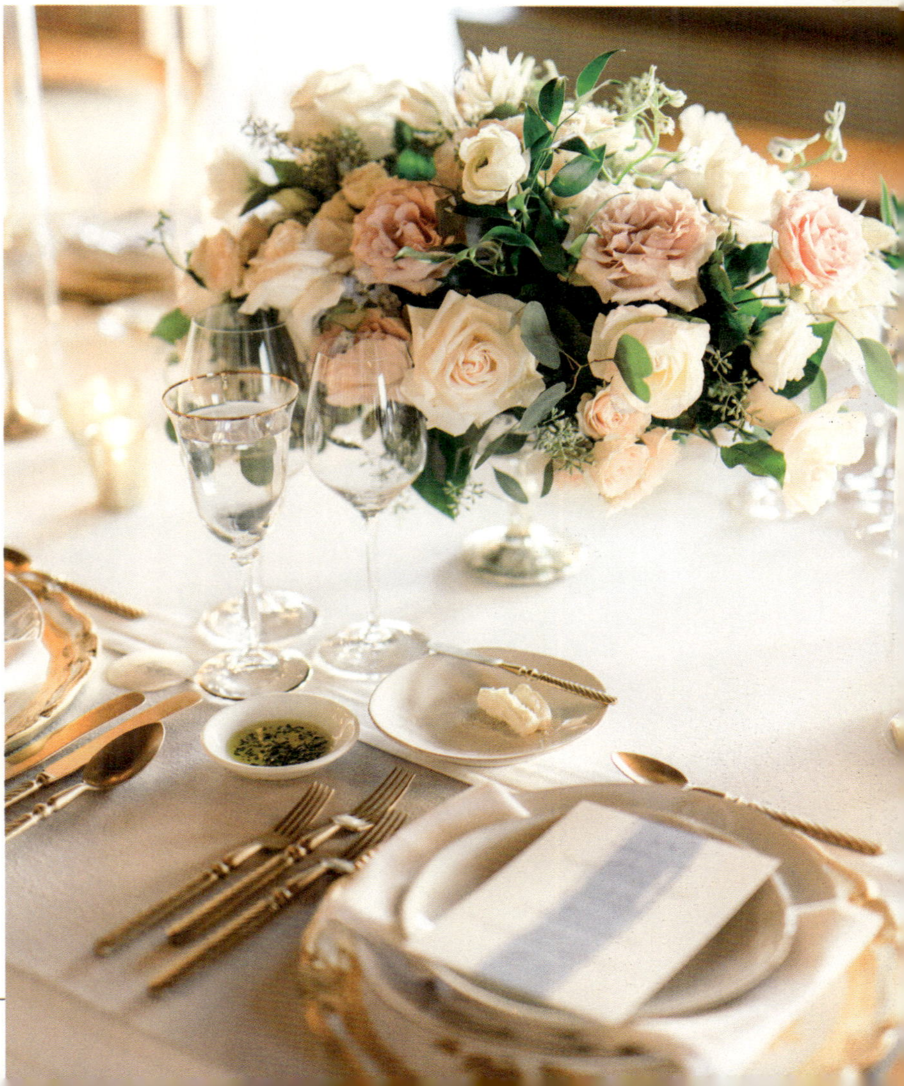

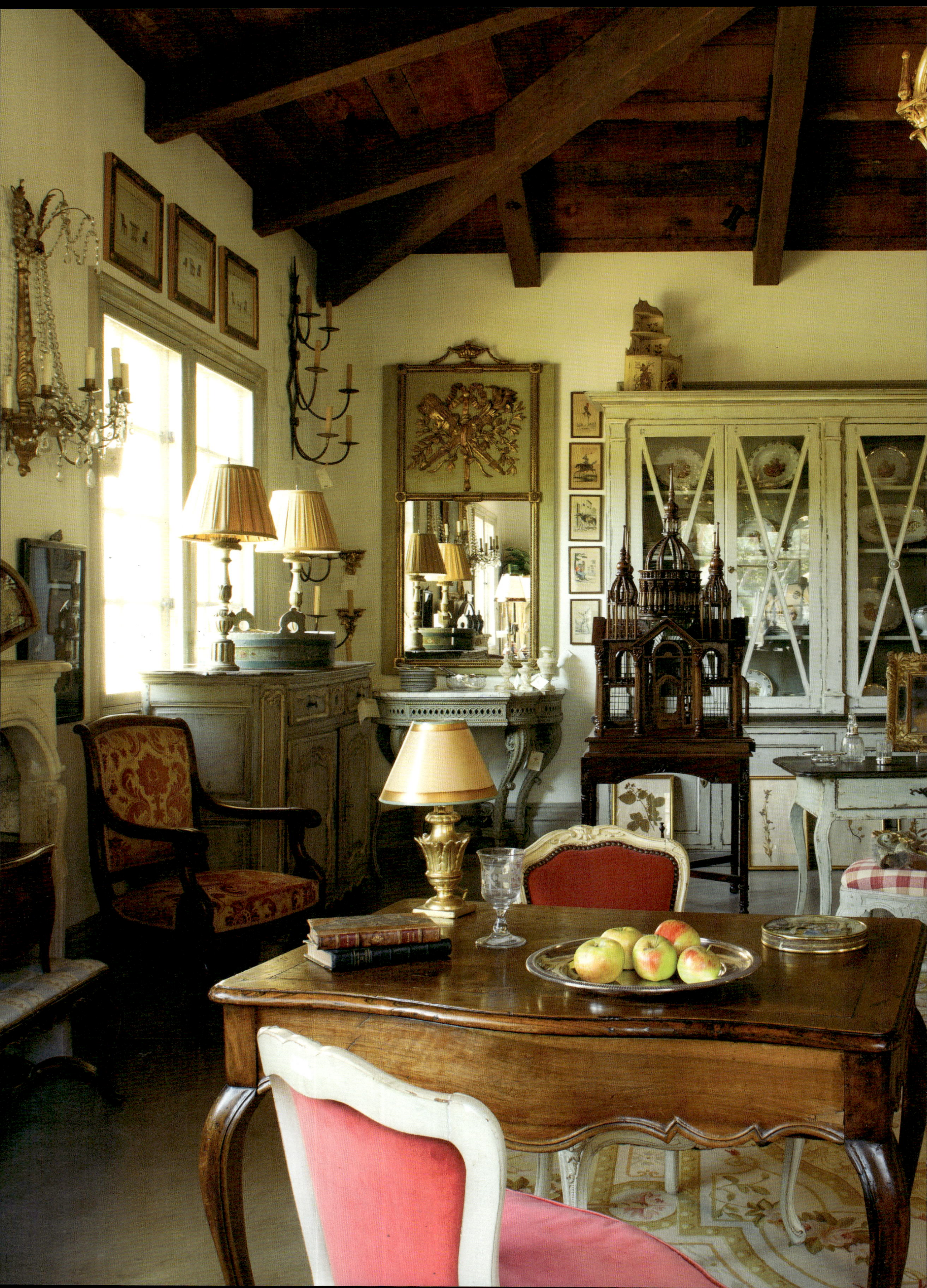

YOUR STAY MAY END

BUT THE CAL-A-VIE EXPERIENCE DOESN'T HAVE TO.

WHEN GUESTS COME TO CAL-A-VIE, WE WANT THEM TO ENJOY LIFE AND LUXURY

in a manner that no place else in the world can match. Typically, they don't want it to end when their stay is over. So we're always getting the question, "How can we take Cal-a-Vie home with us?"

Well, obviously, this cookbook is one way, offering the nutritious recipes and healthy-eating advice that are so much a part of the Cal-a-Vie experience. But there are a lot of other opportunities to make the retreat part of your day-to-day lifestyle as well.

You can buy our signature teas, for example, whose herbs and natural flavors can satisfy anyone's craving for sweets without the calories or carbs. Additionally, our holistic teas contain specific flowers, herbs, and spices whose therapeutic benefits have promoted healing and wellness for centuries.

And while some people may think chocolate should be avoided, I'm sorry, but we beg to differ. It all depends on how you make it. Our handcrafted, organic, dark chocolate is rich in antioxidants and flavonoids, both of which have a ton of health benefits. In other words, you get all the good stuff, and none of the guilt.

When you first walk through Cal-a-Vie's entryway, one of the things you notice right off the bat is the wonderful aroma coming from the front desk. It's from our Sweet Berry Candle, whose fragrance—fresh scents of pear, rhubarb, and berries—really does capture the essence of the spa. It's always been a guest favorite, and will keep Cal-a-Vie on your mind (and in your senses) long after you've returned home.

We are well known for our beauty treatments, so it's only natural that we would offer the same high-quality products used in the spa. Our Vinotherapie line made from grape skin, pulp, and seeds from our own vineyard is

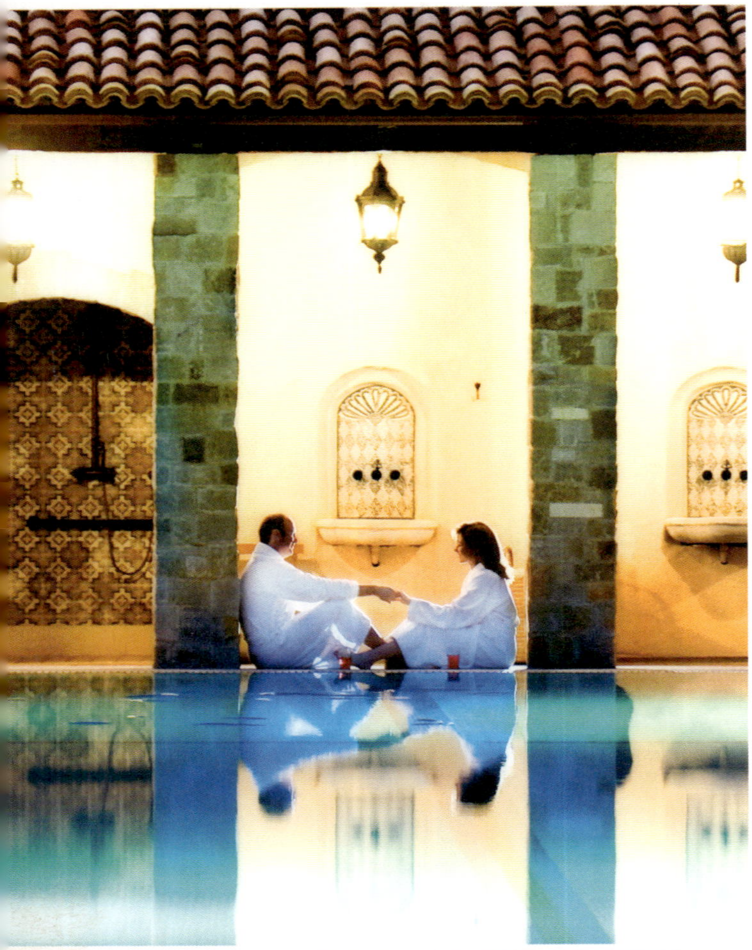

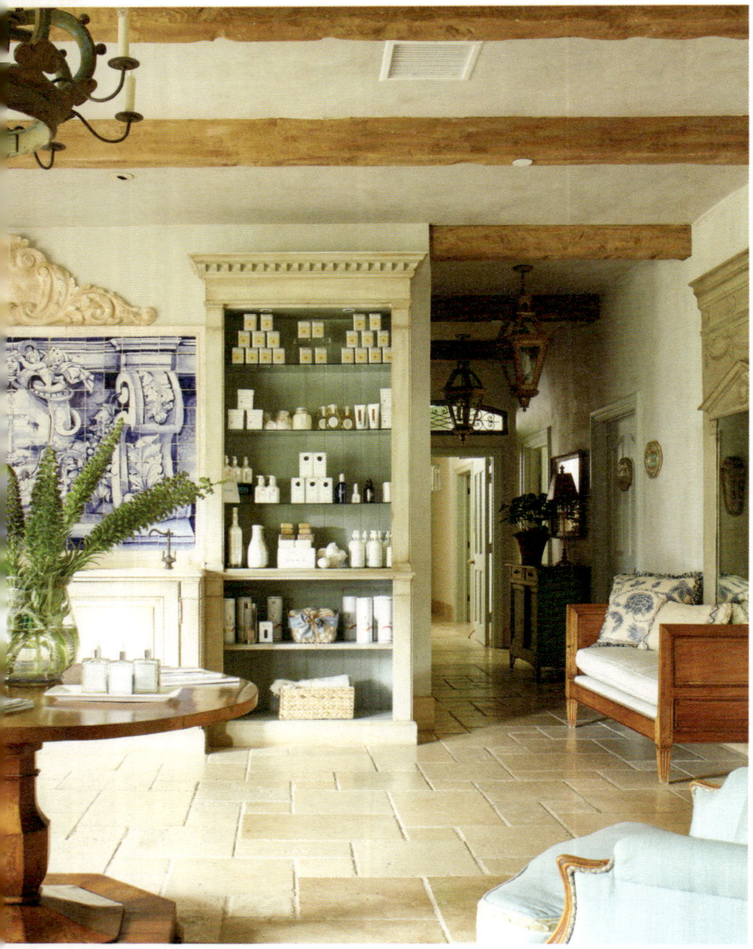

packed full of antioxidants and moisturizers, so you can get that fresh day-spa feeling no matter where you are. Our soothing amenities contain natural ingredients that strengthen and promote healthy skin and hair.

Of course, the décor and décor accessories are very much a part of Cal-a-Vie's character, and we have made sure you can take them with you as well. Cookware, glassware, table linens, pillows, towels—all those and more can be found in our boutique.

Finally, there are the antiques, which reflect the elegance John and I wanted to bring to Cal-a-Vie from Day One. From small trinkets to 18th-century armoires, from crystal chandeliers to French-provincial mirrors, guests can enjoy the spa's casual grace and grandeur right in their own home.

While your stay at Cal-a-Vie may end, we make it easy for the experience to go on.

WHILE YOUR STAY AT CAL-A-VIE MAY END, WE MAKE IT EASY FOR THE EXPERIENCE TO GO ON.

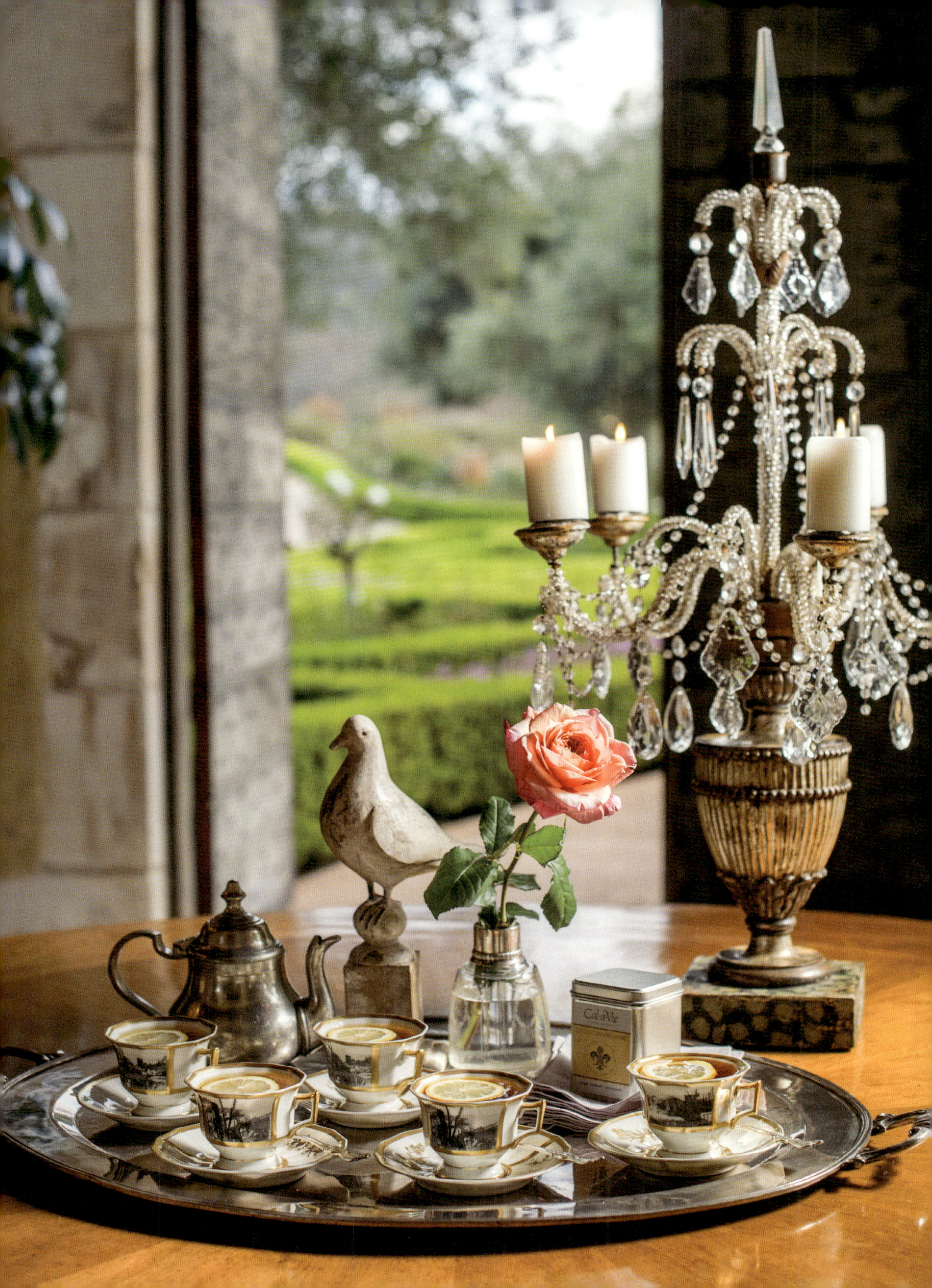
Cal-a-Vie

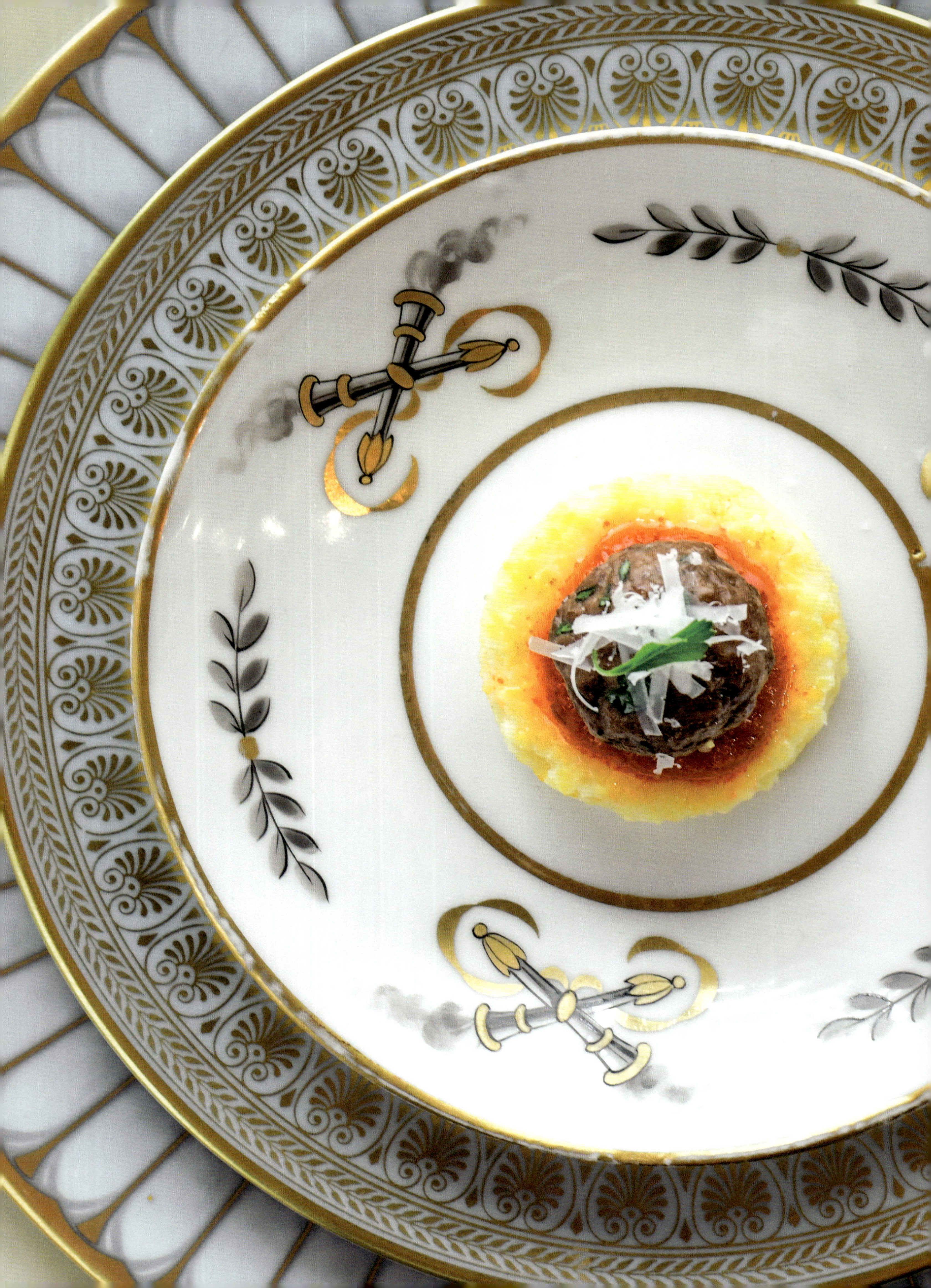

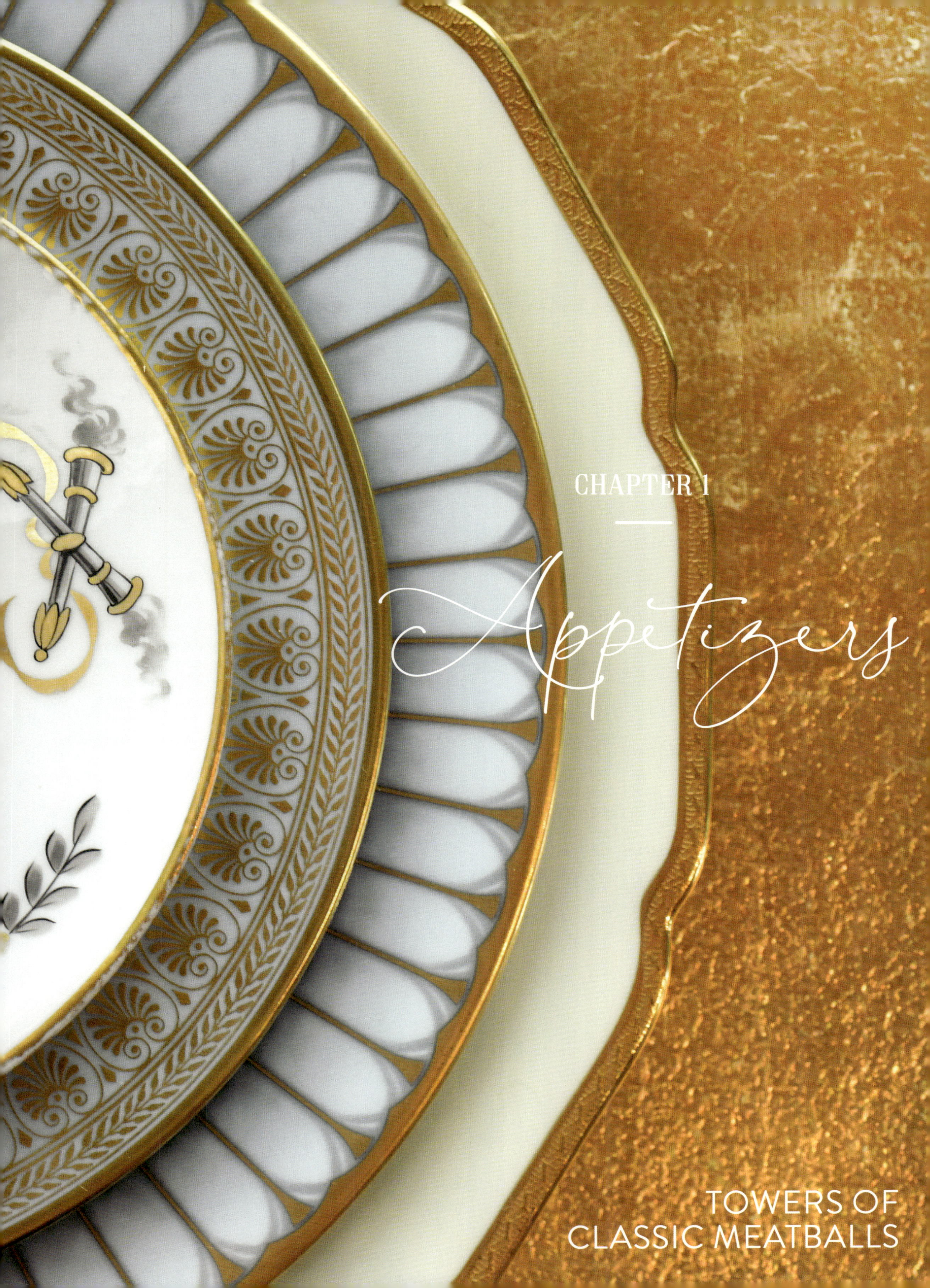

CHAPTER 1

Appetizers

TOWERS OF
CLASSIC MEATBALLS

TOWERS OF CLASSIC MEATBALLS
WITH MARINARA SAUCE AND PARMESAN POLENTA

YIELDS 3 DOZEN TOWERS (36 SERVINGS)

This delicate yet robust appetizer is a nifty spin on ingredients that are usually thought of as parts of a main entree. Pay special attention to the presentation: Small, uniform portion sizes are the key to building a successful meatball tower.

POLENTA

1 cup coarse yellow polenta
4 cups water or chicken stock
kosher or sea salt

Line a baking sheet with parchment paper. In a saucepan over high heat, bring the water or stock to a rolling boil. While whisking, add the polenta gradually to avoid any lumps from forming. Turn the heat down to medium and continue to whisk until the polenta has absorbed all the liquid and is thick and creamy, 12 to 15 minutes. Add salt to taste. Pour the polenta on the baking sheet and smooth out evenly. Place in the refrigerator until cool and firm. Using a small 1½-inch biscuit cutter, cut out 36 rounds. Set aside in refrigerator.

MARINARA SAUCE

YIELDS 1 QUART

2 tablespoons extra-virgin olive oil
1 cup diced yellow onion
3 garlic cloves, minced
1 tablespoon tomato paste
½ cup dry red wine
1 can (28-ounces) whole tomatoes
1 teaspoon fennel seed
¼ teaspoon chili flakes
2 teaspoons sea salt
¼ teaspoon freshly ground black pepper
1 cup fresh basil, leaves torn

In a large saucepan over medium heat, add the olive oil. Add the onions and sauté for about 7 minutes. When the onions start to caramelize, turning a deep brown color, add the garlic and sauté for 1 minute. Add the tomato paste and stir until it turns brick red in color. Deglaze with the red wine, bring to a boil then reduce the heat to a simmer and cook until reduced in half. Add the tomatoes, fennel seed, chili flakes, salt, black pepper, and basil. Simmer for about 30 minutes. Transfer the tomato mixture to a blender and puree until completely smooth. Set aside.

TIP: You'll have plenty of leftover Marinara Sauce, which is delicious on just about any vegetable or protein. It can be stored for three days in the refrigerator or several months in the freezer.

CLASSIC MEATBALLS

- 2 tablespoons ground rice crackers (pulsed in a food processor to resemble bread crumbs)
- 2 tablespoons 2% milk
- 2 teaspoons extra-virgin olive oil
- ½ cup minced yellow onion
- 1 garlic clove, minced
- 1 pound ground beef (we recommend 80/20 grass-fed)
- 1 egg
- 1 tablespoon freshly chopped parsley
- 1 teaspoon garlic powder
- 1 teaspoon onion powder
- ½ teaspoon freshly ground black pepper
- 1 teaspoon sea or kosher salt

Preheat the oven to 350°F. In a small bowl, mix the rice cracker crumbs with the milk to make a thick paste. (This will help to keep the meatballs moist.) Set aside.

In a sauté pan over medium heat, add the olive oil. Add the onions and sauté until translucent, then add the garlic and continue to cook for one minute. Remove from the heat and cool. In a large bowl, add the ground beef, rice cracker mixture, sautéed onion mixture, egg, parsley, garlic powder, onion powder, black pepper, and salt. Gently mix until all of the ingredients are thoroughly incorporated. Using your hands, roll out 36 1-inch meatballs. Arrange on a baking sheet and bake for 10 minutes. Remove from the oven, keep warm and set aside.

TIP: Ground beef labeled 80/20 refers to the make-up of the meat, not its nutritional content—80 percent lean beef to 20 percent fat.

ASSEMBLY

- Polenta rounds
- Marinara Sauce
- Classic Meatballs
- Parmesan cheese for garnish

Preheat the oven to 200°F. To build each meatball tower: Place a round of polenta on a baking sheet lined with parchment paper. Add a half teaspoon of Marinara Sauce. Place one meatball on the marinara, pressing down to ensure it is firmly on the polenta round. You can slice the meatball, on the bottom, to create a flat surface to sit on the polenta. Place in the oven to warm right before serving. Using a microplane, grate some Parmesan cheese and sprinkle on top to garnish.

TIP: The meatballs can also be rolled larger and served with pasta or spaghetti squash as a main course.

NUTRITION PER SERVING	Cal 83	Fat 4g	Protein 4g	Carbs 6g	Sugar 1g	Fiber 1g	Sod 162mg

POACHED SHRIMP WITH PERSIMMON SALSA AND AIOLI IN ENDIVE BOATS

SERVES 6

Poaching shrimp in a brine is a terrific method of adding flavor to shellfish without relying on a heavy sauce. This light and refreshing appetizer is great in the summer when persimmon is in season.

POACHED SHRIMP

- 2 quarts water
- 1 teaspoon whole allspice berries
- 1 star anise, whole
- 1 tablespoon kosher salt
- 1 fresh bay leaf
- ½ teaspoon whole black peppercorns
- 1 large lemon, halved
- 1 large orange, halved
- 8-10 large shrimp, (U10), peeled, tails removed, and deveined

Prepare a bowl of ice water. Set aside.

In a 4-quart saucepan, add the water and spices. Squeeze the lemon and orange into the pan to release the juices and then drop in the pieces of fruit. Bring the brine to a boil, turn down to just below a simmer, and allow the ingredients to steep for 10 minutes. Add the shrimp and poach for 5 minutes. Remove the shrimp and plunge them into a bowl of ice water. When cool, cut the shrimp crosswise into 1-inch pieces, creating large chunks. Set aside in the refrigerator.

TIP: We use U10 shrimp which means Extra Colossal or about 10 shrimps per pound.

PERSIMMON SALSA

- ½ cup finely diced Fuyu persimmon (you can substitute mango)
- ½ cup finely diced Roma tomatoes
- ¼ cup finely diced red onions
- 1 tablespoon finely diced jalapeño
- 1 tablespoon fresh, minced cilantro
- 1 tablespoon fresh lime juice
- kosher salt

In a small mixing bowl, add all of the ingredients and mix well. Season with salt to taste. Set aside in the refrigerator.

ESPELETTE AIOLI

- 1 egg yolk
- 2 teaspoons fresh lemon juice
- 1 teaspoon water
- ¼ teaspoon minced garlic
- 1 cup extra-virgin olive oil
- 1 teaspoon Piment d'Espelette spice
- kosher salt

In a food processor, combine the egg yolk, lemon juice, water, and garlic. With the processor running, slowly drizzle in the olive oil. Pulse in the Piment d'Espelette powder and season with salt to taste. The goal is a creamy, mayonnaise-like consistency. If the aioli is too thick, add another teaspoon of water. If it is too thin, turn the processor back on and drizzle in a little more olive oil to tighten it up. Store in the refrigerator until ready to use.

ASSEMBLY

- 1 head Belgian endive

Cut off the root end of the endive and separate the leaves. In a bowl, combine the Poached Shrimp and Persimmon Salsa and mix thoroughly. Using an endive leaf as the "boat," spread 2 teaspoons of Espelette Aioli inside. Add 3 tablespoons of the shrimp mixture to the "boat." Repeat with remaining endive leaves.

TIP: The Espelette Aioli is also great on sandwiches, tuna salad, chicken, or fish.

NUTRITION PER SERVING	Cal 110	Fat 9g	Protein 2g	Carbs 7g	Sugar 1g	Fiber 2g	Sod 256mg

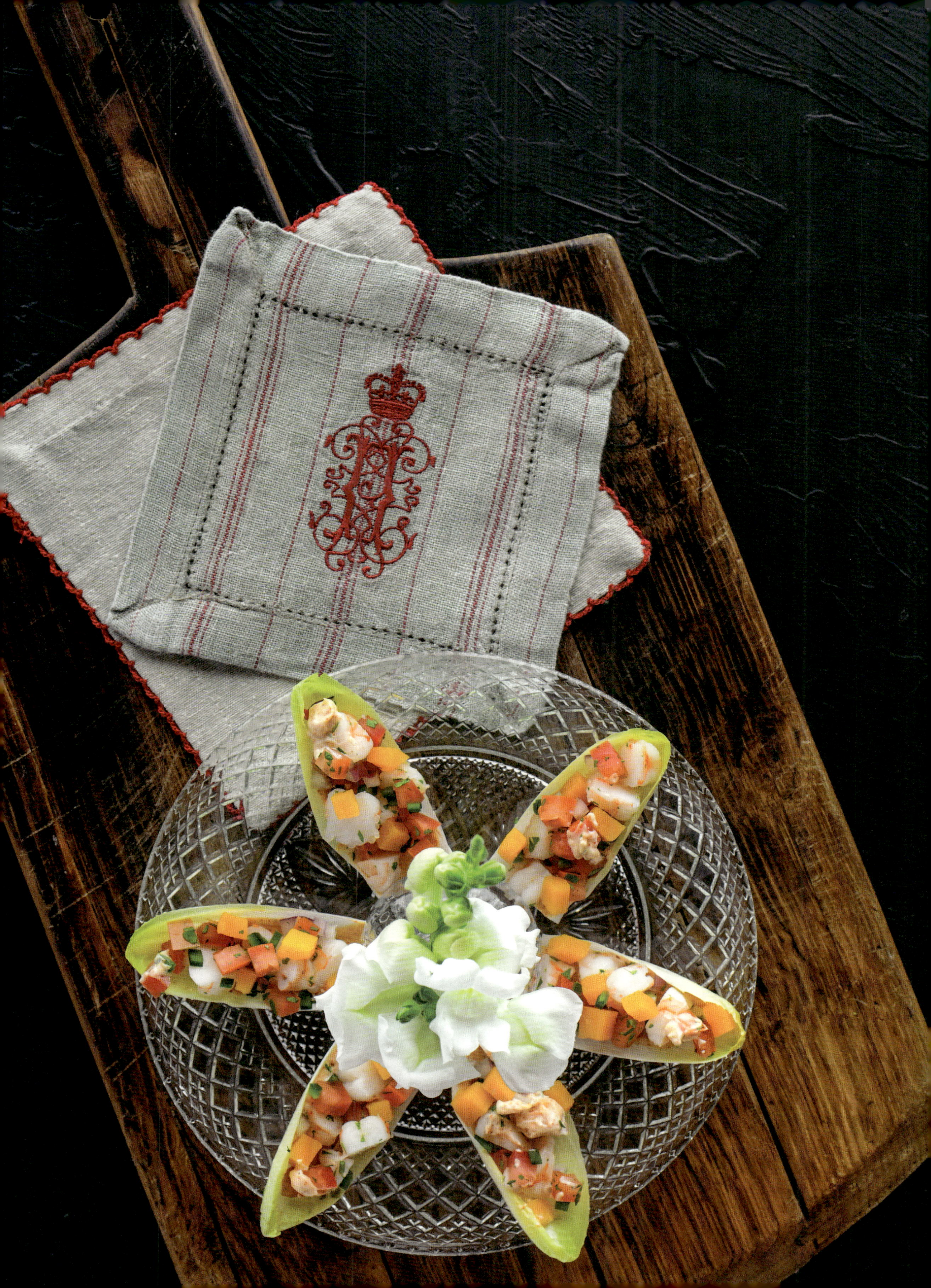

CAVIAR SALMON CUCUMBER CRUDITÉS

YIELDS 24 PIECES (12 SERVINGS)

At first glance, this seems like a complicated appetizer, but the assembly will go smoothly once everything is "mise en place." Think of it as a work of art, with each color and texture working synergistically to create a one-bite masterpiece.

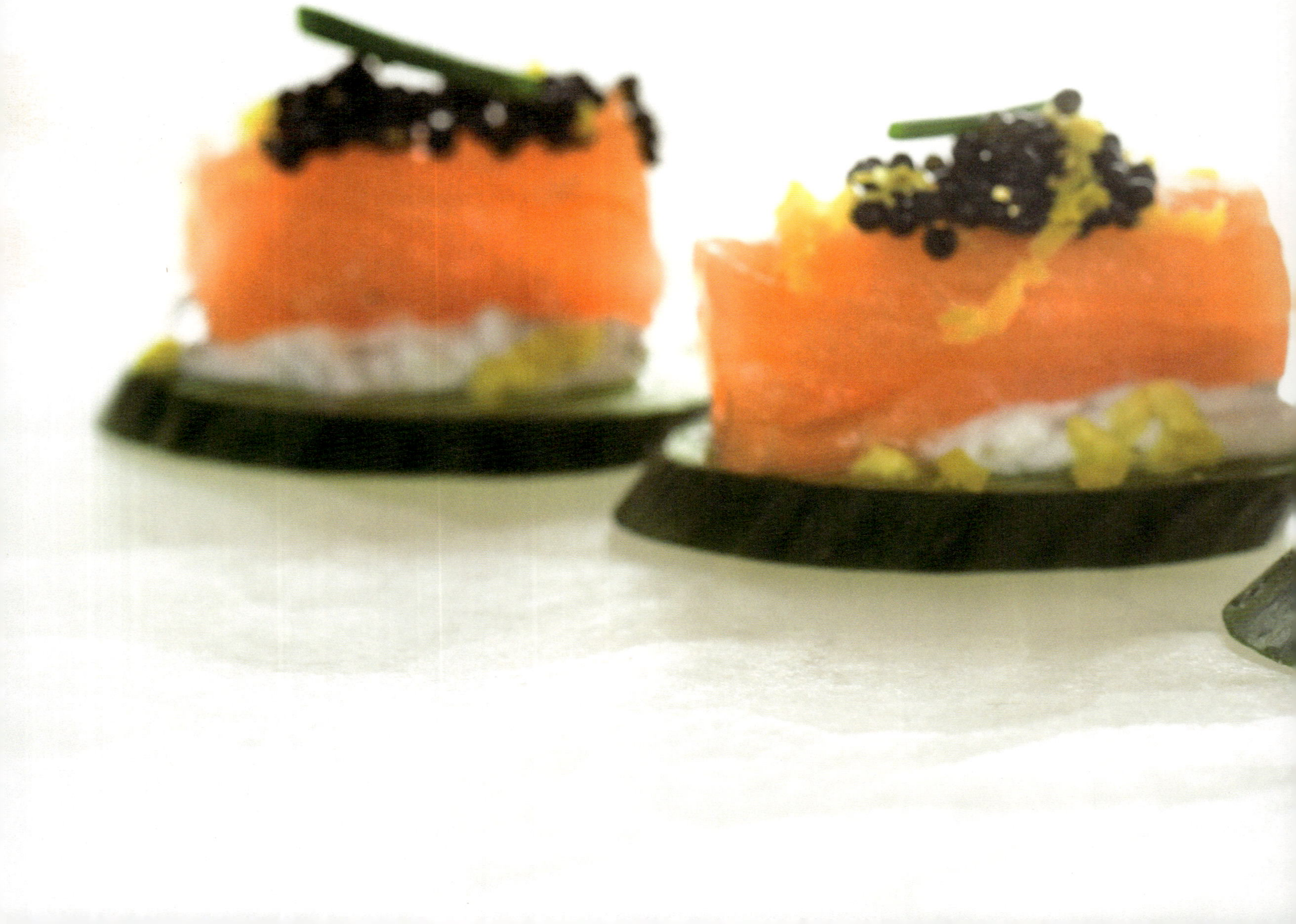

CAPER CREAM

½ cup Tofutti® sour cream (we recommend this dairy-free, vegan sour cream)

3 tablespoons capers, chopped

In a small bowl, combine the Tofutti® sour cream and the capers. Mix well to incorporate and "loosen" up the sour cream. Set aside in the refrigerator.

HARD-BOILED EGGS

1 or 2 eggs

Prepare an ice bath in a bowl, using 50% ice and 50% water. In a medium saucepan, add the eggs and cover with cold water by 4 inches. Over high heat, bring the water and eggs to a rolling boil. Once it reaches this stage, set a timer for 10 minutes. The eggs must cook the entire time at a rolling boil. When the timer goes off, remove the eggs from the pan and immediately submerge them in the ice bath to stop the cooking process. Once the eggs are cool, peel the shells. The eggs should be completely cooked, with bright yellow yolks and no browning. Set aside in the refrigerator.

TIP: You might want to boil a few extra eggs in case one breaks during the cooking process.

SALMON CRUDITÉ ASSEMBLY

1 cucumber, peel on, thinly sliced (about 24 slices)

½ cup Caper Cream

1 pound smoked salmon, thinly sliced and rolled into 1-inch logs (24 pieces)

1 ounce Grade 1 caviar

1 hard-boiled egg yolk

2 tablespoons fresh finely chopped chives

To build each bite, place a cucumber slice on a flat surface, and add a small dollop of Caper Cream. Lay the rolled salmon on top. Place a small pile of caviar on top of the rolled salmon. Using a microplane, shave some cooked egg yolk on top, followed by a sprinkle of chives.

TIP: Caviar comes in two grades. Grade 1 features firm, large, intact eggs with fine color and flavor. Grade 2 is still delicious but less delicate, and the eggs are not as perfectly formed. We recommend splurging on the higher grade.

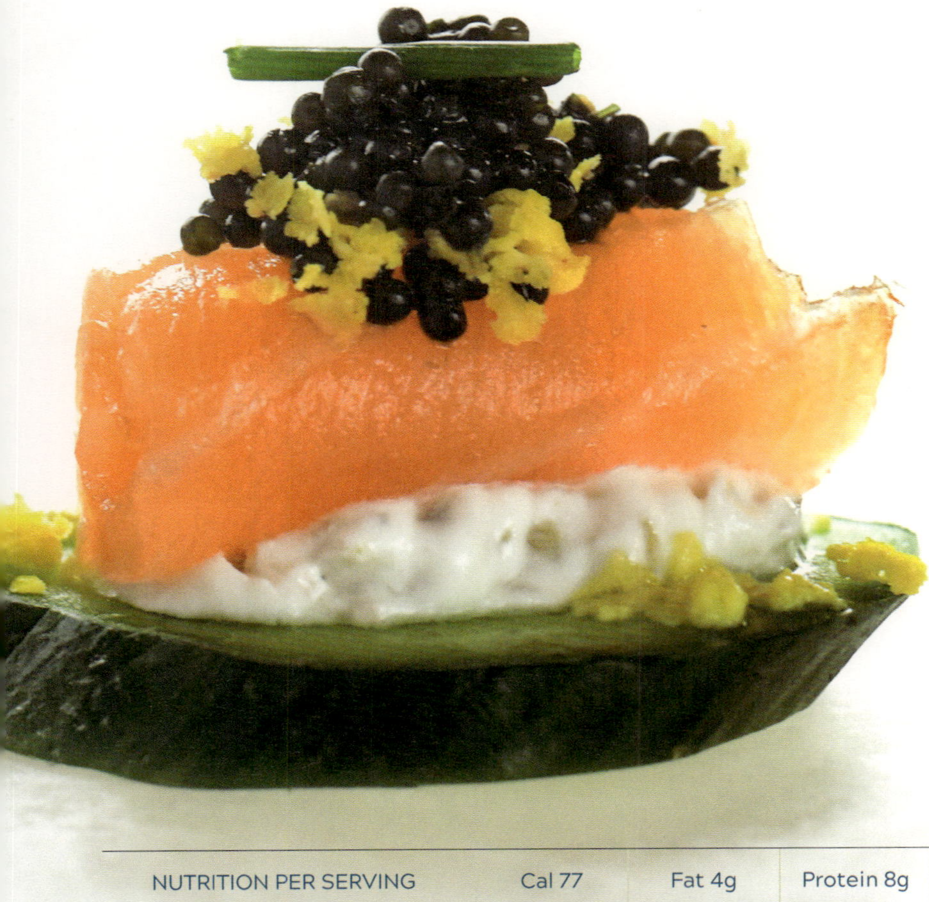

NUTRITION PER SERVING	Cal 77	Fat 4g	Protein 8g	Carbs 1g	Sugar 1g	Fiber 0g	Sod 351mg

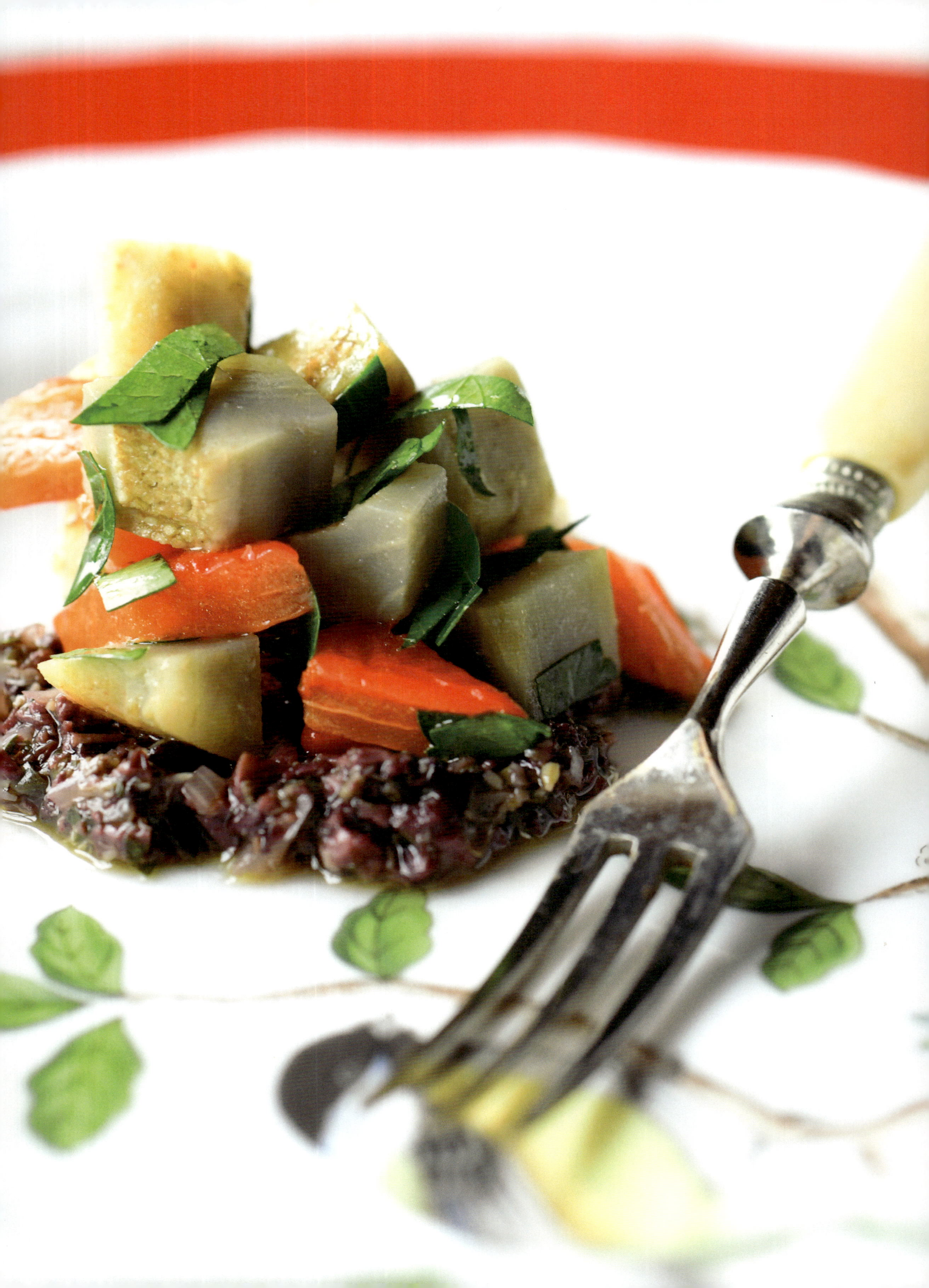

ARTICHOKE AND OLIVE TAPENADE

SERVES 6

We love olives—especially since they're rich in monounsaturated fats, which are plentiful in the health-friendly Mediterranean diet. Artichokes are also part of that diet, and they are another one of our favorites because they're a great source of prebiotic fiber.

POACHED GLOBE ARTICHOKE HEARTS

6 globe artichokes

1 lemon

To clean the artichokes, trim all the leaves until you get to the tender, yellow leaves at the center. Using a peeler, peel the stems. With a serrated knife, cut the rest of the leaves to just where they meet the heart. The goal is to trim the leaves away, exposing the heart (the firm flesh under the leaves). After cleaning the artichokes, place in a pot of simmering water with a squeeze of lemon juice, and cook until just tender, about 5 minutes. Once cooked, remove and plunge into a bowl of ice water. Dice the artichoke hearts and set them aside.

ROASTED RED BELL PEPPER

1 red bell pepper

1 teaspoon extra-virgin olive oil

Preheat the oven to 400°F. Rub a red bell pepper with olive oil, lay it on a baking sheet and place in the oven. Roast for 10 to 12 minutes, turning several times until the skin is blistered and charred. Remove from the oven and cool. Using your fingers, peel the skin from the pepper, remove the seeds and stem, leaving only the flesh. Chop the pepper and set aside.

OLIVE TAPENADE

1 cup Kalamata olives, pitted

1 garlic clove, peeled

1 teaspoon anchovy paste

½ teaspoon fresh chopped rosemary

½ tablespoon capers

¼ cup extra-virgin olive oil

In a food processor, add all of the ingredients and puree until completely smooth. Set aside.

ASSEMBLY

6 chopped Poached Globe Artichoke Hearts

1 cup chopped Roasted Red Bell Pepper

1 tablespoon fresh lemon juice

1 tablespoons extra-virgin olive oil

1 tablespoon freshly minced flat-leaf parsley

kosher or sea salt

4 tablespoons Olive Tapenade

chopped flat leaf parsley, for garnish

In a small mixing bowl, combine the artichokes, bell pepper, lemon juice, olive oil, and parsley, and mix thoroughly. Season with salt and reserve.

On a small appetizer dish, spread two teaspoons of the tapenade. Place about ⅓ cup of artichoke mixture on top and garnish with chopped parsley.

TIP: If you can't find fresh artichokes, use frozen or jarred in water.

NUTRITION PER SERVING	Cal 89	Fat 7g	Protein 2g	Carbs 7g	Sugar 2g	Fiber 3g	Sod 145mg

BABA GANOUSH

YIELDS 4 CUPS (16 SERVINGS)

Cal-a-Vie serves this savory dish in small portions, using shot glasses—proof that less can, indeed, be more delicious. And while we say you should eat 50 percent of your vegetables raw in a given day, eggplant is an exception; it can contain a slightly toxic glycoalkaloid protein called solanine. The cooking process helps to denature this compound and eliminate its negative effects.

- I large eggplant
- ¼ cup extra-virgin olive oil, plus 2 tablespoons, divided use
- ¼ cup tahini
- ⅓ cup fresh lemon juice
- 3 garlic cloves, peeled
- ¼ teaspoon cayenne pepper
- 1 teaspoon sea salt

Preheat the oven to 400°F. Cut the eggplant in half, lengthwise, and rub each cut side with 1 tablespoon of olive oil. Place the eggplant on a baking sheet, cut side down, and roast for 20 minutes or until the flesh is extremely soft. Cool the eggplant. With a spoon, scrape the flesh out of the skin. It should yield about 3 cups. In a food processor, combine the eggplant, ¼ cup oil, tahini, lemon juice, garlic, cayenne pepper and salt, and puree until smooth. Store in the refrigerator.

Serve with Baked Pita Chips (see recipe page 207) or a vegetable crudité.

TIP: For a smoky flavor, grill the eggplant. To prepare, preheat the grill. With a paring knife, pierce the whole eggplant on all sides and place it on the heated grill, turning every 10 minutes until the flesh is extremely soft. Cool, and scrape the flesh from skin.

Eggplant roasted in the oven will be lighter in color than eggplant roasted on the grill.

NUTRITION PER SERVING	Cal	Fat	Protein	Carbs	Sugar	Fiber	Sod
	64	6g	1g	2g	1g	1g	162mg

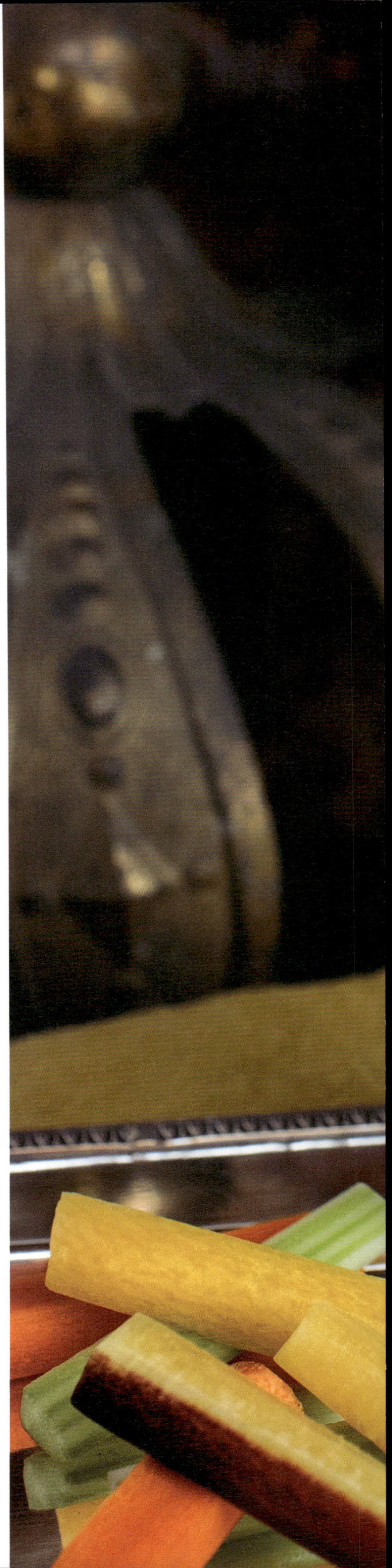

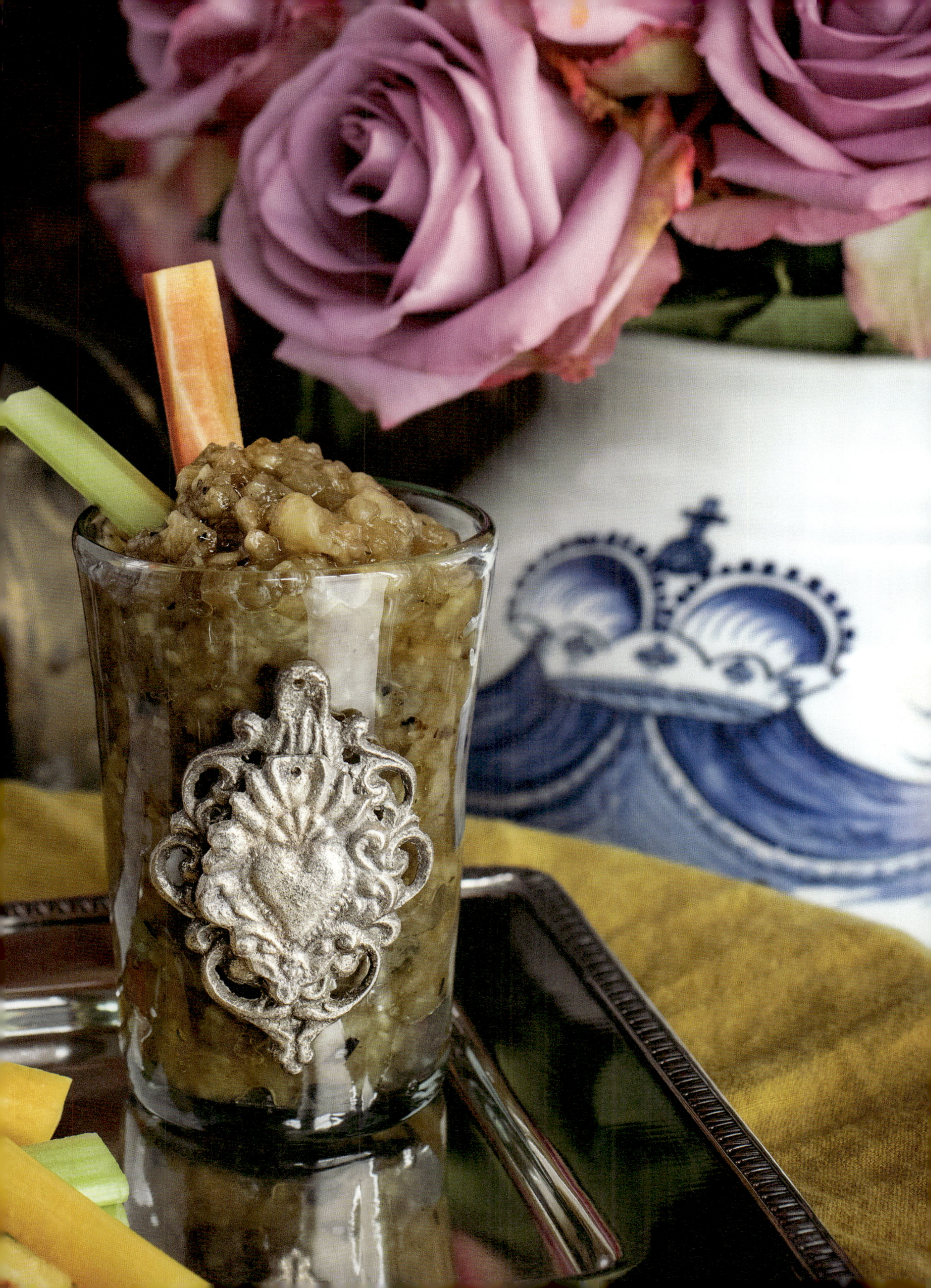

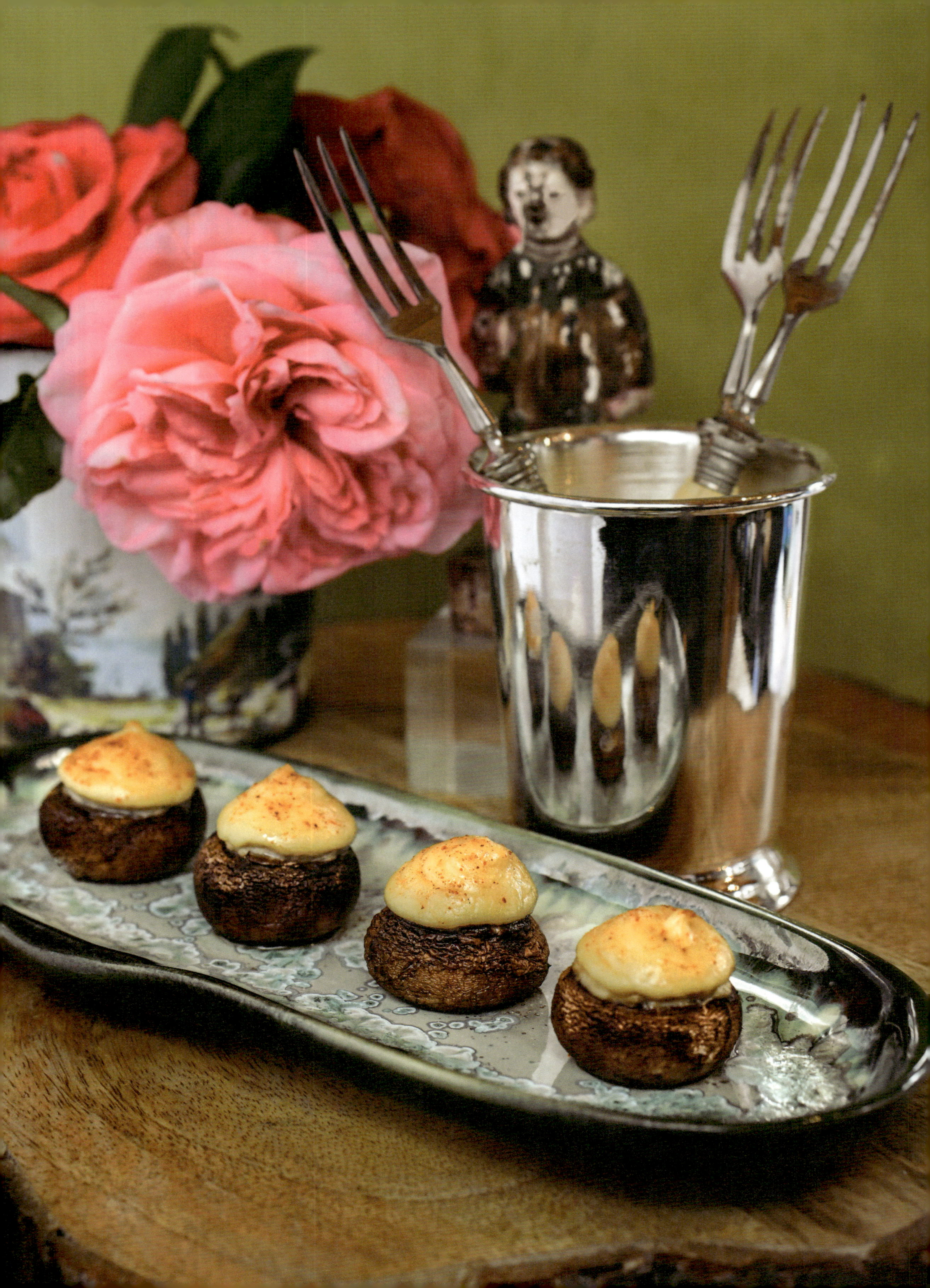

CASHEW-STUFFED MUSHROOMS

8 SERVINGS (2 MUSHROOMS EACH)

We love teaching guests how to make this appetizer in our hands-on cooking demo, and they are always impressed by how versatile cashew cream can be. This recipe works best using raw cashews, as they are sweeter and easier to blend. Nutritional yeast is a tasty vegan condiment that's rich in B vitamins and adds a cheesy, nutty flavor without using any dairy.

CASHEW CREAM

1 cup raw cashews, soaked in water overnight and drained

¼ cup water

¼ cup nutritional yeast (generally found in the specialty or bulk sections of the grocery store)

2 tablespoons fresh lemon juice

2 garlic cloves, peeled

2 tablespoons white wine or apple cider vinegar

1 tablespoon Dijon mustard

sea salt

Add all the ingredients to a blender or Vitamix® and process until smooth. Add more water as needed to achieve a smooth, creamy texture. Add salt to taste. Set aside.

STUFFED-MUSHROOM ASSEMBLY

¼ cup kosher salt

16 cremini mushrooms, de-stemmed

extra-virgin olive oil

1 cup Cashew Cream

smoked paprika

Preheat the oven to 350°F. Prepare a brine by dissolving the salt in 1 quart of water. Submerge the de-stemmed mushrooms into the brine and let sit for 20 minutes. Remove the mushrooms and pat dry. Drizzle a small amount of olive oil into each mushroom cavity. Rub the olive oil around to coat the mushroom. With the Cashew Cream in a piping bag, fill each cavity with the cream. Place the mushrooms on a baking sheet lined with a piece of parchment paper and roast for about 10 minutes. Garnish with smoked paprika.

TIP: The longer the Cashew Cream is blended, the smoother it will become.

NUTRITION PER SERVING	Cal 31	Fat 2g	Protein 1g	Carbs 2g	Sugar 1g	Fiber 0g	Sod 115mg

BUFFALO CAULIFLOWER

SERVES 20 SERVINGS AS AN APPETIZER

This is our healthy spin on the traditional buffalo-wing appetizer. Cauliflower has a surprisingly similar texture to meat when roasted, making it a popular ingredient in vegetarian dishes.

1 cauliflower head, core removed, cut into bite-sized florets (about 5-6 cups)
2 tablespoons grapeseed oil
½ teaspoon kosher salt
2-3 tablespoons Frank's RedHot® sauce
(if unavailable, any other spicy buffalo sauce will work)

Preheat the oven to 350°F. In a large bowl, toss the cauliflower florets with grapeseed oil and salt. Spread evenly onto a baking sheet and roast in the oven for 15 minutes, or until crispy. Remove from the oven, toss in the hot sauce, and return to oven for 10 minutes. Remove and allow to cool.

ASSEMBLY

2 celery stalks, peeled and thinly cut into ¼-inch half moons
1 bunch green onions, trimmed and thinly sliced (using white and green parts)
¾ cup crumbled blue cheese

To serve, plate about ¼ cup roasted cauliflower and top with celery slices, green onions, and crumbled blue cheese. Feel free to add as much hot sauce as you like.

TIP: Not everyone peels celery, but the stringy outside can be tough and hard to eat. Use a regular peeler to remove this fibrous side.

NUTRITION PER SERVING	Cal	Fat	Protein	Carbs	Sugar	Fiber	Sod
	43	3g	2g	2g	1g	1g	104mg

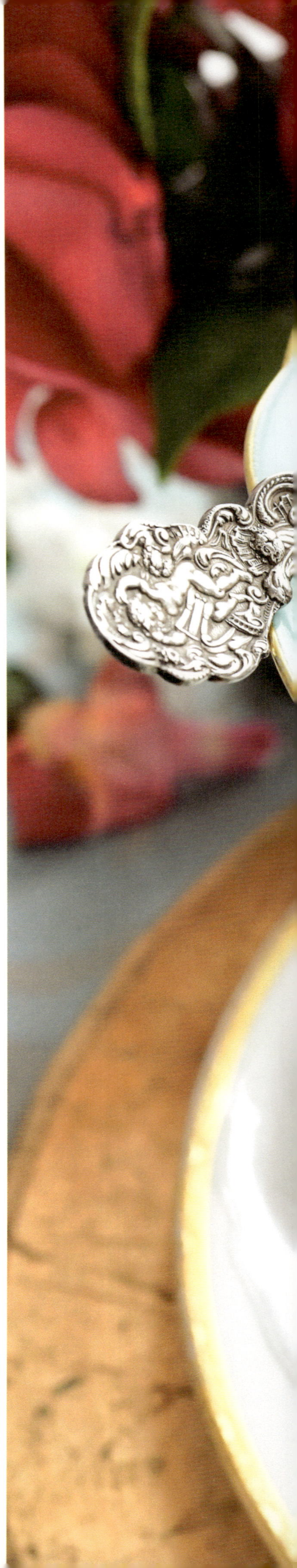

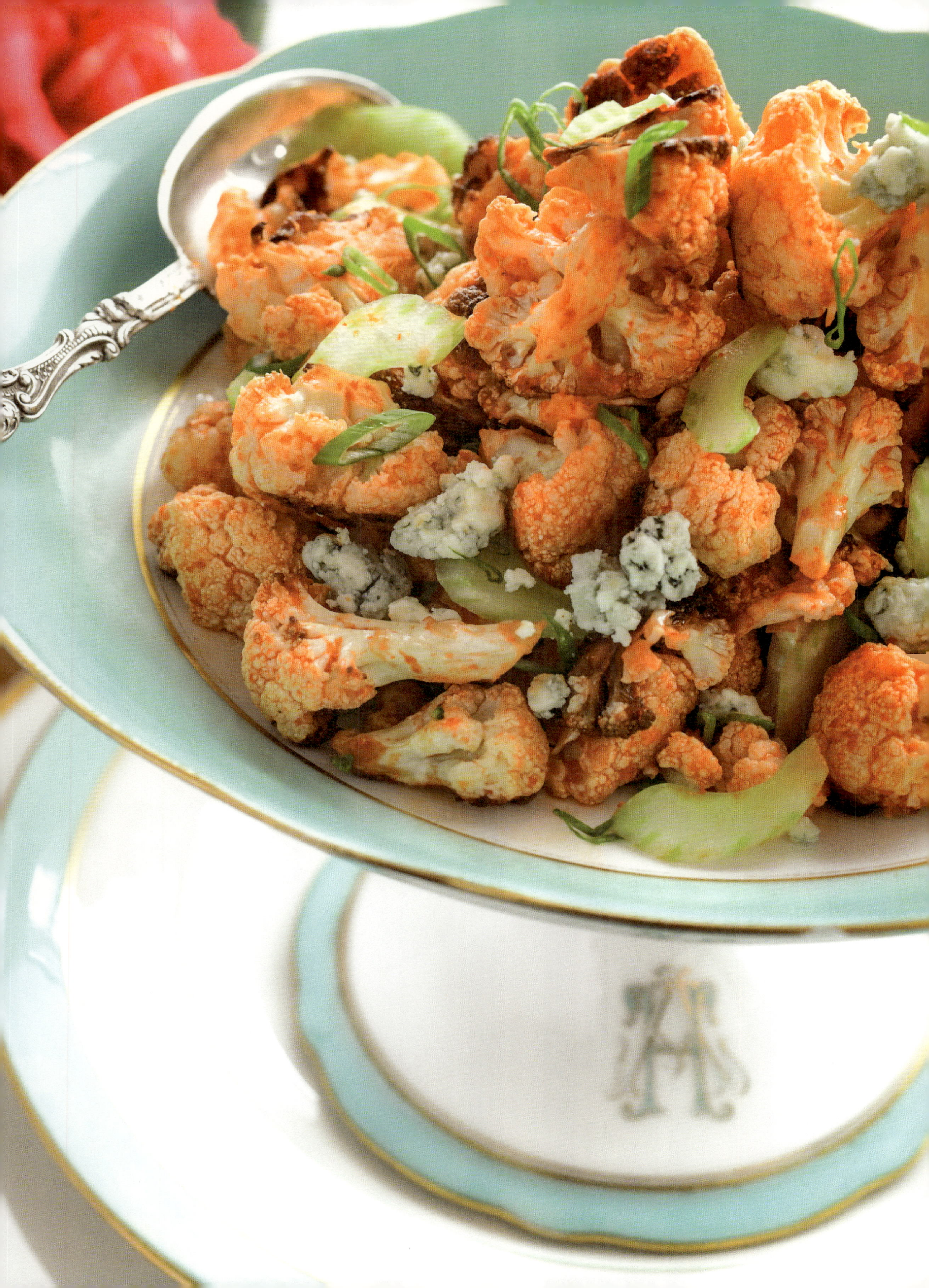

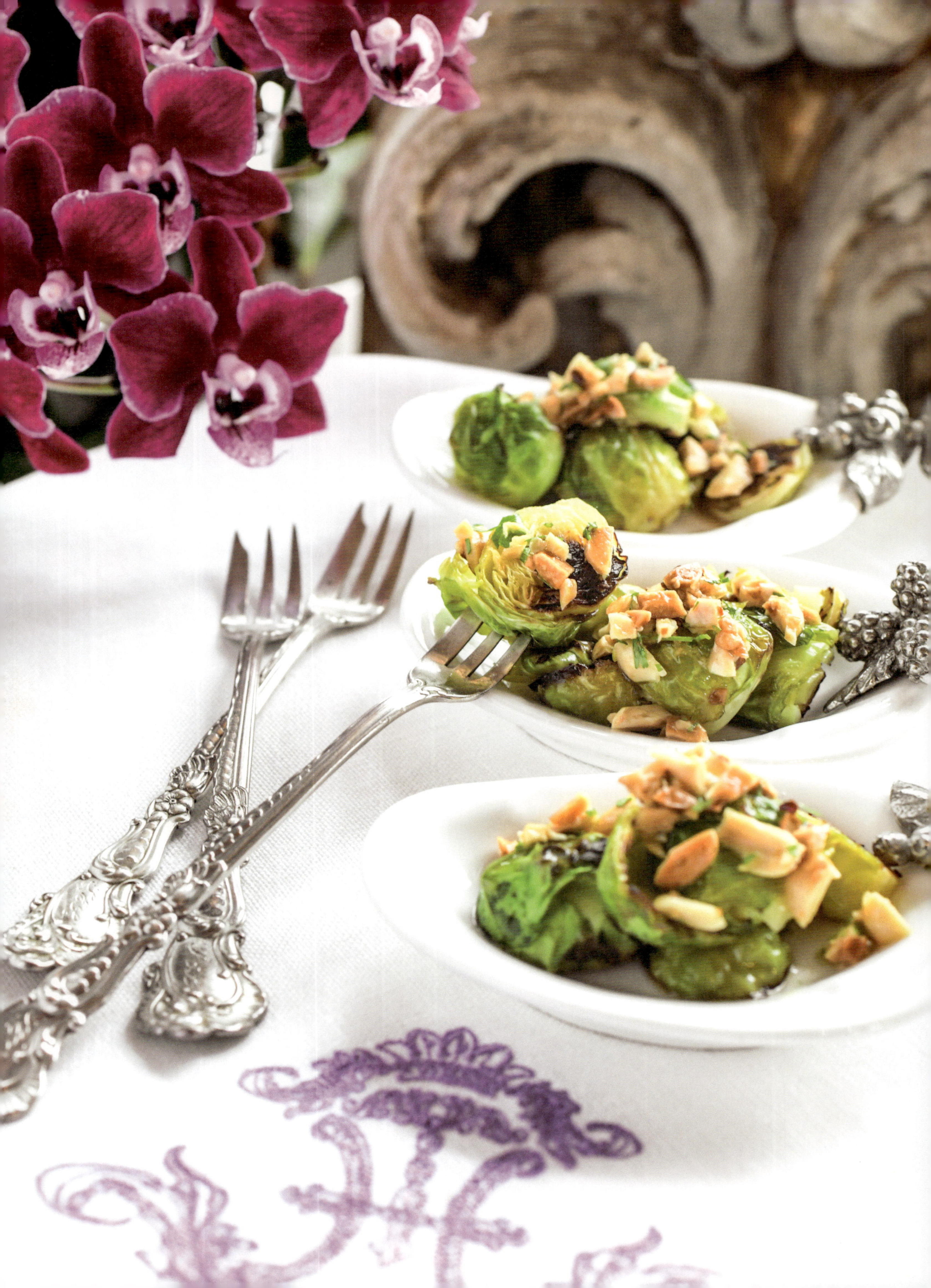

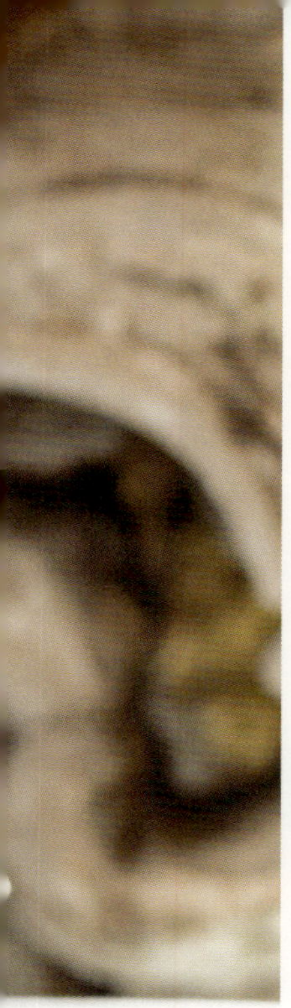

ROASTED BRUSSELS SPROUTS
WITH PEANUT CHILI VINAIGRETTE

SERVES 16

This is another favorite appetizer we serve during the winter. Make sure to watch your Brussels sprouts in the oven, as their cooking time may vary depending on size. For an extra special crunch, gather the Brussels sprouts leaves that fall off when you're cutting them, and roast them separately for about 5 minutes. Toss them in before serving.

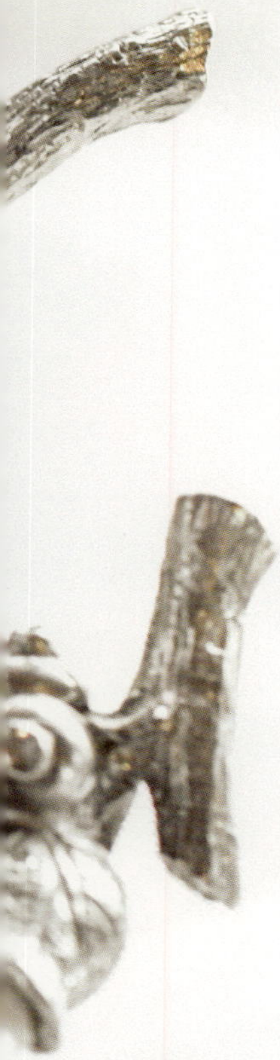

PEANUT CHILI VINAIGRETTE

YIELDS 1 CUP

½ cup white balsamic vinegar
¼ cup peanuts, roasted and chopped
2 tablespoons chili flakes
½ cup olive oil

In a small bowl, add all the ingredients and whisk vigorously to incorporate. Set aside.

ROASTED BRUSSELS SPROUTS

4 cups Brussels sprouts, halved
¼ cup olive oil
kosher or sea salt

Preheat the oven to 400°F. In a large bowl, toss the Brussels sprouts with olive oil and season with salt to taste. Spread the Brussels sprouts evenly on a baking sheet. Place in the oven and roast for 15 minutes. Rotate the sprouts on the tray and return to the oven for 10 more minutes. The Brussels sprouts should be cooked through, with a nice roasted char to them.

Divide the Brussels sprouts between 12-16 small plates (¼- to ⅓-cup portions on each plate). Spoon a couple of teaspoons of the Peanut Chili Vinaigrette over the top of the Brussels sprouts, making sure each portion gets some chopped peanuts.

NUTRITION PER SERVING	Cal 102	Fat 10g	Protein 1g	Carbs 3g	Sugar 2g	Fiber 1g	Sod 92mg

TOMATO BROCCOLI FLATBREAD

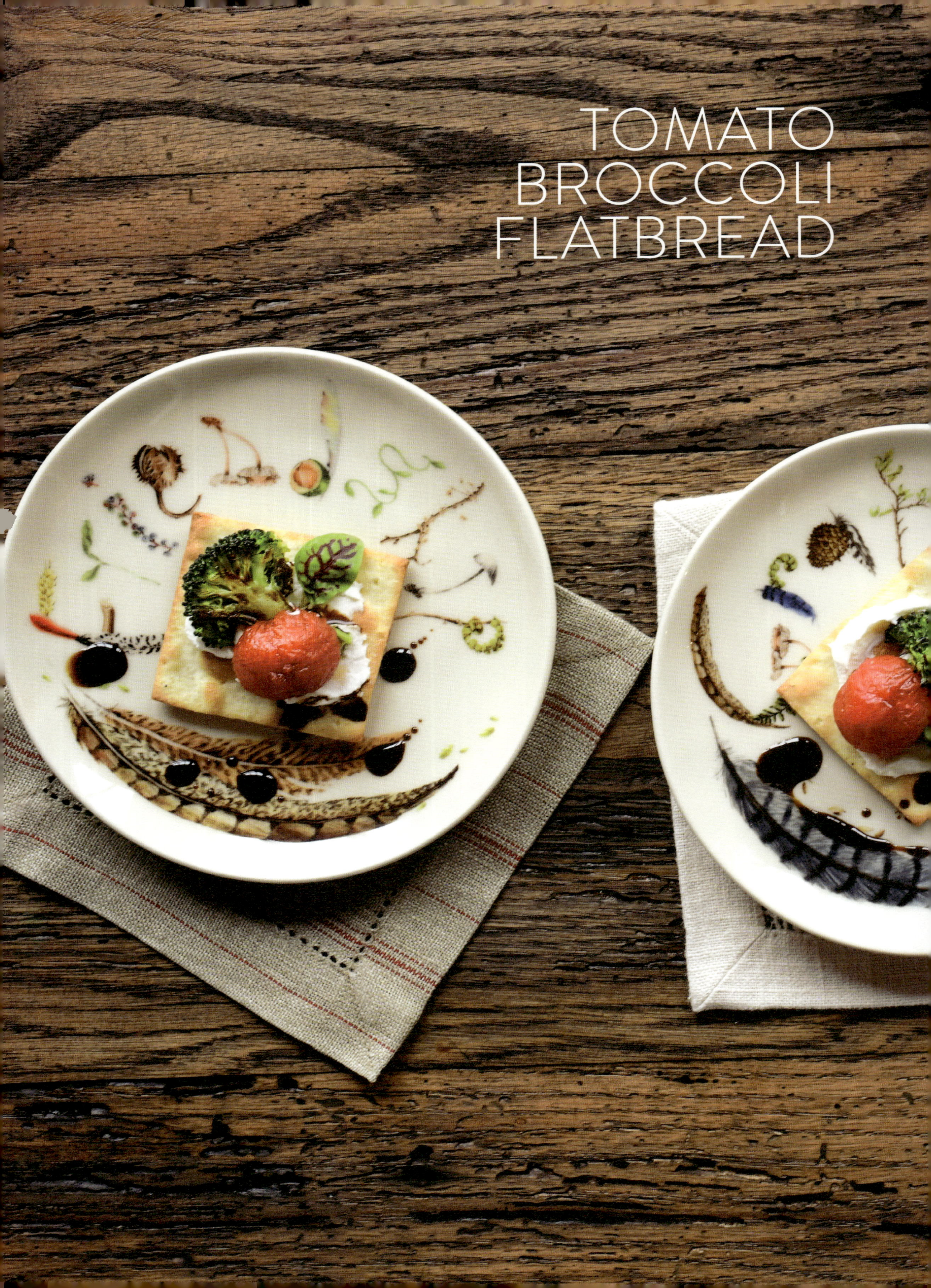

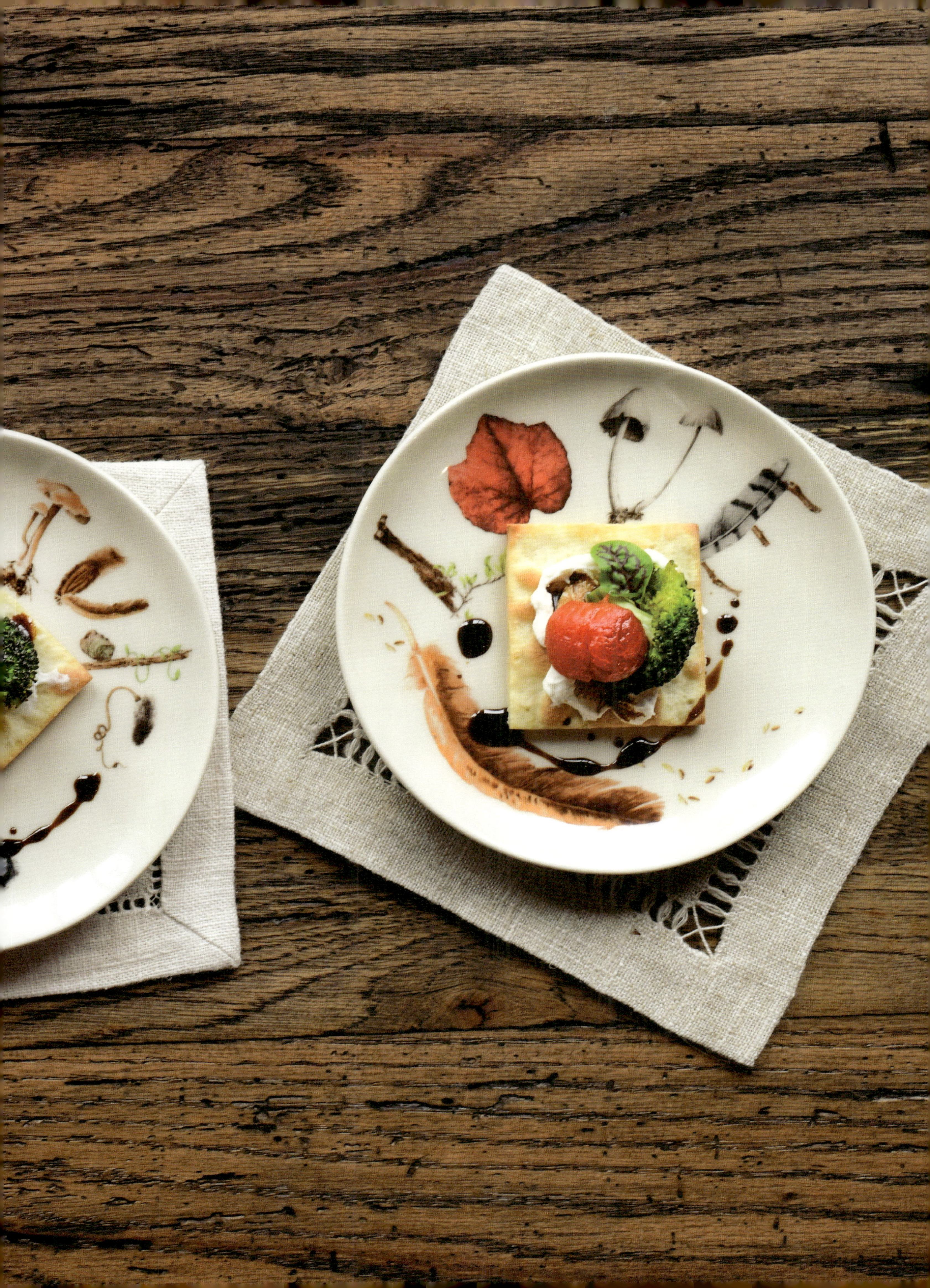

TOMATO BROCCOLI FLATBREAD

SERVES 18

This flatbread is a beautiful, gluten-free appetizer that's perfect for entertaining—or for pairing with a salad or soup for a light lunch. The homemade Garlic Oil and acidic-yet-sweet Balsamic Syrup create a symphony of flavors in your mouth. One serving will be sure to satisfy.

GARLIC OIL

1 cup olive oil

6 garlic cloves, peeled

Preheat the oven to 350°F. In a small oven-safe saucepan or small baking dish, add the olive oil and the garlic cloves. The garlic should be submerged in the olive oil. Cover with foil. Bake for 30 minutes or until the garlic is soft. Set aside to cool, then chill in the refrigerator.

BALSAMIC SYRUP

1 cup balsamic vinegar

¼ cup honey

In a small saucepan, bring the vinegar and honey to a boil. Reduce the heat and allow the mixture to simmer until a light syrup consistency is achieved. Cool down and set aside. Store in the refrigerator.

ROASTED CHERRY TOMATOES AND BROCCOLI

1 cup cherry tomatoes, halved

½ cup small broccoli florets

2 tablespoons olive oil, divided use

kosher salt

Preheat the oven to 350°F. Toss the tomatoes and the broccoli, separately, with 1 tablespoon of olive oil and lightly season with salt. Keep the broccoli and tomatoes separate on a baking sheet and place in the oven to roast for about 5 minutes or until lightly toasted. Remove from the oven and set aside.

ASSEMBLY

1 package Udi's® gluten free pizza crusts (2 8-ounce crusts)

1 tablespoon Garlic Oil

½ cup ricotta cheese

1 cup roasted cherry tomatoes

½ cup roasted broccoli

¼ cup Balsamic Syrup

Preheat the oven to 350°F. Brush the flatbread crusts with the Garlic Oil, then spread with ricotta. Bake in the oven for 5 to 7 minutes, or until the ricotta is bubbling and lightly toasted.

Remove from the oven and cut into 2-inch by 2-inch squares. Top each square with a tomato and a piece of broccoli. Place back into the oven to warm. Remove just before serving, place on a platter, and drizzle the Balsamic Syrup over each piece.

TIP: Balsamic Syrup can also be used on fish and chicken dishes as a sauce that's drizzled on top in small amounts. The extra Garlic Oil can keep in the refrigerator for several weeks, and can be brushed on any vegetables you are roasting in the oven.

NUTRITION PER SERVING	Cal 102	Fat 4g	Protein 2g	Carbs 15g	Sugar 4g	Fiber 1g	Sod 66mg

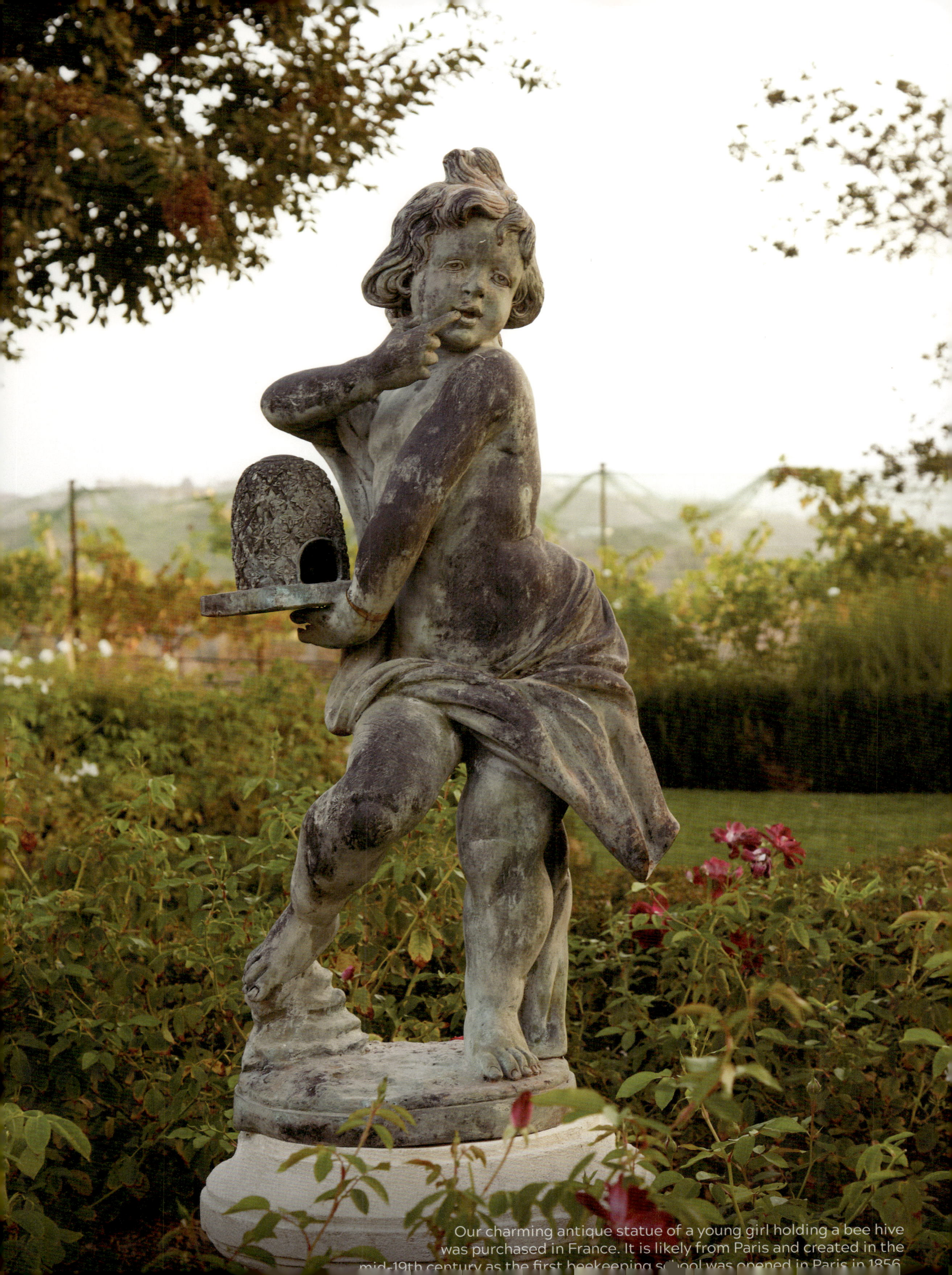

Our charming antique statue of a young girl holding a bee hive was purchased in France. It is likely from Paris and created in the mid-19th century as the first beekeeping school was opened in Paris in 1856.

WATERMELON, CUCUMBER, AND TOMATO SKEWERS WITH VANILLA-HONEY GASTRIQUE

SERVES 6 (2 SKEWERS PER SERVING)

Watermelon and cucumber are cool and healthy ways to chill out during the summer. Watermelon is 92 percent water and contains only about 9 grams of sugar per cup when diced. So you can put it on a skewer and enjoy—without worrying about sugar overload. And cucumber is 96 percent water, letting you rehydrate and refresh at once.

VANILLA-HONEY GASTRIQUE

¼ cup honey

¼ cup white wine vinegar

½ vanilla bean,
split and scraped

In a small saucepan, combine the honey, white wine vinegar, and vanilla bean paste. Bring to a simmer and cook until reduced by half. Remove from the heat and cool. You should have a light syrup. Set aside.

WATERMELON CUCUMBER TOMATO SKEWERS

12 bamboo skewers (4½ inches long)

12 1-inch cucumber cubes, skin-on

24 mint leaves (extra for garnish)

6 cherry tomatoes (yellow or red), halved

12 1-inch watermelon cubes

½ cup Vanilla-Honey Gastrique

To build a skewer: start with a cucumber cube, followed by a mint leaf, then a tomato half, another mint leaf and a cucumber cube, and finally a watermelon cube. Repeat this process for the remaining skewers. Place the skewers on your favorite platter and drizzle with some of the Vanilla-Honey Gastrique. Garnish with additional mint leaves, if desired.

NUTRITION PER SERVING	Cal	Fat	Protein	Carbs	Sugar	Fiber	Sod
	24	0g	0g	3g	3g	0g	2mg

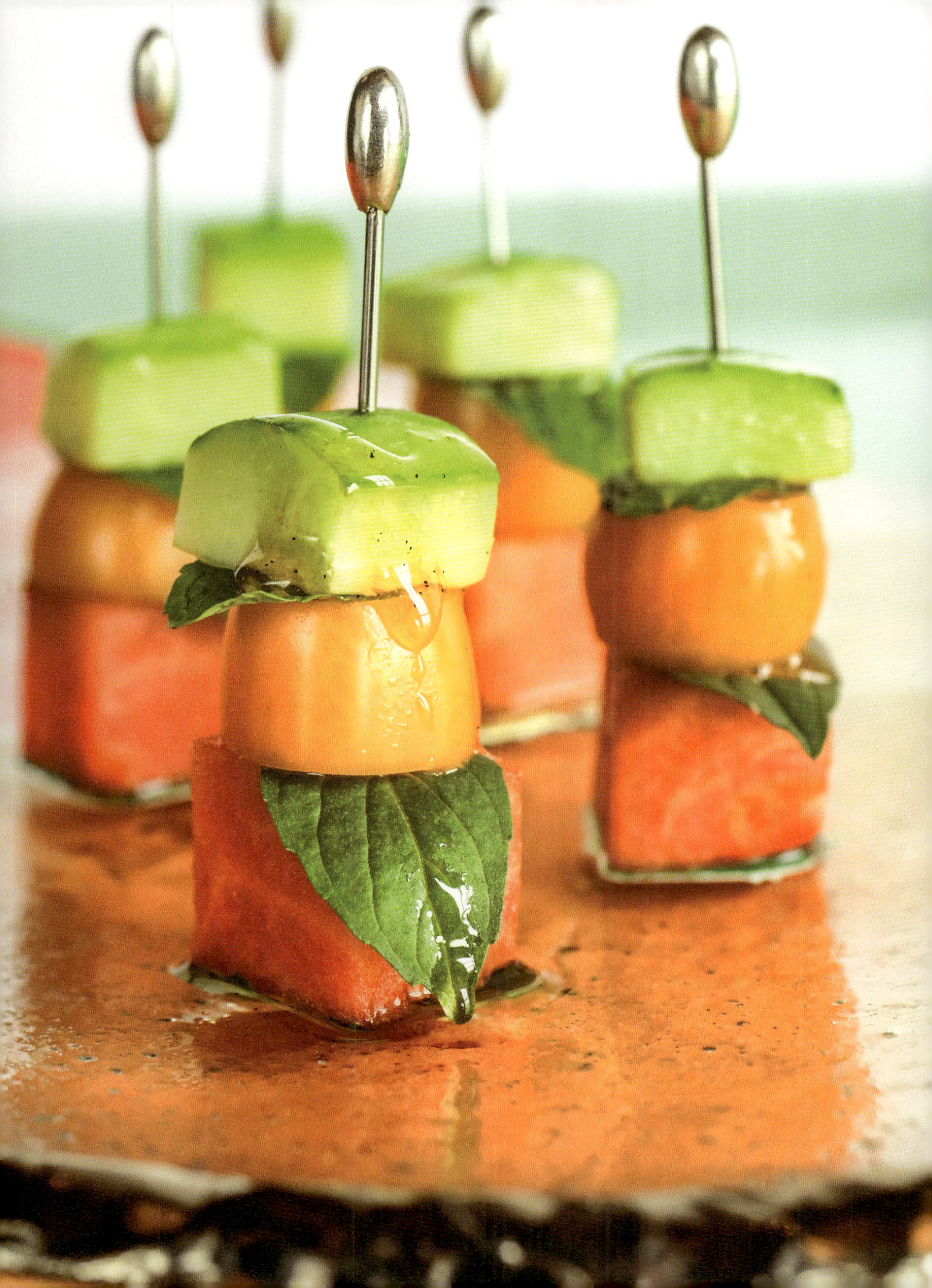

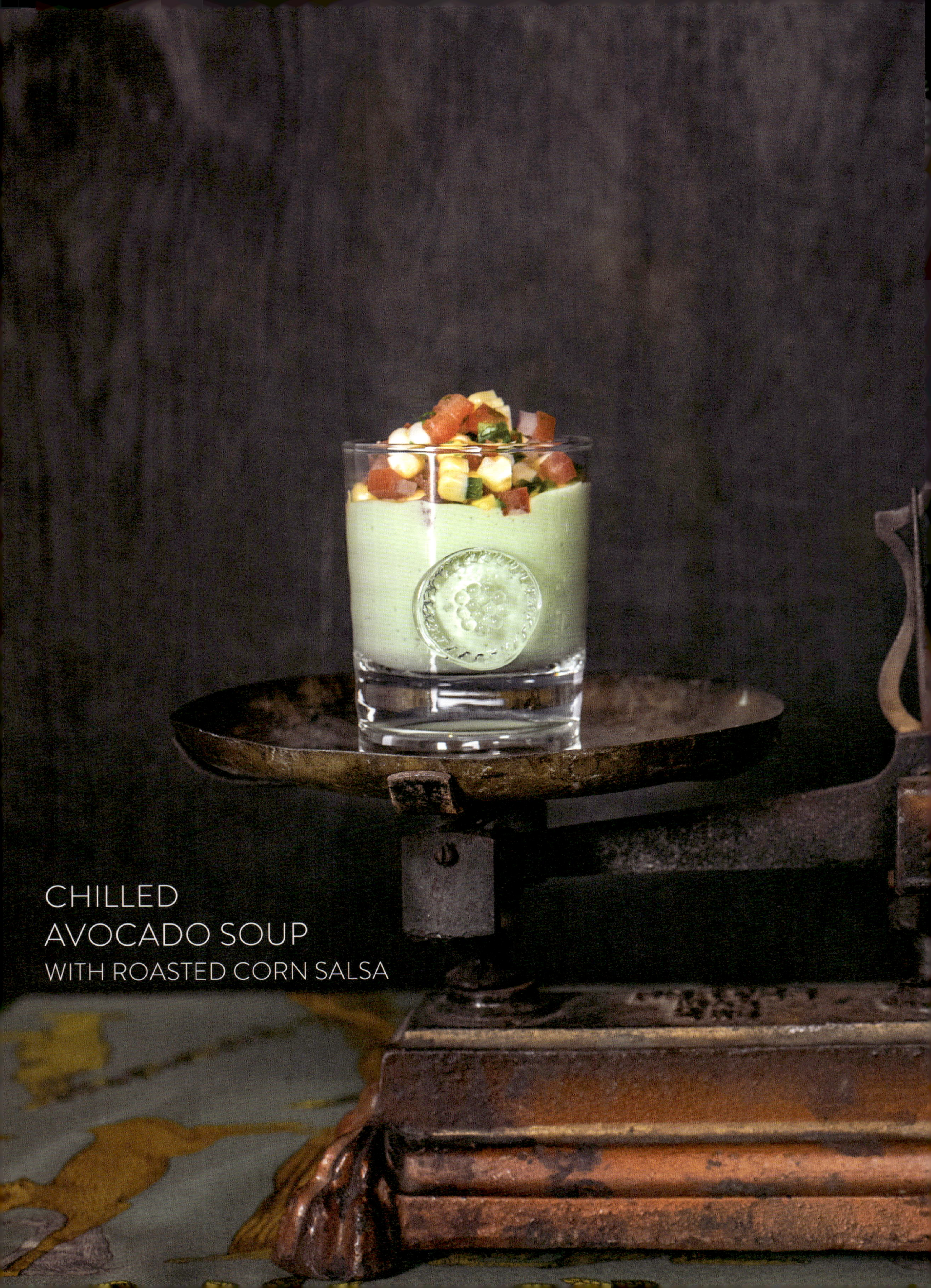

CHILLED AVOCADO SOUP
WITH ROASTED CORN SALSA

CHAPTER 2

Soups

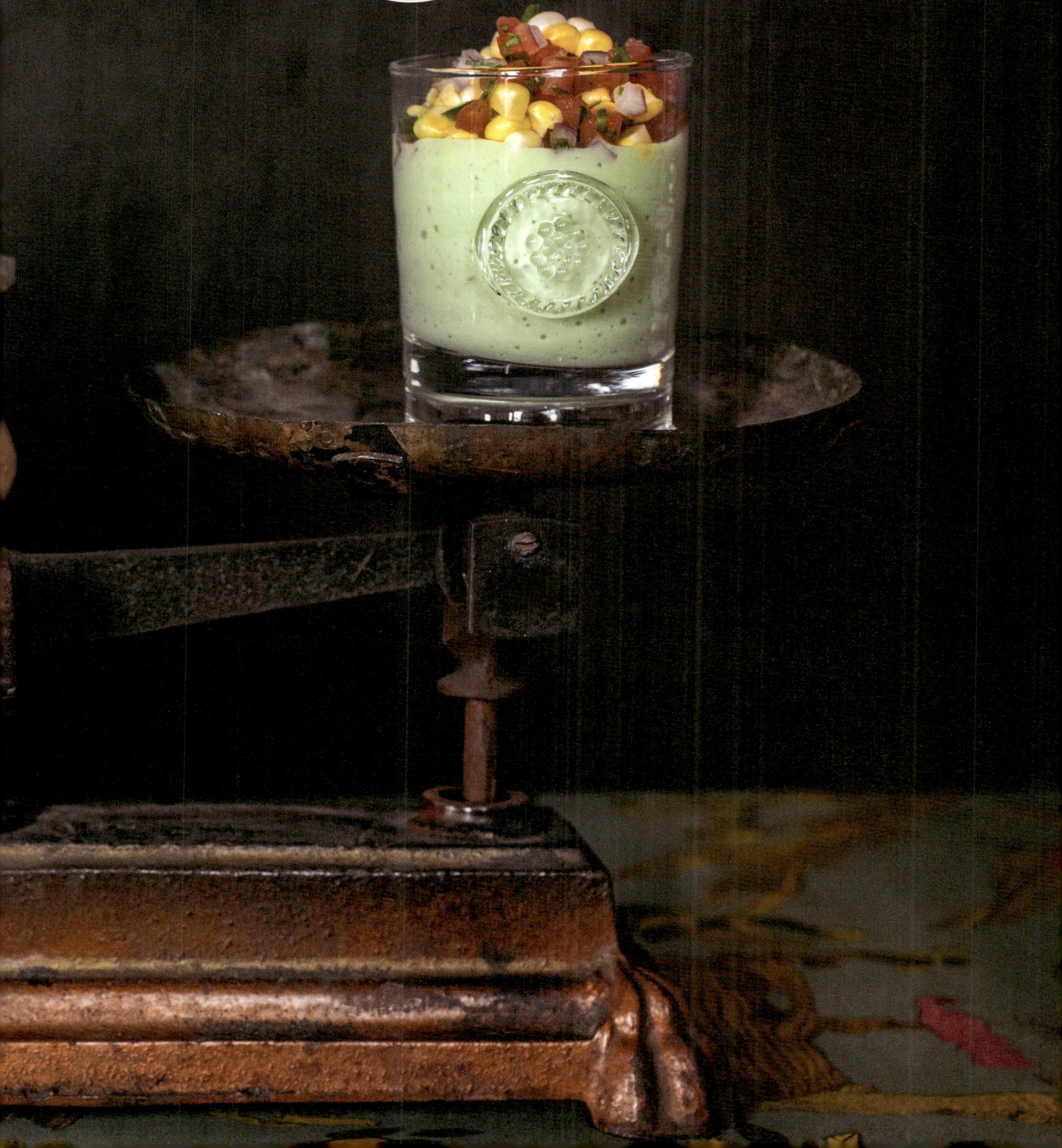

CHILLED AVOCADO SOUP
WITH ROASTED CORN SALSA

SERVES 8

We often serve this colorful soup as an hors d'oeuvre before dinner. Avocado adds potassium, soluble fiber, and monounsaturated fat to this soup, along with amazing mouthfeel. It's one of those dishes everyone wants to know how to make. You'll have to decide if you want to share the secret.

ROASTED CORN SALSA

1 cup fresh corn (approximately 3-4 large ears), husked

1 tablespoon grapeseed oil

1 cup diced tomato

1 jalapeño, seeded and minced

¼ cup minced red onion

juice of 1 lime

1 tablespoon chopped fresh cilantro

Preheat the oven to 350°F. Lightly brush the oil on the ears of the corn, wrap in foil and place on a baking sheet. Roast for 15 minutes until corn is soft. Remove from the oven and allow to cool. Using a sharp knife, slice down along the cob to remove the kernels. Add to a medium bowl along with the remaining ingredients. Mix well. Refrigerate until ready to use.

AVOCADO SOUP

2 avocados, halved, pitted, and peeled

1½ cups low-fat buttermilk

2½ cups water

1 teaspoon kosher salt

dash of Tabasco®

In a high-speed blender, combine all the ingredients and puree until completely smooth. Cover and refrigerate. When ready to serve, pour the soup into small bowls and garnish with a spoonful of Roasted Corn Salsa.

TIP: When selecting ripe, perfect avocados, go by feel rather than color. A ready-to-eat avocado should feel slightly soft, but not overly soft or mushy.

TIP: Serve this soup in glass bowls or shooter glasses, where the lime color and corn salsa make an impressive presentation. If you want to develop a brown, charred look to the corn, after baking for 15 minutes, remove the foil and raise the oven temperature to broil. Keep an eye on it, and after 5 minutes it should have a slightly blistered look.

NUTRITION PER SERVING	Cal 106	Fat 8g	Protein 3g	Carbs 7g	Sugar 3g	Fiber 4g	Sod 336mg

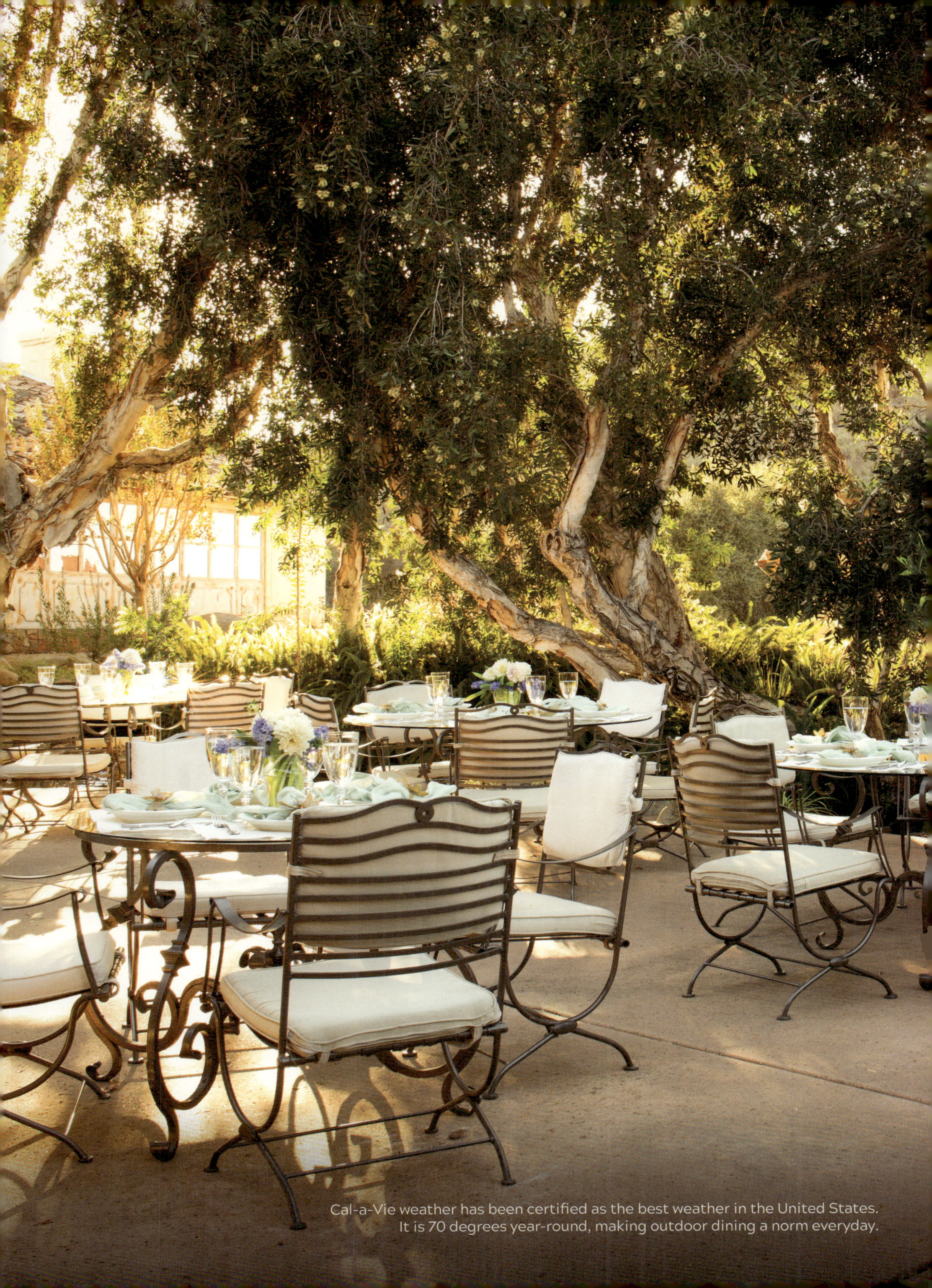

Cal-a-Vie weather has been certified as the best weather in the United States.
It is 70 degrees year-round, making outdoor dining a norm everyday.

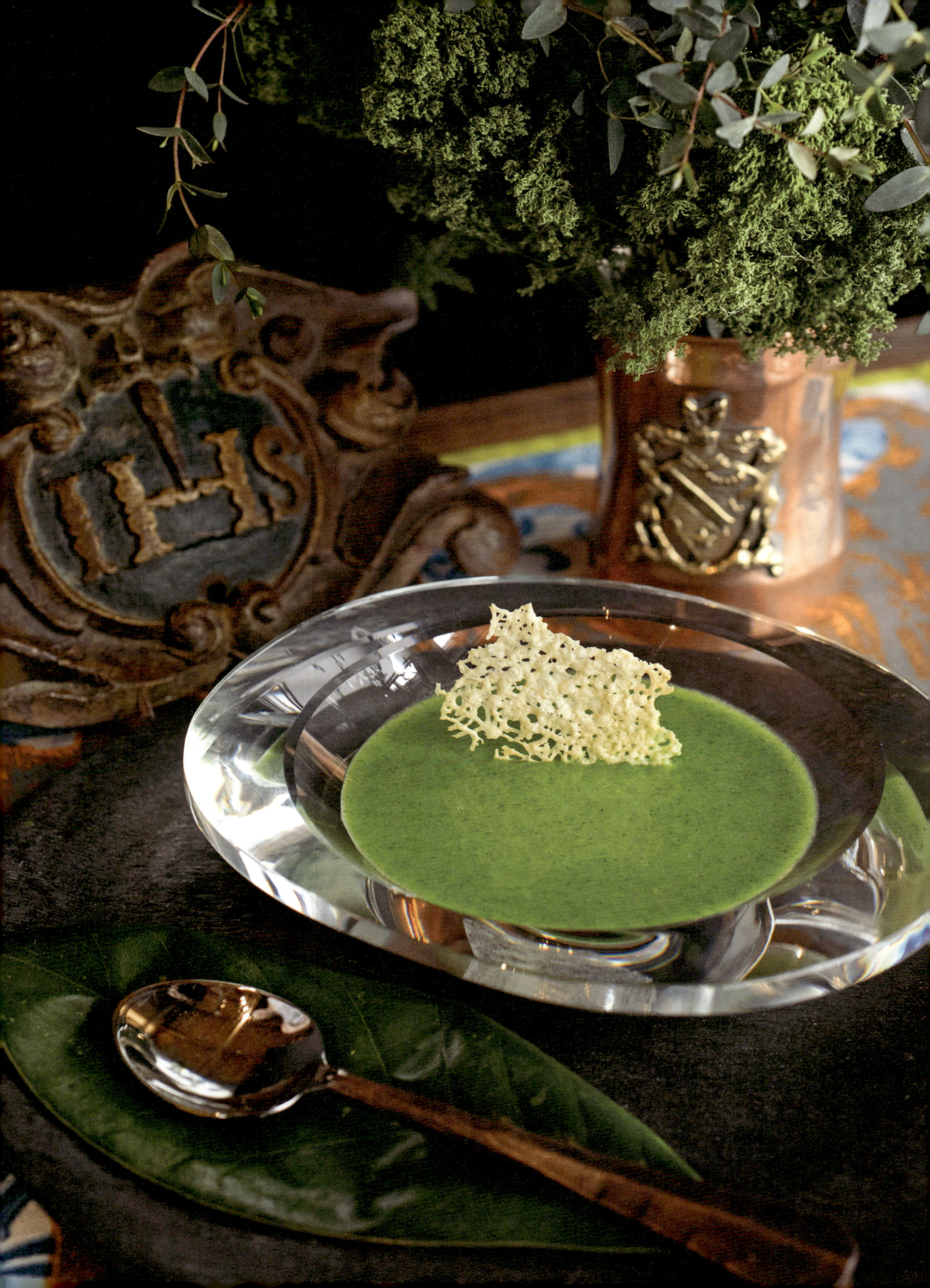
IHS

BROCCOLI SOUP
WITH PARMESAN CRISPS

SERVES 8

We love to serve broccoli at Cal-a-Vie because it's part of the brassica family, a cancer-fighting group of plants. Rich in Vitamins A and C, broccoli is also a great source of sulfur (which explains that less-than-pleasant smell that comes with cooking it). Odor aside, sulfur is critical for the production of glutathione—the most important detoxifying antioxidant in your body.

BROCCOLI STOCK

- 4 broccoli stalks (save the florets for the soup)
- ½ yellow onion, sliced
- 2 celery stalks, sliced
- 1 bay leaf
- 3 black peppercorns
- 4 cups water

In a large stock pot, add all the ingredients. Bring to a boil, then reduce the heat and simmer for 45 minutes. Strain through a fine-mesh sieve, preserving all the liquid stock and discarding the solids. Set the Broccoli Stock aside.

BROCCOLI SOUP

- 8 cups broccoli florets
- Broccoli Stock
- 2 teaspoons sea salt

In a large stock pot, bring 3 quarts of water to a rolling boil. In a large bowl, prepare an ice bath with 60 percent ice and 40 percent water. Working in small batches, add one-third of the broccoli florets to the boiling water and cook for 2-3 minutes. Remove broccoli from the boiling water and immediately plunge into the ice bath to stop the cooking and preserve its deep, bright-green hue. The goal is to keep the broccoli as soft and green as possible. Continue until all of the broccoli is cooked and completely chilled in the ice bath.

In a high-speed blender, also working in batches, add the broccoli florets and ¼ cup of Broccoli Stock. Puree on high until completely smooth. Additional stock may be needed to achieve the desired consistency each time you add broccoli and stock to the blender. Return the soup to a stock pot, and gently bring it up to serving temperature over medium heat. Season with salt.

PARMESAN CRISPS

- 1 cup grated Parmesan

Preheat the oven to 400°F. Spread the grated Parmesan on a baking sheet lined with a silicone mat and pat down. Bake for about 5 minutes or until the Parmesan is bubbly and golden brown. Remove from the oven and let sit for a few minutes until cool. Break into 8 large pieces and use for garnish on top of the soup.

TIP: You can start this recipe earlier in the day by preparing the Broccoli Stock and broccoli florets and storing them separately in the refrigerator in covered, airtight containers. Add them to the blender shortly before heating and serving.

But remember: The key to a vibrant broccoli soup is to make sure not to overcook your florets and to use an ice bath. If you cook the broccoli for too long, it will lose its beautiful green color.

NUTRITION PER SERVING	Cal 95	Fat 4g	Protein 8g	Carbs 7g	Sugar 2g	Fiber 2g	Sod 303mg

BLOODY MARY GAZPACHO

SERVES 6

Our Bloody Mary Gazpacho is the perfect soup to serve on a hot, summer day. The addition of Lime Salt gives the soup a sweet, zesty twist. If you don't have a spice grinder to make the lime salt, use a mortar and pestle to infuse the sea salt with the lime. Try adding our optional Cipollini Cucumber Salsa to garnish the top of the soup.

2 pounds heirloom tomatoes, blanched, peeled, and chopped

1 large cucumber, peeled and chopped

1 green bell pepper, seeded and chopped

3 garlic cloves

1 tablespoon sherry vinegar

1 tablespoon Worcestershire sauce

1 teaspoon sea salt

1 teaspoon celery seed

1 teaspoon Tabasco®

⅓ cup extra-virgin olive oil

sea salt, to taste

In a high-speed blender, combine all of the ingredients except the olive oil and puree until completely smooth. While the blender is on, slowly add the olive oil until completely incorporated. Add salt to taste. Chill in the refrigerator until ready to serve.

LIME SALT

3 limes, zested

2 teaspoons sea salt

In a spice grinder, combine the lime zest and salt and puree until fully incorporated. Set aside.

CIPOLLINI CUCUMBER SALSA (OPTIONAL TOPPING)

1 pint baby heirloom tomatoes, halved

1 cucumber, seeded, quartered, and cut into diamonds

1 green bell pepper, seeded and diced

Cipollini onion leaves

¼ cup chopped celery hearts

1 tablespoon extra-virgin olive oil

Lime Salt to taste

In a medium bowl, combine all of the ingredients and toss. Chill in the refrigerator.

When ready to serve, ladle the soup into serving bowls and top with a scoop of the garnish.

TIP: Cipollini onions used to be hard to find in grocery stores, but now many produce sections carry this small, chunky, round onion. These little darlings are delicious roasted whole or sautéed and will literally melt in your mouth.

NUTRITION PER SERVING	Cal 183	Fat 13g	Protein 3g	Carbs 18g	Sugar 9g	Fiber 5g	Sod 365mg

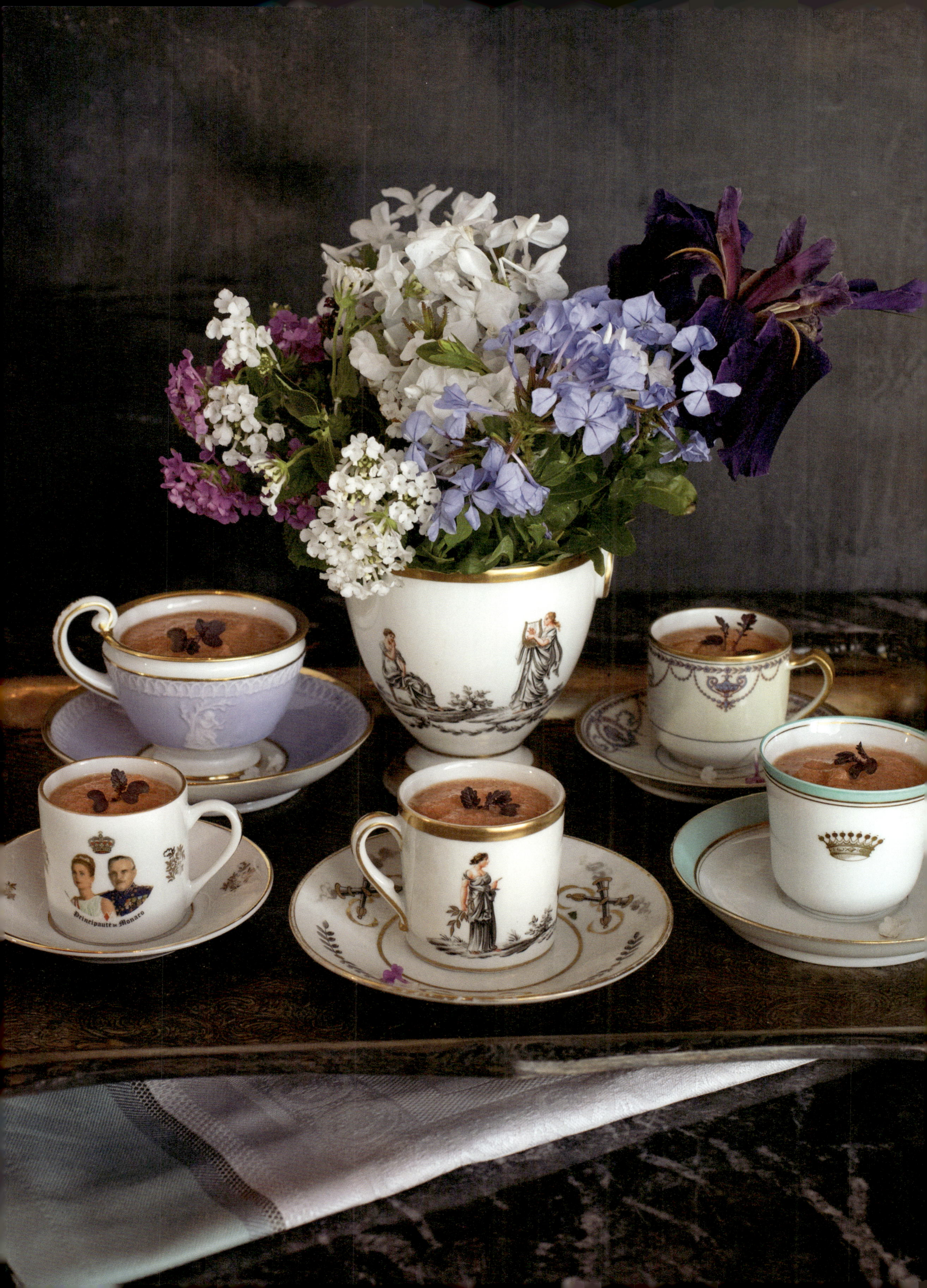
Principauté de Monaco

CARROT COCONUT SOUP

SERVES 8

Many guests compliment us on this classic Cal-a-Vie soup, which is often on the menu during a typical week's stay. You'll be amazed at how easy it is to make! Don't be afraid to use full-fat coconut milk; it helps to add to the richness of this deeply satisfying soup. Coconut milk is a great source of medium-chain triglycerides, which are easy to digest, especially for anyone who has a sluggish liver or issues with their gallbladder.

1 teaspoon grapeseed oil
2 shallots, sliced
3 garlic cloves, smashed
2 stalks lemongrass, sliced into 4-inch pieces
4 cups trimmed, peeled, and chopped carrots
1¼ cups unsweetened coconut milk
4 cups vegetable stock
salt and freshly ground black pepper, to taste

In a large saucepan over medium heat, add the grapeseed oil and sweat the shallots, garlic, and lemongrass, stirring often until they become soft but not brown. Add the carrots, coconut milk, and vegetable stock. Bring to a boil, then reduce heat to a simmer. Cook about 20 minutes until the carrots are soft. Remove the lemongrass stalks. Strain the solids over a bowl to reserve the liquid. Using a blender or a Vitamix® machine, transfer in batches some of the carrot mixture and the liquid and puree until smooth. Add additional liquid to create a soup consistency. Add salt and pepper to taste. Serve immediately.

TIP: Leftover soup will keep in an airtight container in the refrigerator for up to 5 days. It will store in the freezer for about a month.

NUTRITION PER SERVING	Cal	Fat	Protein	Carbs	Sugar	Fiber	Sod
	117	8g	2g	11g	5g	2g	72mg

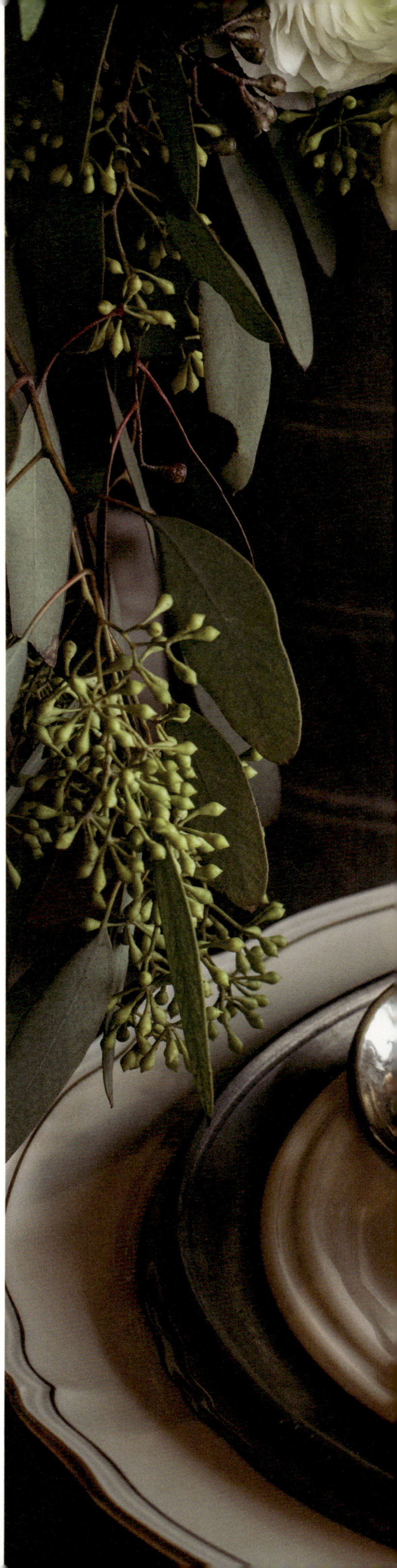

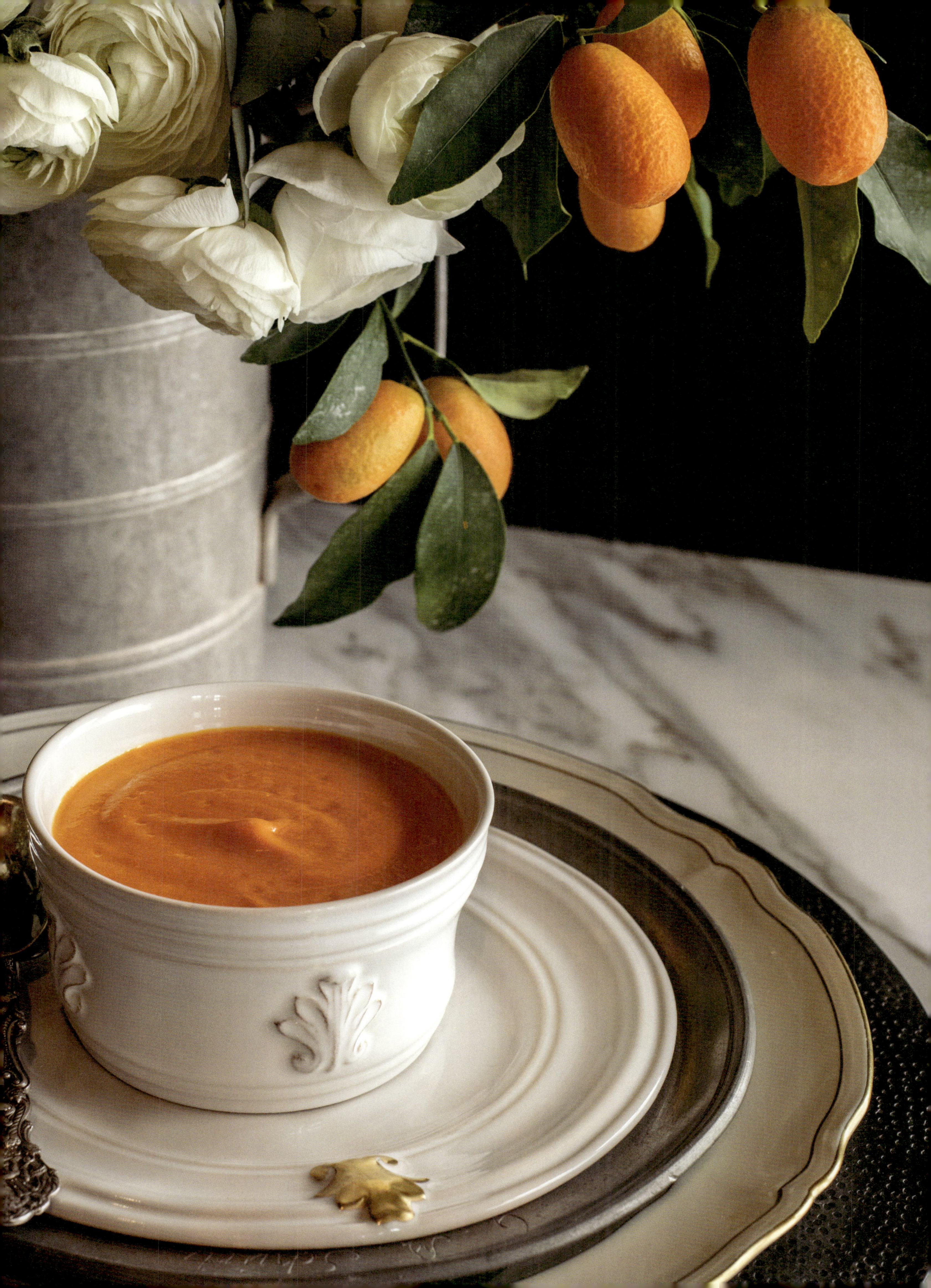

GARDEN PUMPKIN SOUP
WITH GOAT CHEESE CREMA AND SALTED PEPITAS

SERVES 12

It feels like fall when you serve up a bowl of our Garden Pumpkin Soup, even if it's a balmy 75 degrees outside. Surprisingly, pumpkins are very sensitive to cold weather, which is why they thrive in our organic garden here in lovely Southern California. We start planting them around June because they require a long growing season; sometimes it takes up to 100 days before they are ready to be harvested. The deep orange color of pumpkin paired with the brightness of turmeric make for a nutritiously beautiful soup.

SALTED PEPITAS

- 1 teaspoon salt
- 2 tablespoons water
- ½ cup pepitas (pumpkin seeds)

Preheat the oven to 350°F. In a small saucepan, add the salt and water. Bring to a boil to dissolve the salt. Remove from the heat. In a small bowl, mix the pepitas and the salt water. Spread on a baking sheet and bake for 5-7 minutes. Remove and set aside.

GOAT CHEESE CREMA

- ½ cup goat cheese, softened
- ¼ tablespoons 2% milk

In a high-speed blender, combine the goat cheese and milk and puree until completely smooth. Refrigerate until ready to use.

PUMPKIN SOUP

- 1 garden pumpkin (about 3 pounds)
- 1 tablespoon olive oil
- 1 tablespoon grapeseed oil
- 1 cup chopped yellow onion
- ½ cup chopped carrots
- 2 smashed garlic cloves
- 1 tablespoon sea salt
- 2 teaspoons turmeric
- 1 herb sachet (2 bay leaves and 3-4 fresh thyme sprigs wrapped in cheesecloth and tied with butcher's twine)
- ½ cup white wine (we recommend using Chardonnay)
- 2 quarts vegetable stock
- 2 tablespoons honey

Preheat the oven to 400°F. Cut the pumpkin in half and scoop out the seeds. Rub the inside of the pumpkin with olive oil and place on a baking sheet cut-side down. Roast the pumpkin for 30 minutes, or until extremely soft. Scoop the pumpkin meat from the skins and reserve for making the soup. The cooked pumpkin should equal about 6 cups.

In a large stock pot over medium heat, warm the grapeseed oil. Add the onions, carrots, garlic, and sea salt and sauté for 4-6 minutes, or until the onions have become translucent. Add the turmeric and thyme-bay leaf sachet and deglaze with white wine, stirring to pick up the flavorful bits of food stuck to the bottom of the pot. Simmer until the wine is reduced by half. Add the roasted pumpkin, vegetable stock, and honey. Simmer for about 30 minutes. Remove the herb sachet and strain the solids (pumpkin and vegetables) from the liquid, reserving both to puree in small batches.

In a high-speed blender, add a third of the pumpkin mixture and just enough of the reserved stock to cover. Puree until completely smooth. Repeat this process until all of the soup is pureed and the desired consistency is achieved. Strain the pureed soup through a fine-mesh sieve. Return to the stock pot and warm. Adjust the seasoning with salt to taste. Serve each bowl with a dollop of Goat Cheese Crema and a few Salted Pepitas sprinkled on top.

TIP: Although this recipe doesn't use them, it's not necessary to throw away your pumpkin guts. They can be prepared into stock and used for just about any other soup.

NUTRITION PER SERVING	Cal 106	Fat 5g	Protein 3g	Carbs 13g	Sugar 7g	Fiber 1g	Sod 821mg

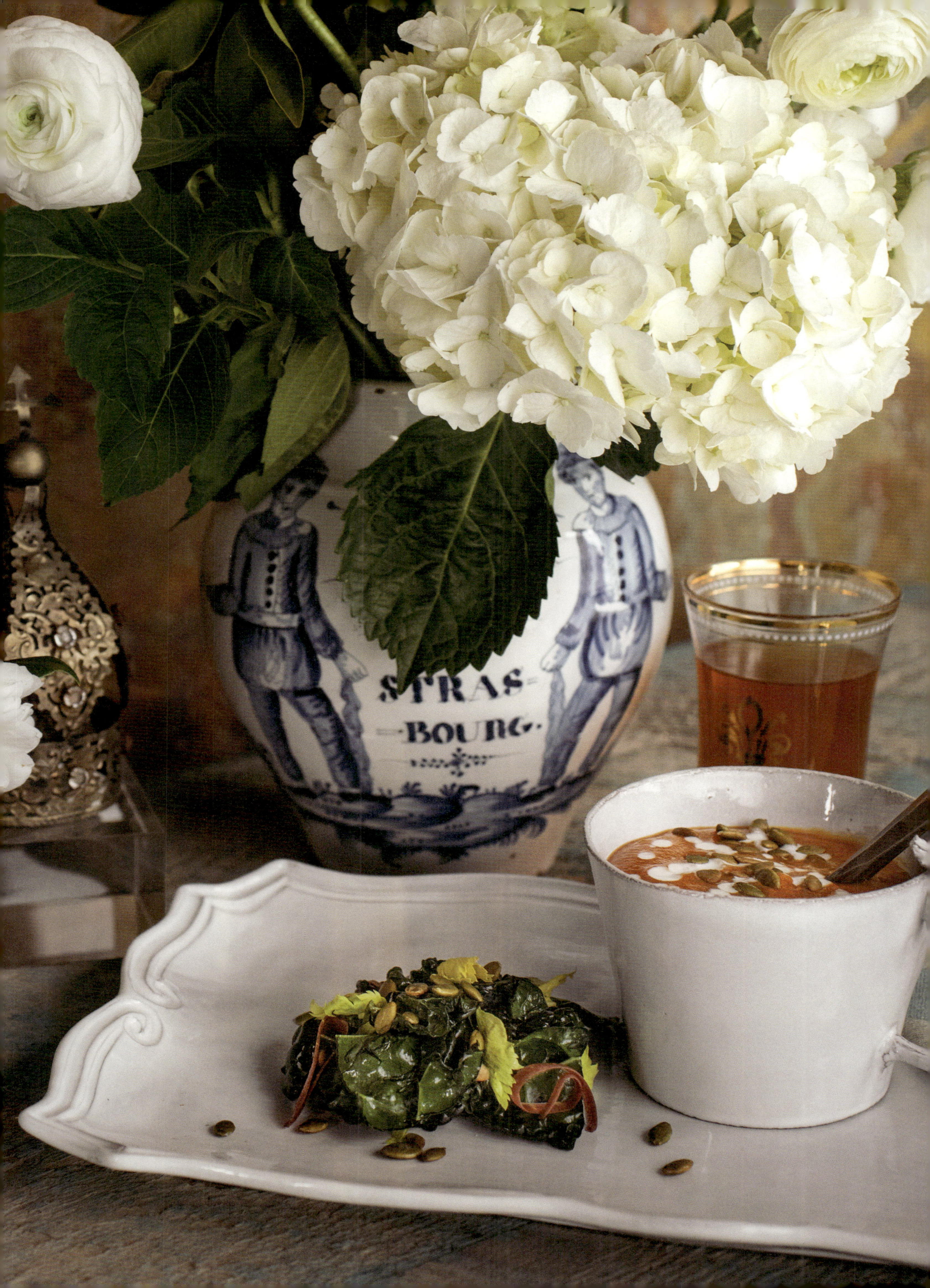
STRAS-
-BOURG.

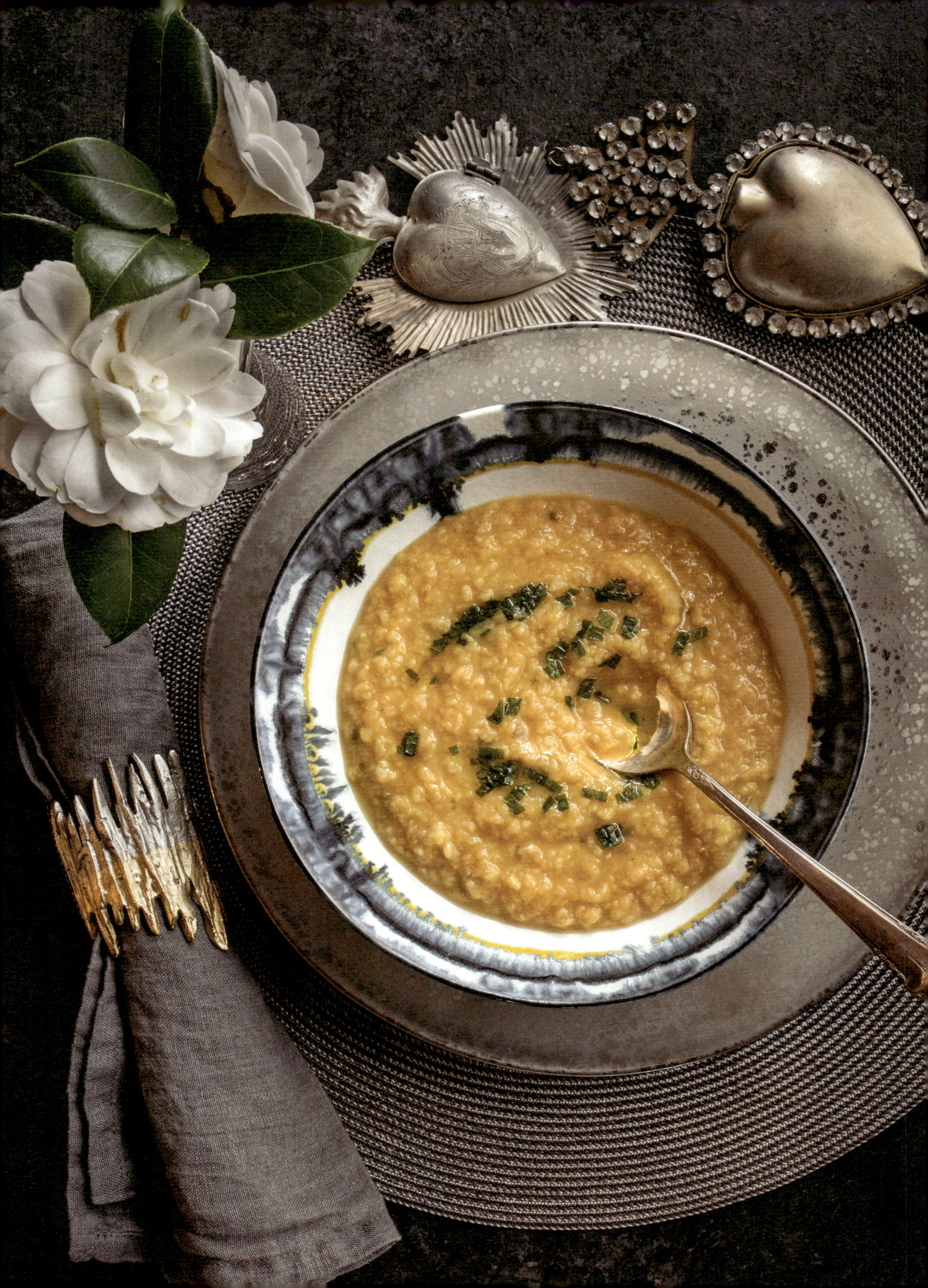

GOLDEN LENTIL SOUP

SERVES 8

This soup is packed with spices that deliver nutrition as well as a ton of flavor. Mustard, cumin, and coriander seeds are good for everything from aiding your digestive and bronchial systems to purifying your blood. Garlic, ginger, and turmeric are all known for their anti-inflammatory and immune-boosting properties.

- 1 teaspoon whole cumin seeds
- 1 teaspoon whole mustard seeds
- ½ teaspoon whole coriander seeds
- 1 tablespoon grapeseed oil
- 1 cup diced onion
- 1 jalapeño, seeded and diced
- 4 garlic cloves, minced
- 1 tablespoon fresh ginger, peeled and minced
- ½ teaspoon smoked paprika
- 1 teaspoon turmeric
- 1 cup yellow lentils (If they are not with the other beans, look for yellow lentils in the international or bulk supply sections of your grocery store.)
- 6 cups vegetable stock
- kosher salt, to taste
- chopped fresh chives for garnish

Place a small skillet over medium heat. Once hot, add the cumin seeds, mustard seeds, and coriander seeds and shake the pan for 1-2 minutes until toasted and fragrant. Remove from the heat and allow to cool slightly. Wrap the toasted spices in cheesecloth and tie with butcher's twine. In a medium pot over medium heat, add the grapeseed oil. Once warm, add the onion, jalapeño, garlic, and ginger. Sauté until the onions are translucent in color, about 3 minutes. Add the smoked paprika and turmeric and stir for 30 seconds. Add the lentils, cheesecloth with toasted spices, and vegetable stock. Bring to a boil and then reduce the heat to a simmer. Cook uncovered until the lentils are completely softened and the soup is a thick consistency, about 45 minutes. Allow to simmer longer or add more stock if necessary until desired consistency is achieved. Add salt to taste. Top with chopped chives. Serve immediately.

TIP: Most store-bought vegetable stock is dark in color and will produce a darker soup; however, you can often find clear vegetable stock in the international section of the grocery store.

Yellow lentils come in many sizes and from all parts of the globe. Any yellow lentil will work in this recipe, but it may take longer for the lentils to soften depending on their size and variety.

The trick to giving this soup its creamy texture is to let the lentils get extra soft, to the point that they blend together.

NUTRITION PER SERVING	Cal 117	Fat 2g	Protein 6g	Carbs 19g	Sugar 2g	Fiber 3g	Sod 40mg

KALE AND VEGGIE SOUP

SERVES 10

Kale has made it up the ranks over the years from merely a garnish to a staple vegetable in every health-conscious cook's kitchen—and with good reason! Kale is a super food in the brassica family, chock full of beta-carotene and fiber. Paired with butternut squash and black-eyed peas, this soup makes for a hearty first course at dinner or a delicious lunch the next day.

1 tablespoon extra-virgin olive oil
¼ cup diced onion
¼ cup diced celery
¼ cup diced fennel
1 cup diced carrots
2 garlic cloves, minced
2 quarts chicken stock
1 cup cooked black-eyed peas (if using canned, rinsed and drained)
1 cup diced butternut squash (or any root vegetable)
2 cups kale, cut into 1-inch pieces
2 teaspoons sea salt
¼ teaspoon freshly ground black pepper

In a large saucepan over medium heat, warm the olive oil. Add the onion, celery, fennel, and carrots, and sauté for about 5 minutes. Add the garlic and continue to cook for one minute. Add the chicken stock and bring to a boil, then lower the heat to simmer. Add the black-eyed peas and butternut squash and continue simmering for 3 to 5 minutes. Add the kale, salt, and pepper and simmer for an additional 2 minutes. Serve immediately.

TIP: Substitute vegetable stock for chicken stock and this soup becomes a vegetarian version.

TIP: Most grocery stores now carry butternut squash already cubed, making this soup easy and fast to prepare. If using fresh black-eyed peas, soak them overnight in water, then drain and rinse. Boil for 30-60 minutes depending on how soft you like them. Drain again and use in our Kale and Veggie Soup.

NUTRITION PER SERVING	Cal 111	Fat 4g	Protein 6g	Carbs 13g	Sugar 5g	Fiber 2g	Sod 574mg

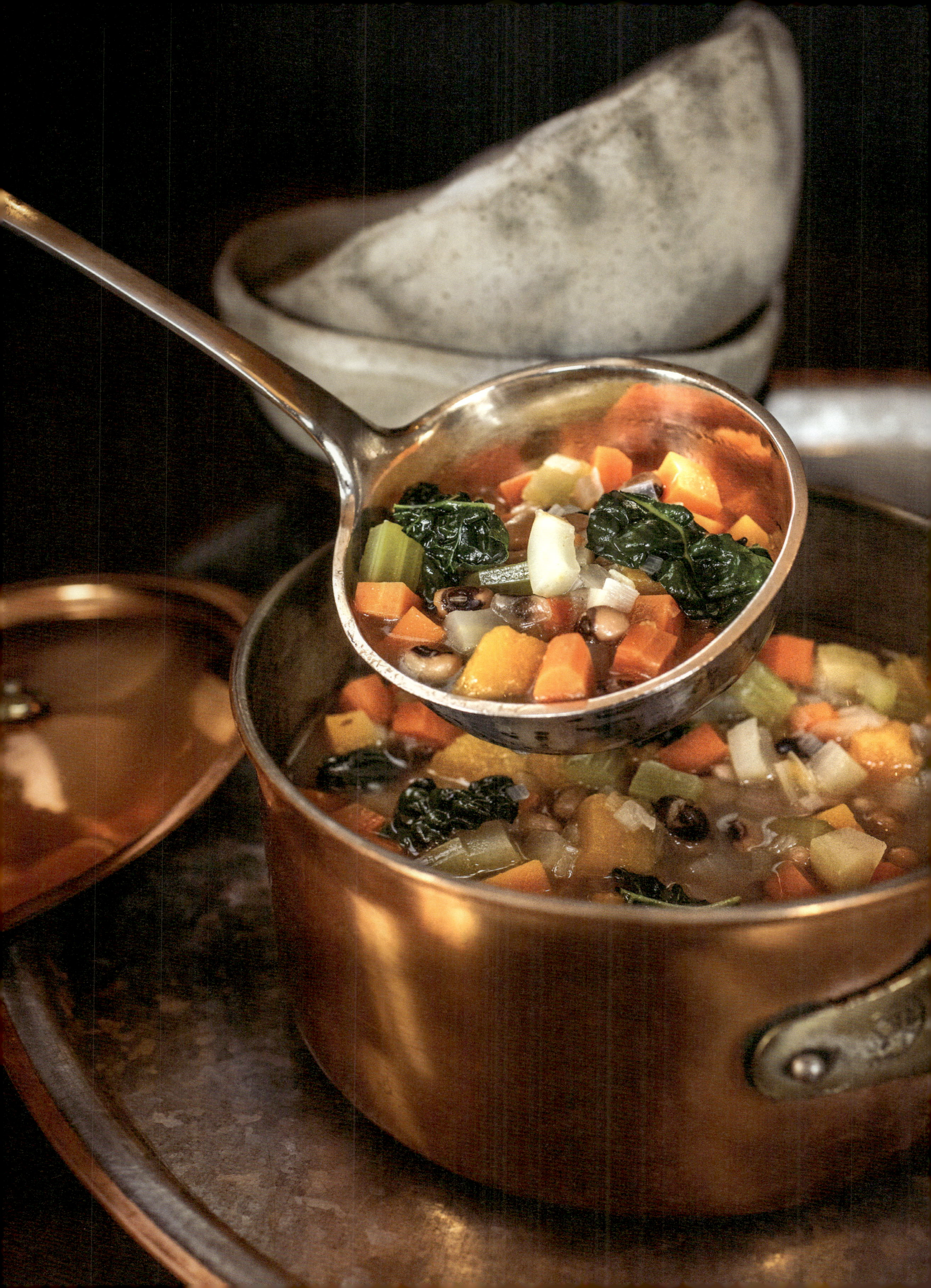

PARSNIP-APPLE SOUP

SERVES 10

Most root vegetables like parsnips are starches—a kind of carbohydrate that the body breaks down into glucose for energy. Parsnips are also higher in fiber and lower in calories than potatoes. Scratch the outer surface of your parsnip to check for wax, which helps to extend its shelf life. If it's waxed, make sure to peel it, even if it's organic.

1 tablespoon extra-virgin olive oil
1 onion, sliced
3 pounds parsnips, peeled and chopped (about 6 medium parsnips)
1 garlic clove, smashed
1 pound Gala apples, peeled, cored, and chopped (about 2 large apples)
½ cup dry white wine (we recommend using Chardonnay)
2 quarts vegetable stock
4 sprigs fresh thyme
1 bay leaf
salt and freshly ground pepper, to taste
2 cups 2% milk

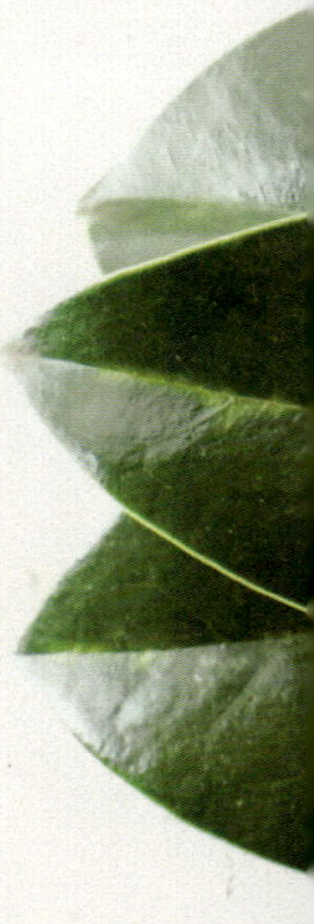

In a large soup pot over medium heat, add the olive oil. When warm, add the onions and parsnips. Sauté about 8 minutes until soft and beginning to turn brown. Add the garlic and stir about 1 minute. Add the apples, wine, vegetable stock, thyme, and bay leaf. Bring to a boil and then reduce the heat to simmer for about 45 minutes or until apples and parsnips are soft enough to smash with a fork on the side of the pot. Remove from heat and discard the thyme sprigs and bay leaf.

Using a blender, puree in batches while adding the milk to create the correct soup texture. Return to the pot and reheat. Add salt and pepper to taste.

TIP: If you can't find parsnips at your grocery store, try substituting other root vegetables such as rutabagas or turnips.

NUTRITION PER SERVING	Cal	Fat	Protein	Carbs	Sugar	Fiber	Sod
	116	2g	1g	23g	9g	5g	77mg

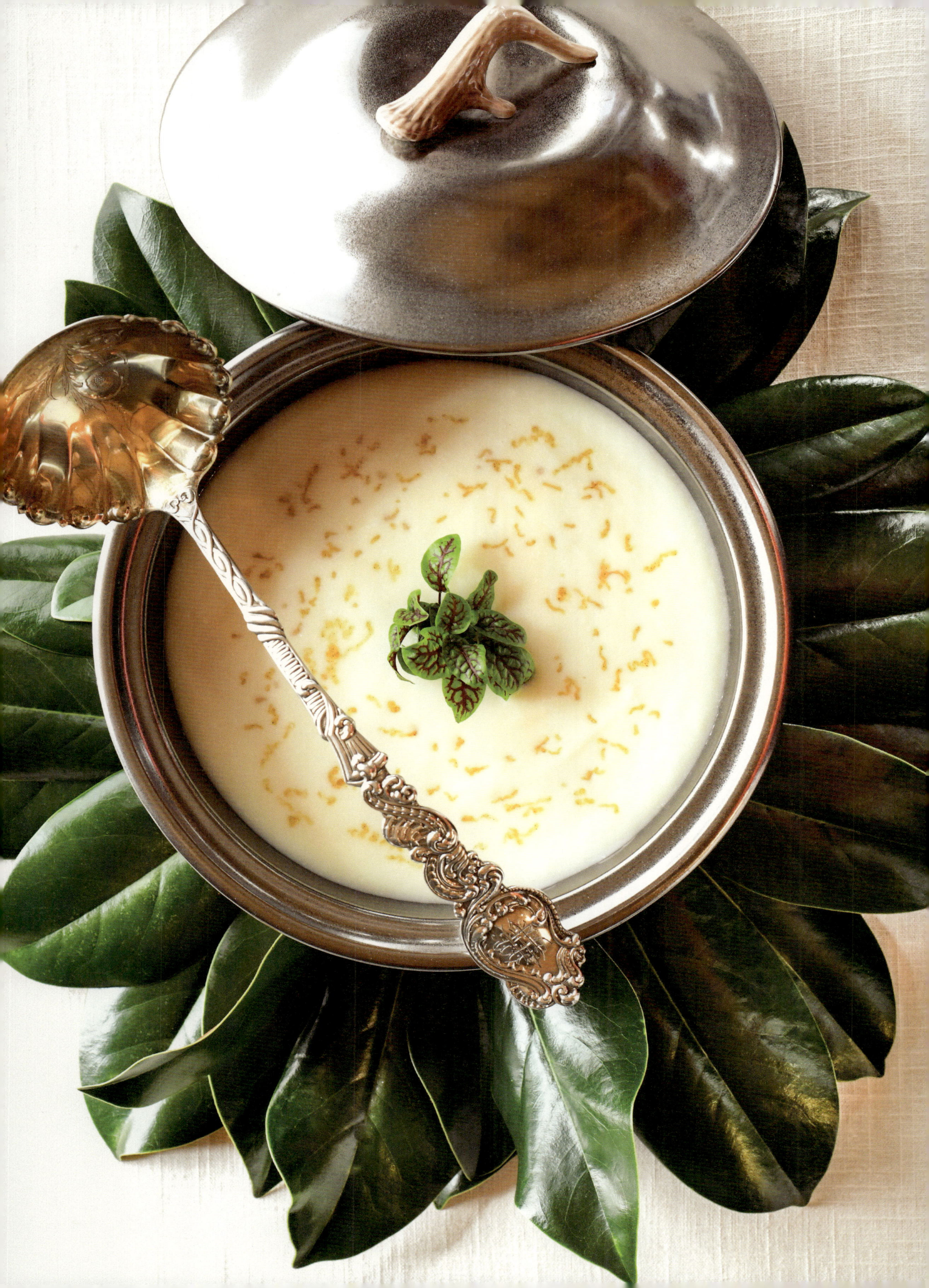

ROASTED CAULIFLOWER SOUP

WITH CURRY OIL

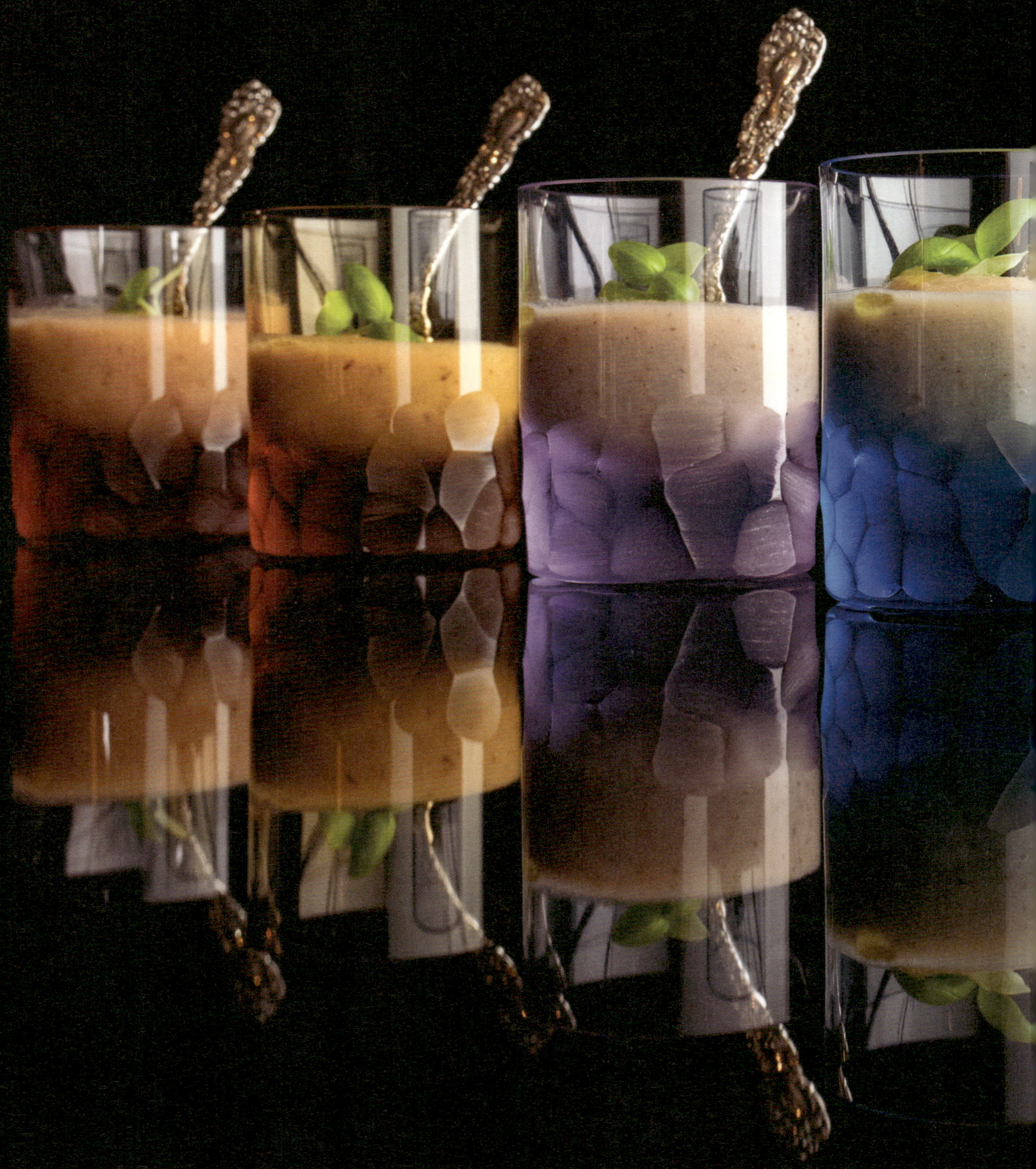

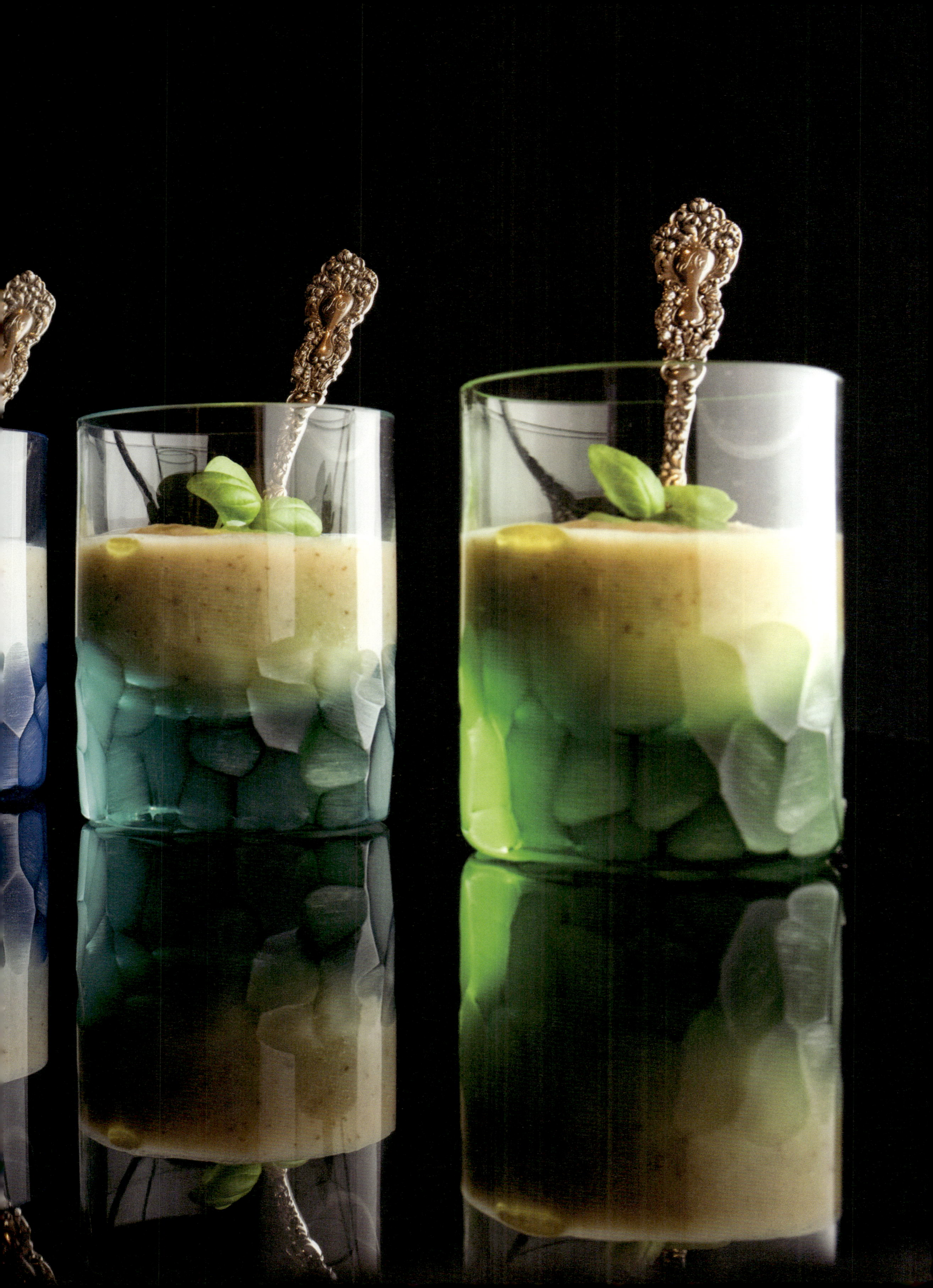

ROASTED CAULIFLOWER SOUP
WITH CURRY OIL

SERVES 8

Quick and easy to make, our Roasted Cauliflower Soup will become a family favorite. Roasting cauliflower florets caramelizes them into lightly browned, sweet, and savory pieces. Cauliflower adds creaminess and body to this soup, even though it's low in carbohydrates. It's also as nutritious as broccoli and kale, providing fiber and lots of potassium, both of which are great for anyone with cholesterol or blood pressure issues.

CURRY OIL

- 2 teaspoons Madras curry powder
- ⅓ cup grapeseed oil

Combine the powder and oil in a small sauce pot. Using a food thermometer, heat to 160°F. Remove from the heat and let steep for 20 minutes. Strain out the solids and set the oil aside.

ROASTED CAULIFLOWER SOUP

- 2 heads cauliflower, core removed, florets cut into 2-inch pieces
- 3 tablespoons extra-virgin olive oil, divided use
- 1 cup diced onion
- 1 garlic clove, minced
- 2 quarts vegetable stock
- 1 teaspoon cumin seeds
- 1 herb sachet (3 sprigs fresh thyme and 1 bay leaf wrapped in cheesecloth and tied with butcher's twine)
- 1 teaspoon sea salt

Preheat the oven to 350°F. In a large bowl, toss the cauliflower florets with 2 tablespoons of olive oil. Spread evenly onto a baking sheet and roast in the oven for 30 minutes, or until tender and golden brown. Set aside.

In a large stock pot, heat the remaining tablespoon of olive oil over medium heat and add the onion and garlic. Sauté about 10 minutes until translucent in color. Add the roasted cauliflower florets, vegetable stock, cumin seeds, and herb sachet. Bring to a boil and then reduce the heat and simmer for 10 minutes. Turn off the heat and remove the herb sachet. Using a blender, working in batches, puree the soup to achieve the desired consistency. Return to the stove over medium heat. Season with sea salt to taste.

When ready to serve, pour the soup into bowls and top with a small amount of Curry Oil.

TIP: To prepare the cauliflower, use a sharp knife to trim the bottom, then quarter it into four wedges. Slice off the inner core from each quarter, then cut the pieces into florets, keeping them similar in size so they roast evenly.

NUTRITION PER SERVING	Cal 152	Fat 12g	Protein 3g	Carbs 10g	Sugar 4g	Fiber 3g	Sod 437 mg

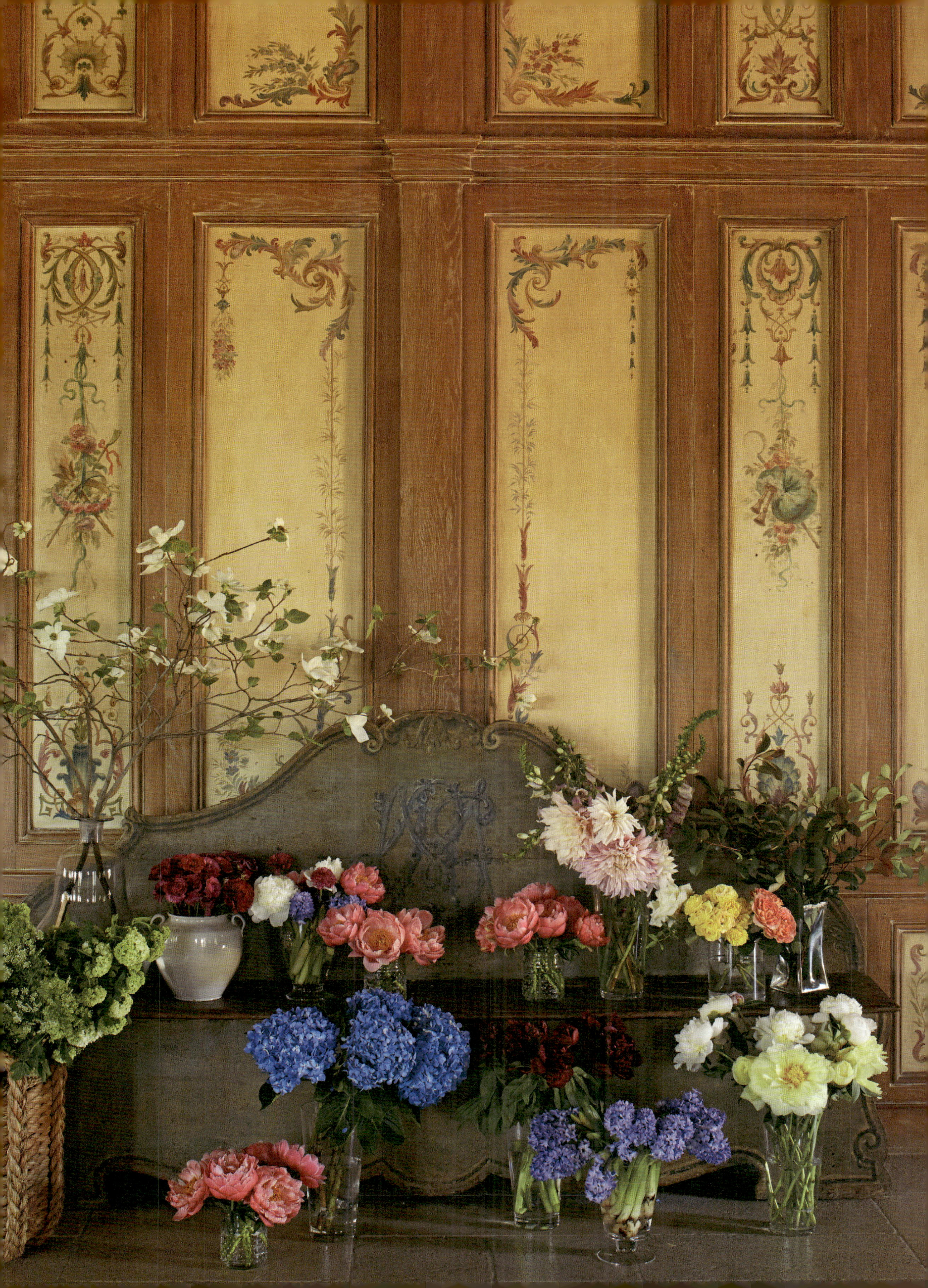

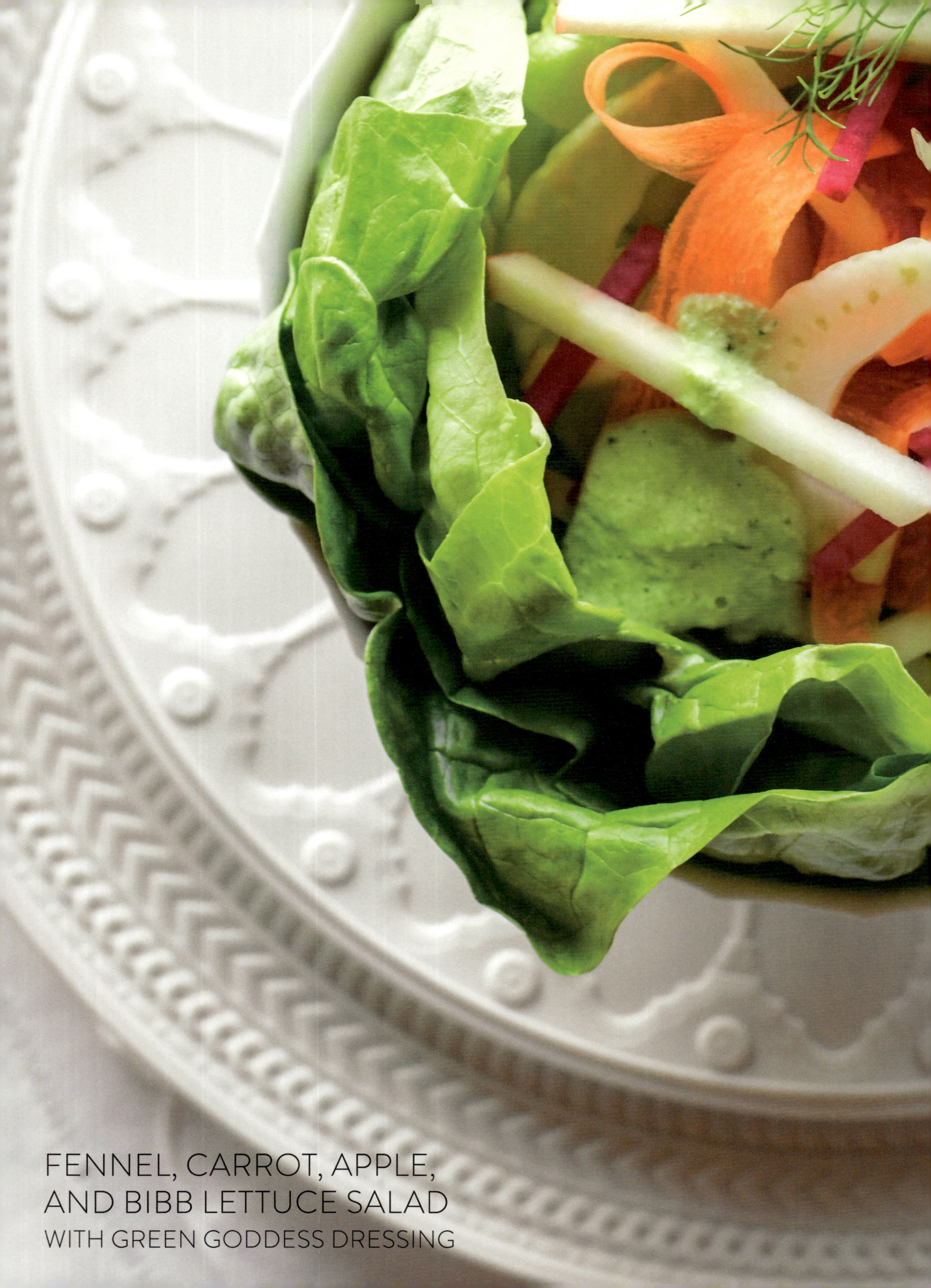

FENNEL, CARROT, APPLE, AND BIBB LETTUCE SALAD

WITH GREEN GODDESS DRESSING

CHAPTER 3

Salads

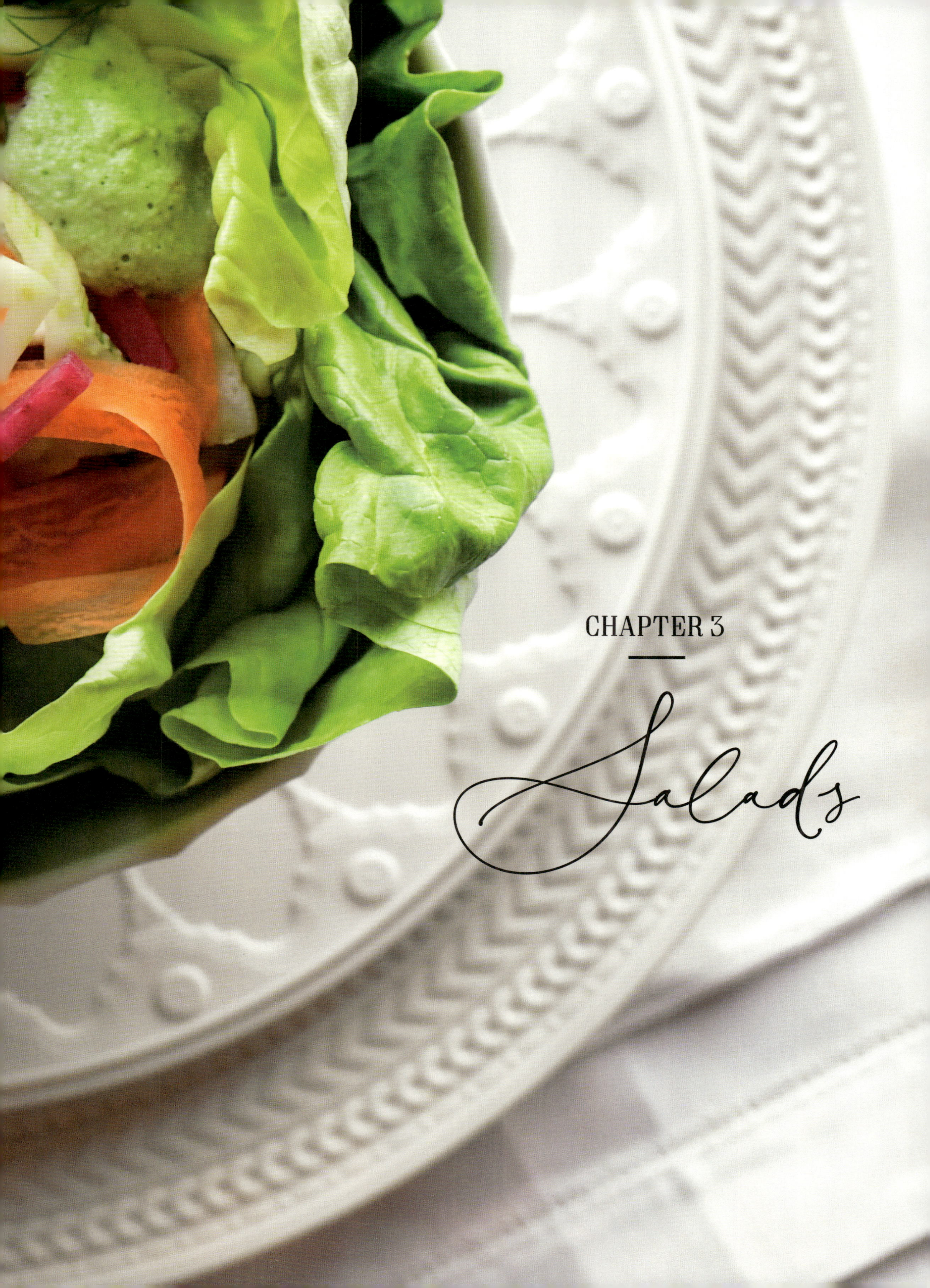

FENNEL, CARROT, APPLE, AND BIBB LETTUCE SALAD
WITH GREEN GODDESS DRESSING

SERVES 4

A Green Goddess Dressing typically contains mayonnaise and sour cream, but the Cal-a-Vie version of this classic dressing is high in flavor and extremely low in calories. Once you've created the dressing our way, we guarantee you will never go back. Use it over all sorts of salads and vegetables. It's Paleo and vegan friendly, too.

GREEN GODDESS DRESSING

1 cup raw cashews, soaked overnight in water, drained, and stored in refrigerator

½ cup fresh parsley leaves

2 tablespoons fresh tarragon leaves

¼ cup chopped fresh chives

½ teaspoon sea salt

½ tablespoon fresh lemon juice

1¼ cups water, divided use

In a blender, combine cashews, parsley, tarragon, chives, sea salt, lemon juice, and 1 cup of water. Puree on high until all the ingredients are completely smooth. Adjust the consistency with the remaining ¼ cup of water. Strain through a mesh sieve, pressing with a spoon to release all the liquid. Refrigerate until ready to use.

SALAD ASSEMBLY

1 cup thinly sliced fennel

1 cup julienned carrots

1 cup julienned red apples (we recommend Pink Lady or Honeycrisp)

½ cup thinly sliced red radishes

½ cup Green Goddess Dressing

2 heads Bibb lettuce, core removed and leaves separated

In a large bowl, combine the fennel, carrots, apples, and radishes. Toss together with the dressing to coat the vegetables and apples.

In 4 small bowls, layer the Bibb lettuce leaves around the sides and place a spoonful of the apple-vegetable mixture in the middle. Drizzle a little extra dressing over the lettuce.

TIP: The extra dressing can be stored in the refrigerator for a week. Butter, Boston, and Bibb lettuces are almost identical greens if you need to use one of them as a substitute.

NUTRITION PER SERVING	Cal 92	Fat 4g	Protein 3g	Carbs 13g	Sugar 7g	Fiber 4g	Sod 99mg

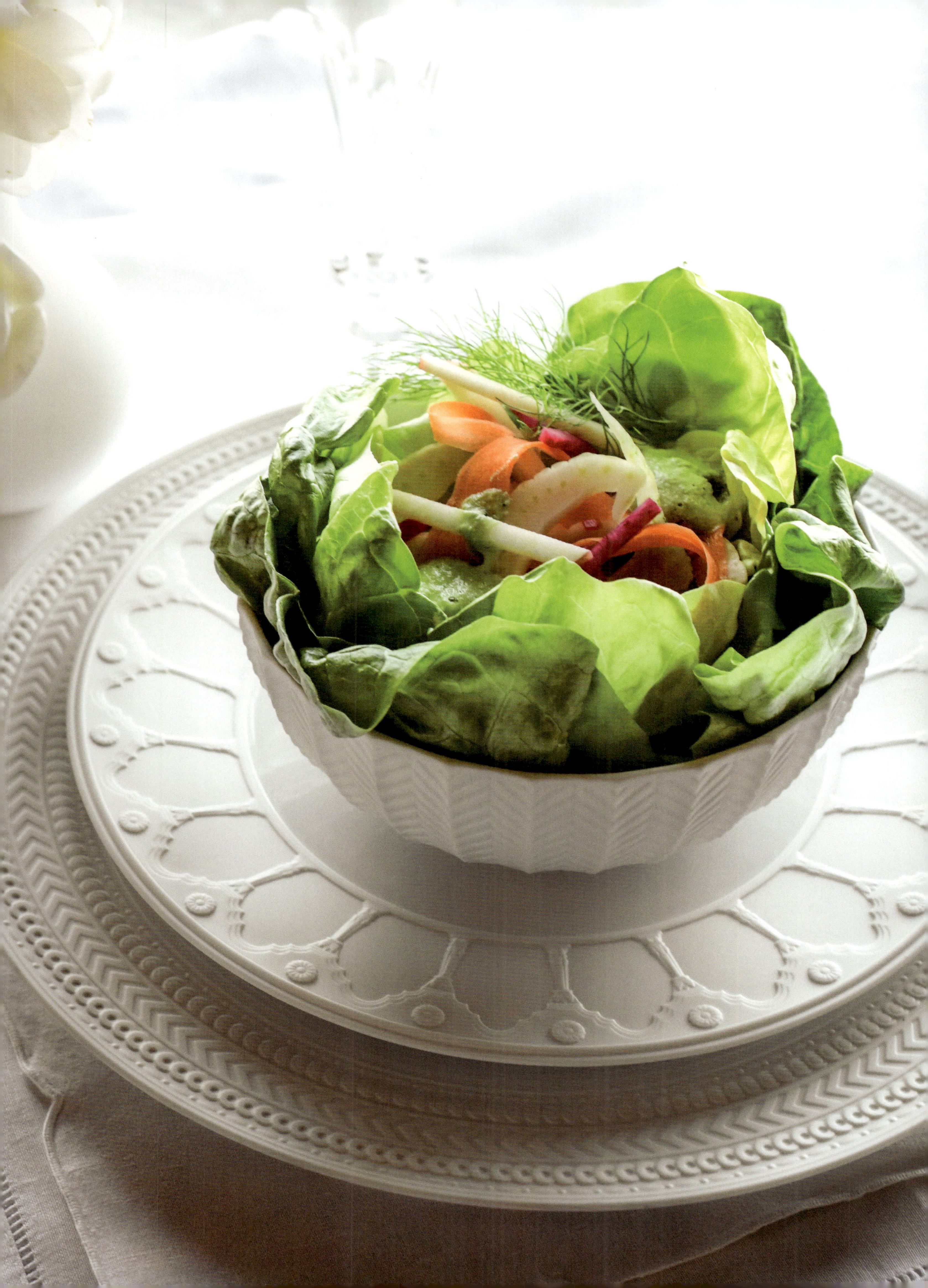

ARUGULA WITH STRAWBERRIES AND VANILLA CHAMPAGNE VINAIGRETTE

SERVES 4

This crisp and light salad makes a perfect addition to a spring or summer meal. Pickled shallots are a delicious homemade condiment that is easy to make and delivers a pop of flavor. Pickling is a form of fermentation, which nourishes the digestive tract with healthy probiotics.

PICKLED SHALLOTS

1 cup champagne vinegar
½ cup sugar
1 tablespoon sea salt or kosher salt
2 cups thinly sliced shallots

In a small saucepan, add the vinegar, sugar, and salt. Bring to a boil. Remove from the heat and pour over the sliced shallots. Cool and then place in the refrigerator for at least 4 hours.

VANILLA CHAMPAGNE VINAIGRETTE

1 cup champagne vinegar
¼ cup honey
2 tablespoons Dijon mustard
1 teaspoon sea salt
1 vanilla bean, scraped
½ cup water
1½ cups grapeseed oil

In a blender, combine the vinegar, honey, mustard, salt, vanilla bean scraping, and water. Blend on high. While blending, slowly add the oil until completely emulsified. Set aside in the refrigerator.

SALAD ASSEMBLY

4 cups arugula
1 cup strawberries, hulled and quartered
1 cup cherry tomatoes, halved
¼ cup Pickled Shallots
¼ cup crumbled goat cheese
¼ cup slivered almonds, toasted
¼ cup Vanilla Champagne Vinaigrette

In a large bowl, combine all the ingredients and toss. Divide among 4 plates.

NUTRITION PER SERVING	Cal 158	Fat 12g	Protein 5g	Carbs 10g	Sugar 6g	Fiber 3g	Sod 94mg

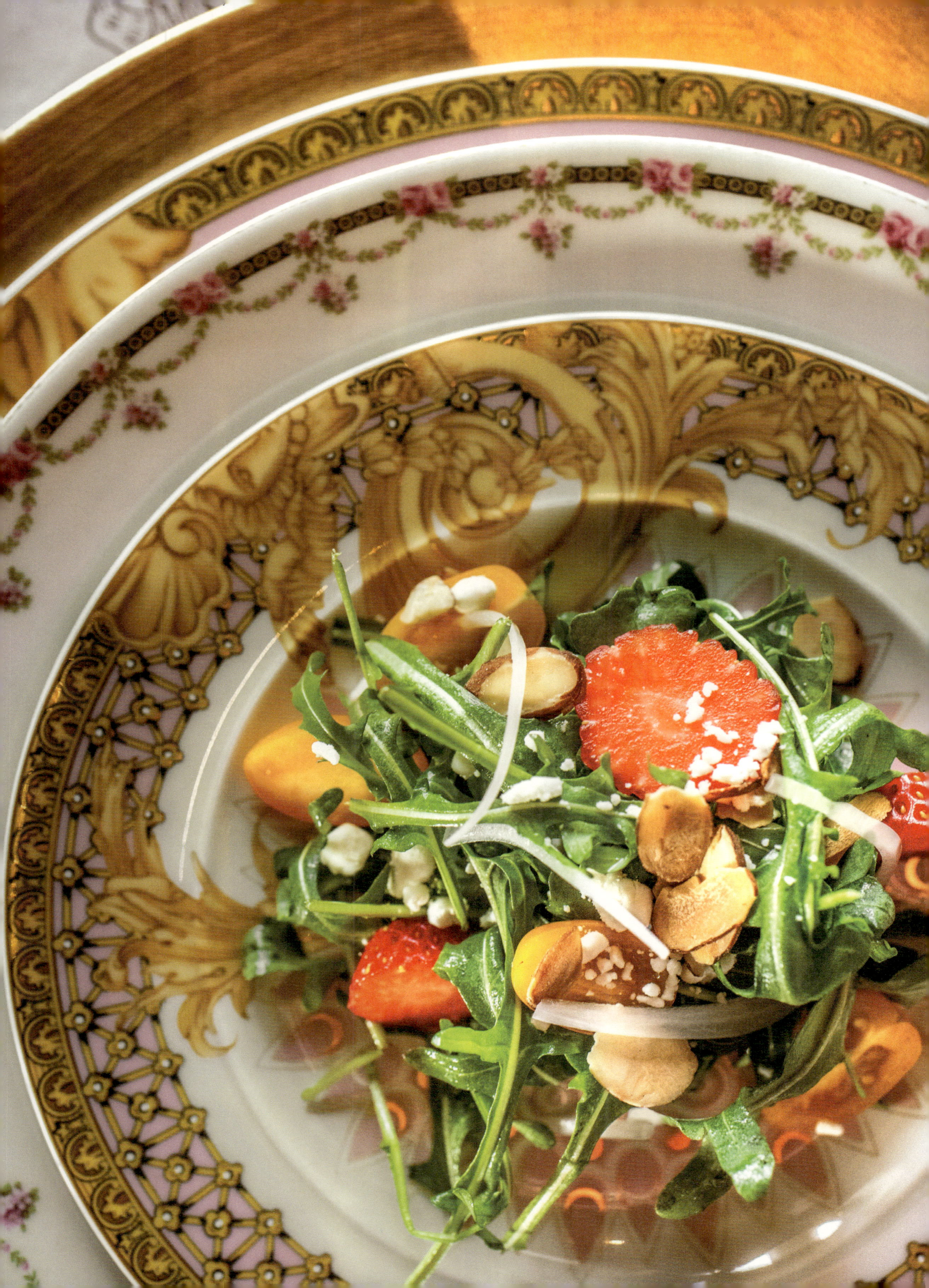

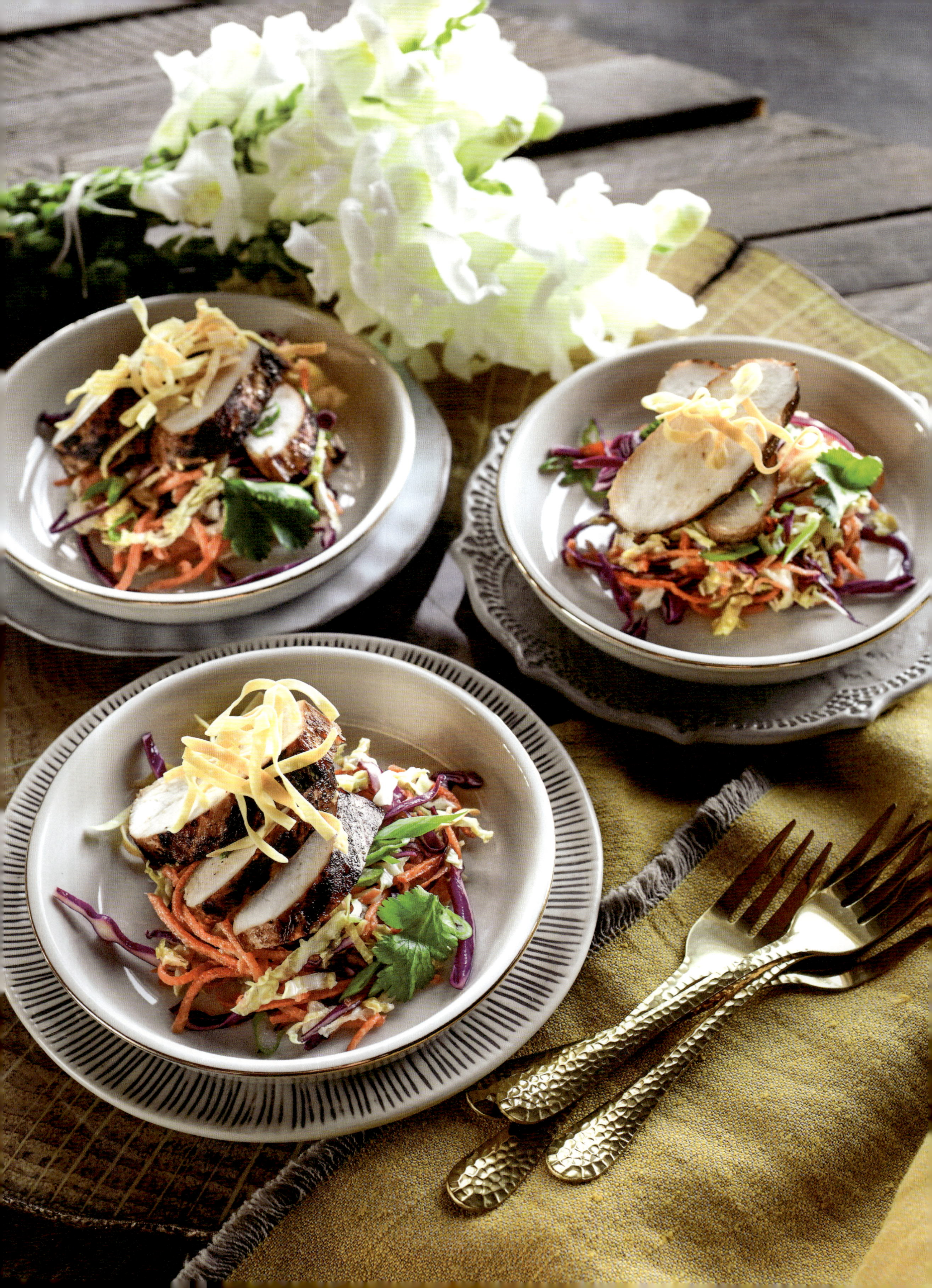

ASIAN CHICKEN SALAD

SERVES 12

This salad is a vibrant reflection of our nutrition philosophy. It combines a spectrum of colors and flavors that offer an array of beneficial phytonutrients. Cabbage is rich in sulforaphane, which acts as a potent antioxidant by scavenging for free radicals and safely converting hydrogen peroxide into water in the body. Add in crisp beta-carotene-rich carrots to create a salad that is a masterpiece of visual appeal and healthy eating.

MARINATED CHICKEN

1 cup tamari sauce
½ cup honey
¼ cup thinly sliced green onion
3 tablespoons fresh minced ginger
3 tablespoons minced garlic
2 tablespoons sesame oil
1 tablespoon sambal sauce
6 6-ounce skinless chicken breasts, cut in half to make 3-ounce portions

In a small bowl, combine all the ingredients except the chicken breasts. In a large shallow pan, lay the chicken breast down and pour over the marinade. Cover and allow the chicken to marinate for 4 to 24 hours in the refrigerator.

CHILI-LIME VINAIGRETTE

2 jalapeños, seeded and minced
1 cup grapeseed oil
¾ cup fresh lime juice
½ cup tamari sauce
6 tablespoons honey
1 tablespoon fish sauce
1 tablespoon fresh grated ginger

In a small bowl, whisk all the ingredients together until combined. Set aside in the refrigerator.

BAKED WONTON STRIPS

10-12 sheets square wonton wrappers, each sheet cut into very thin strips
extra-virgin olive oil spray

Preheat the oven to 350°F. Place the wonton strips on a large baking sheet. Spray with olive oil spray and bake for about 10 minutes until golden brown. Remove from the oven, let cool and set aside.

GRILLED CHICKEN AND SALAD ASSEMBLY

12 (3 ounces each) Marinated Chicken breasts
4 cups thinly sliced napa cabbage
2 cups thinly sliced red cabbage
2 cups shredded carrots
1 cup thinly sliced green onions
1 cup fresh cilantro leaves
2 cups cashews, lightly toasted
1 cup Baked Wonton Strips
1 cup Chili-Lime Vinaigrette

Preheat the grill to high heat. Remove the chicken from the refrigerator and drain off the marinade and discard. When the grill is ready, place the chicken breasts in a line and cook for 2 minutes. Then turn the chicken 45 degrees for another 2 minutes. That creates crosshatch grill marks on the top side. Flip the chicken over for another 2 minutes and turn 45 degrees for another 2 minutes. Test the chicken with a meat thermometer to make sure it has reached 168°F and remove from the grill. Let rest 2 minutes before slicing into even strips.

In a large bowl, toss the cabbage, carrots, green onions, cilantro leaves, and cashews with the Chili-Lime Vinaigrette. Place a large helping of the cabbage on each plate, top with wontons and sliced chicken. Drizzle a little more dressing on top. Extra Chili-Lime Vinaigrette will keep in an airtight container in the refrigerator for about a week.

NUTRITION PER SERVING	Cal 319	Fat 18g	Protein 23g	Carbs 19g	Sugar 8g	Fiber 3g	Sod 338mg

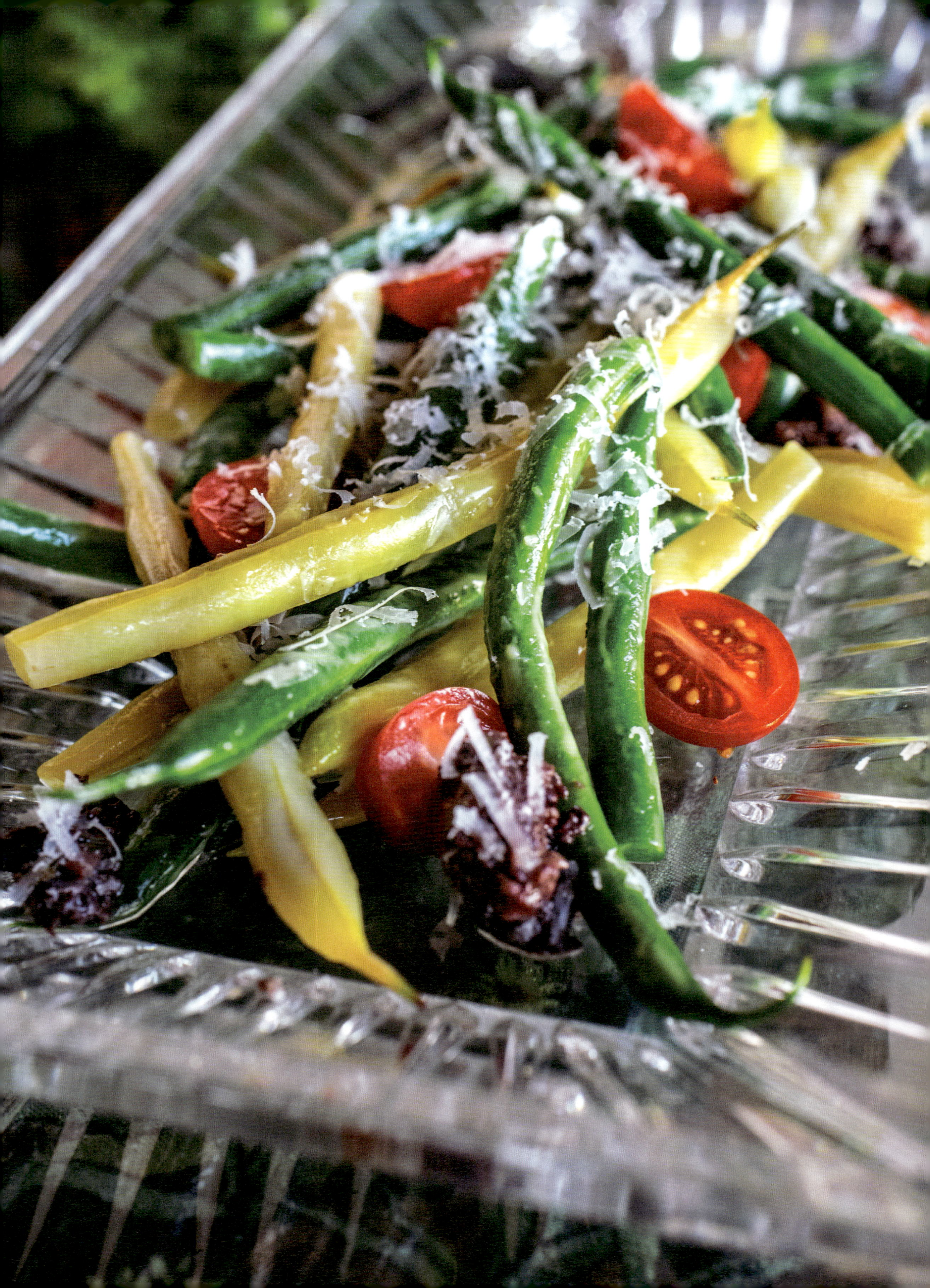

GREEN AND YELLOW BEAN SALAD
WITH HEIRLOOM TOMATOES, OLIVE TAPENADE, AND GRAPEFRUIT VINAIGRETTE

SERVES 6

Our fresh bean salad is the Cal-a-Vie take on a typical Mediterranean diet, which is generally rich in monounsaturated fats and high in fiber. Filled with fruits, vegetables, fish, and olive oil, this diet makes for a heart-healthy style of eating. The Mediterranean lifestyle also encourages dining with family, and friends, making meals a social experience!

BEANS

3 cups haricot verts, trimmed

3 cups yellow wax beans, trimmed

Prepare a large bowl of ice water (half ice and half water). In a large pot, over high heat, bring 4 quarts of water to a rolling boil. Add the haricot verts and let them cook for about 3 minutes. Remove the haricot verts from the boiling water and plunge into the ice bath. Allow the beans to completely cool before removing them from the ice bath. Remove the beans and dry on a towel. Repeat this process for the yellow wax beans. Set the beans aside in the refrigerator.

OLIVE TAPENADE

2 cups Kalamata olives, pitted

2 garlic cloves

2 teaspoons anchovy paste

1 teaspoon chopped fresh rosemary

1 tablespoon capers

½ cup olive oil

In a food processor, add all the ingredients and puree until completely smooth. Set aside.

GRAPEFRUIT VINAIGRETTE

1 cup grapefruit juice

2 tablespoons white balsamic vinegar

¼ cup honey

2 tablespoons Dijon mustard

½ cup water

1 teaspoon sea salt

1½ cups grapeseed oil

In a blender, combine all of the ingredients except for the grapeseed oil. While the blender is turned on high, slowly add the grapeseed oil until it is completely emulsified. Set aside.

SALAD ASSEMBLY

3 cups blanched haricot verts

3 cups blanched yellow wax beans

⅓ cup Grapefruit Vinaigrette

⅓ cup Olive Tapenade

2 cups cherry tomatoes, halved

¼ cup grated Parmesan cheese

In a large bowl, toss the beans with the Grapefruit Vinaigrette. On 6 separate plates, smear 1 to 2 tablespoons of the Olive Tapenade. Add about a cup of the dressed beans onto the center of each plate. Place 6 to 8 cherry tomato halves on top of the beans. Sprinkle each salad with about a tablespoon of Parmesan cheese and drizzle with additional dressing. The extra vinaigrette and Olive Tapenade will store in an air tight container in the refrigerator for a week.

NUTRITION PER SERVING	Cal 163	Fat 12g	Protein 4g	Carbs 12g	Sugar 5g	Fiber 4g	Sod 193mg

KALE SALAD
WITH PERSIAN CUCUMBERS, SALTED PEPITAS, AND WHOLE GRAIN MUSTARD VINAIGRETTE

SERVES 12

The deep green color of curly leaf kale is such a treat to the eyes when you are eating this salad. We always say that color equals vitamins and minerals and this is certainly no exception. Persian cucumbers are small, sweet, and essentially seedless. We love to eat them in salads right out of our garden.

SALTED PEPITAS

2 tablespoons water

2 teaspoons sea salt

1 cup pepitas (pumpkin seeds)

Preheat the oven to 350°F. In a small sauté pan, add the water and salt. Bring to a boil and toss in the pepitas. Transfer to a baking sheet lined with a piece of parchment paper. Bake for 7 minutes or until toasted. Remove and let cool. Set aside.

WHOLE GRAIN MUSTARD VINAIGRETTE

½ cup fresh lemon juice

2½ tablespoons whole grain mustard

½ tablespoon Dijon mustard

2½ tablespoons honey

½ teaspoon sea salt

1 cup extra-virgin olive oil

In a bowl, whisk all the ingredients together to fully incorporate them. Set aside.

SALAD ASSEMBLY

12 cups curly leaf kale, stems discarded, cut into bite-sized pieces

2 cups Persian cucumbers, sliced

3 apples, thinly sliced (we recommend Pink Lady or Honeycrisp)

¾ cup Whole Grain Mustard Vinaigrette

¾ cup Salted Pepitas

¾ cup manchego cheese, shredded on a microplane

In a large bowl, toss the kale, cucumbers, and apples with the Whole Grain Mustard Vinaigrette. Garnish the top with the Salted Pepitas and shredded manchego cheese.

NUTRITION PER SERVING	Cal	Fat	Protein	Carbs	Sugar	Fiber	Sod
	175	13g	5g	11g	7g	2g	71mg

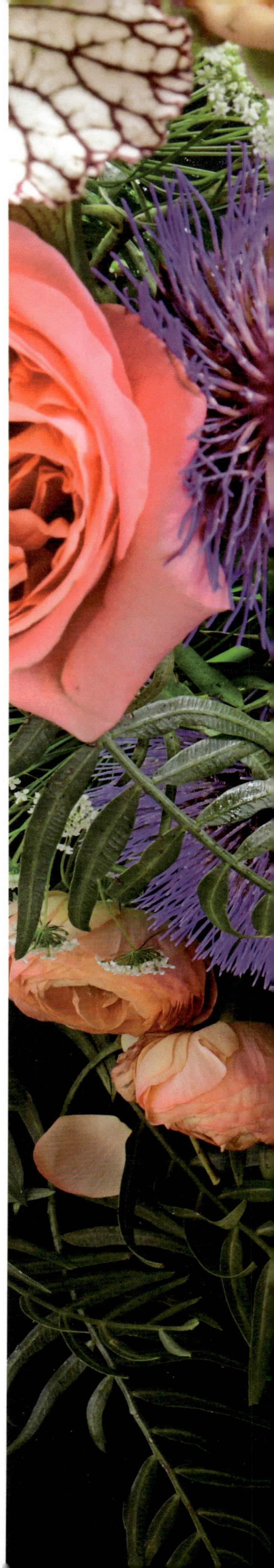

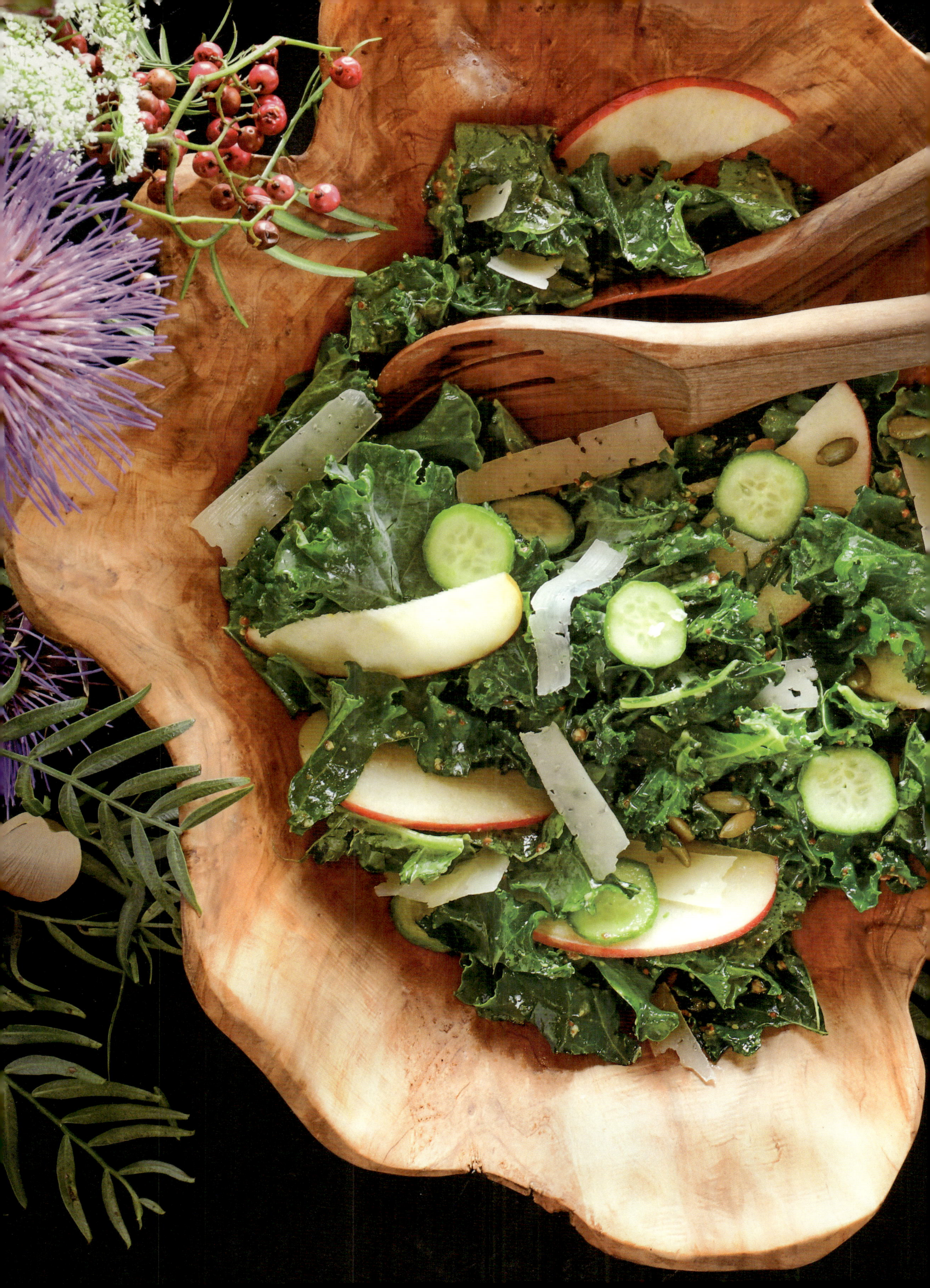

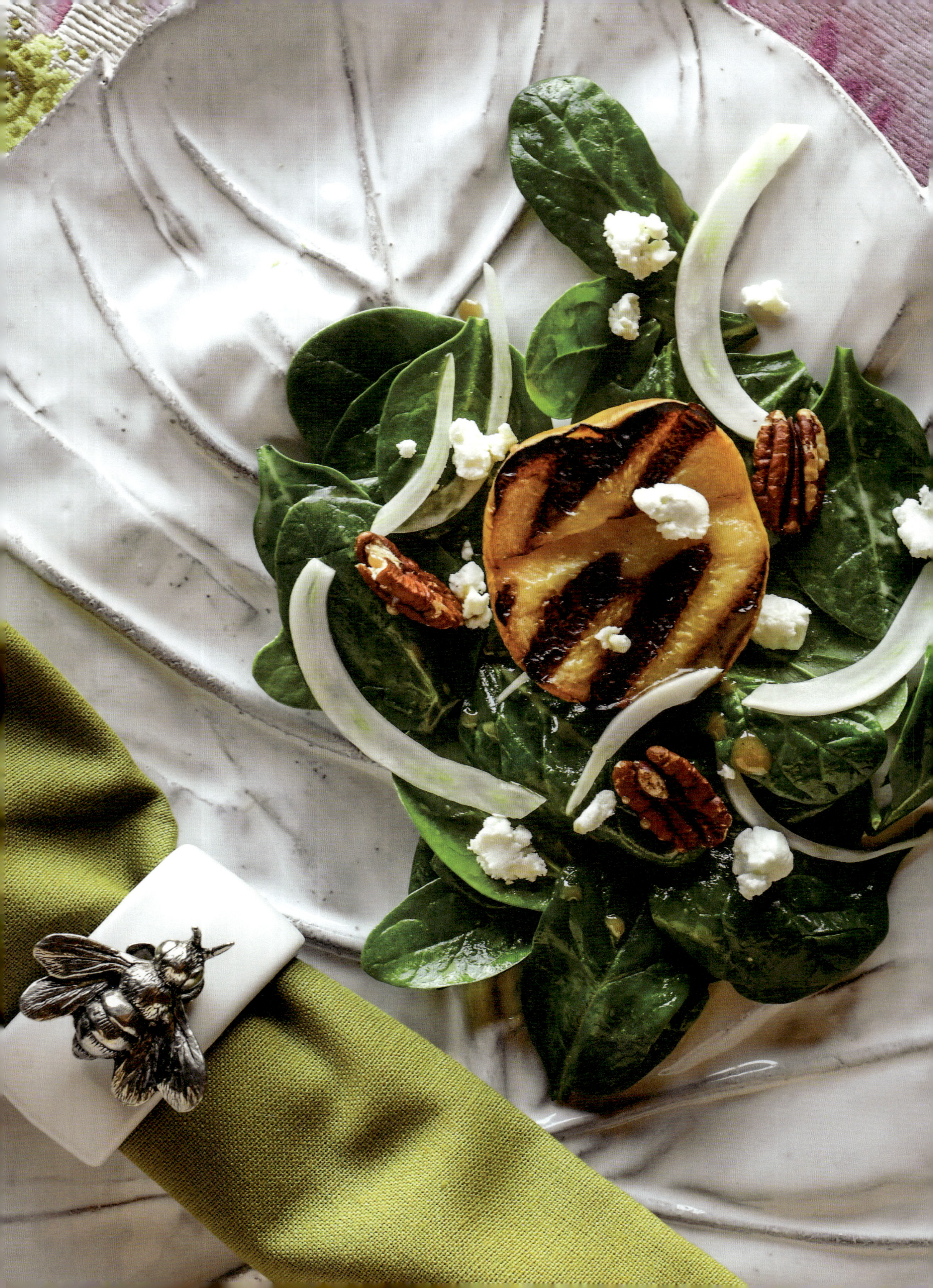

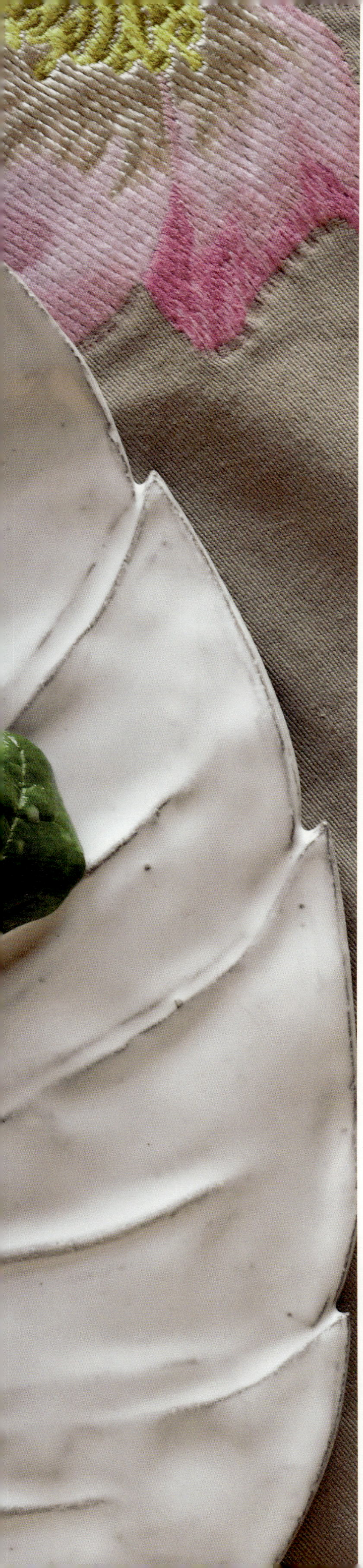

PEACH SALAD
WITH SPINACH, TOASTED PECANS, AND WHITE BALSAMIC VINAIGRETTE

SERVES 6

Peaches in the summertime are perfectly sweet from the moment they're picked. Shop at your local farmers market for "tree-ripened" peaches. The difference in flavor is day and night compared to store-bought peaches that are harvested prematurely and shipped far distances. Also, since they are on the "Dirty Dozen" list of produce (see page 276) with the highest concentration of pesticides, try to make sure your peaches are organic.

GRILLED PEACHES

3 peaches, quartered, pit removed

2 tablespoons extra-virgin olive oil

2 teaspoons sea salt

Preheat the grill to medium-high heat. Toss the quartered peaches with olive oil and salt. Place peaches on the grill. Leave for 2 to 3 minutes to achieve grill marks. Remove and set aside to cool.

MAPLE GASTRIQUE

1 cup maple syrup

½ cup sherry vinegar

1 vanilla bean, split and seeds scraped

In a small saucepan, combine all of the ingredients and place over medium heat. Bring to a simmer and reduce the maple mixture until it coats the back of a spoon. Remove from the heat and cool completely.

SALAD ASSEMBLY

6 cups baby spinach

1 fennel bulb, thinly sliced

¼ cup pecans, toasted

⅓ cup crumbled goat cheese

¼ cup White Balsamic Vinaigrette (see the recipe page 124)

2 tablespoons Maple Gastrique

3 Grilled Peaches

In a large bowl, toss the spinach and fennel with the vinaigrette. Divide among 6 plates and top with pecans, goat cheese, and Grilled Peaches. Drizzle the extra Maple Gastrique and some of the White Balsamic Vinaigrette over the toppings and peaches.

NUTRITION PER SERVING	Cal 146	Fat 8g	Protein 4g	Carbs 16g	Sugar 12g	Fiber 3g	Sod 402mg

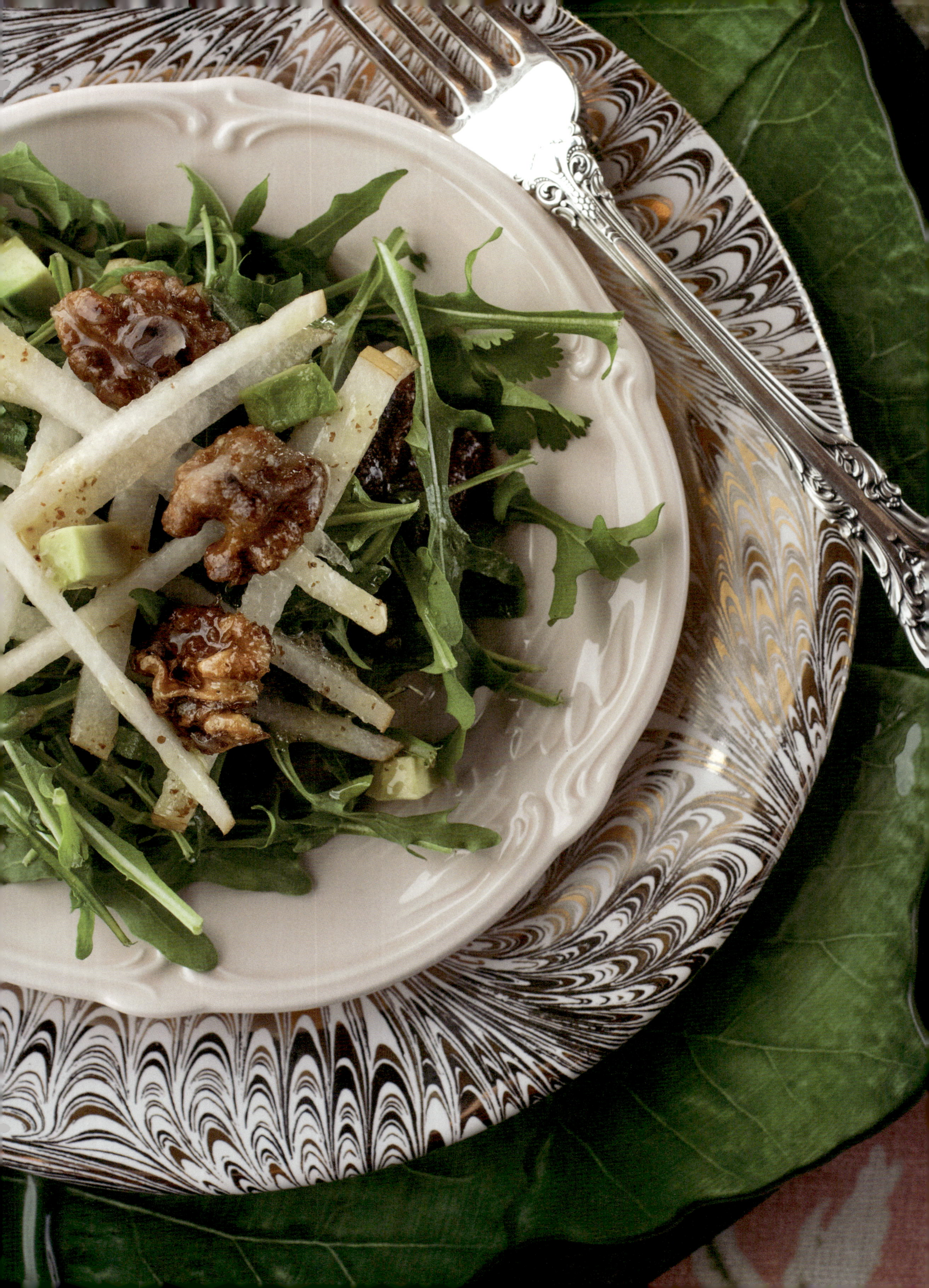

PETITE ARUGULA SALAD
WITH PEARS AND CANDIED WALNUTS

SERVES 4

This salad has a winning combination of flavor and textures: the sweetness of pear, the crunchiness of walnuts, the creaminess of avocado, the bitterness of arugula, and the tartness of citrus. The health benefits of arugula are impressive; they include weight loss, healthy bones, and improved eyesight.

CANDIED WALNUTS

⅓ cup organic, unrefined cane sugar

1 teaspoon water

1 cup walnuts

Preheat the oven to 350°F. In a small saucepan over medium heat, add the sugar and the water. Stir occasionally until the sugar is melted and remove from the heat. Toss the melted sugar with the walnuts and transfer to a baking sheet covered with a piece of parchment paper. Roast in the oven for about 7 to 8 minutes. Remove from the oven and cool.

ORANGE VINAIGRETTE

1 cup orange juice

2 tablespoons white balsamic vinegar

¼ cup honey

2 tablespoons Dijon mustard

½ cup water

1 teaspoon sea salt

1½ cups grapeseed oil

In a blender, combine all the ingredients except for the grapeseed oil. With the blender on high, slowly add the oil in a steady stream to emulsify. Set aside in the refrigerator.

SALAD ASSEMBLY

4 cups petite arugula

1 Asian pear, peeled, cored, and julienned

Candied Walnuts as a garnish, sprinkle what you like on top

1 avocado, pitted, peeled, and diced

¼ cup Orange Vinaigrette

In a large bowl, combine the arugula, pear, avocado, and Candied Walnuts. Gently toss together with the vinaigrette and divide between 4 plates.

Store the extra dressing in an airtight container in the refrigerator no longer than a week.

NUTRITION PER SERVING	Cal 186	Fat 15g	Protein 2g	Carbs 15g	Sugar 7g	Fiber 5g	Sod 42mg

ROASTED BEET SALAD
WITH TOASTED HAZELNUTS AND CITRUS VINAIGRETTE

SERVES 4

Beets aren't everyone's favorite vegetable, but they are worth trying if you prepare them correctly. The comment we get the most is that they taste "earthy." Taking the skin off after roasting can definitely help. Beets are rich in arginine, which helps to promote good cardiovascular circulation. They can also give you an instant boost of energy after you eat them.

ROASTED BEETS

3 baby golden beets
3 baby red beets
3 candy-stripe beets
9 garlic cloves
9 sprigs of fresh thyme
2 tablespoons extra-virgin olive oil

Preheat the oven to 350°F. It's important to try to get beets that are similar in size so they roast evenly, but if that's not possible, make sure to trim the large beets to be closer in size to the small ones. Cut the tops off the beets. Keeping all the colors separate, toss the beets in olive oil, then wrap them loosely in aluminum foil with a clove of garlic and a few sprigs of thyme in each foil packet. Place on a baking sheet and roast for about 45 minutes, depending on the size of the beets. The best way to tell if they are done is to pierce the beet with a small knife. If the tip of the knife easily makes it to the center of the beet with no resistance, it's done.

When the beets have cooled enough to handle, use your fingers to peel off the outside skin. Cut into wedges and keep warm or at this point they can be chilled in the refrigerator. Keep the colors separate until ready to serve.

CITRUS VINAIGRETTE

1 tablespoon white balsamic vinegar
2 tablespoons honey
1 tablespoon Dijon mustard
6 tablespoons orange juice
1 tablespoon fresh lemon juice
½ teaspoon sea salt
¼ cup water
¾ cup grapeseed oil

In a blender, combine the vinegar, honey, mustard, orange juice, lemon juice, salt, and water. While blending, slowly add the oil until completely emulsified. Set aside in refrigerator.

TOASTED HAZELNUTS

½ cup raw hazelnuts, coarsely chopped

Preheat the oven to 350°F. Place the hazelnuts on a baking sheet and toast for 5 to 7 minutes or until golden brown.

SALAD ASSEMBLY

4 cups mixed greens
wedges from 9 Roasted Beets
¼ cup Citrus Vinaigrette
2 tablespoons Toasted Hazelnuts
¼ cup crumbled goat cheese

In a large bowl, toss the greens with the Citrus Vinaigrette. Divide the greens between 4 plates and garnish with the beets, hazelnuts, and goat cheese. Drizzle some of the extra Citrus Vinaigrette over the beets.

TIP: The extra Citrus Vinaigrette can be stored in the refrigerator for about two weeks.

NUTRITION PER SERVING	Cal 133	Fat 11g	Protein 4g	Carbs 7g	Sugar 4g	Fiber 3g	Sod 115mg

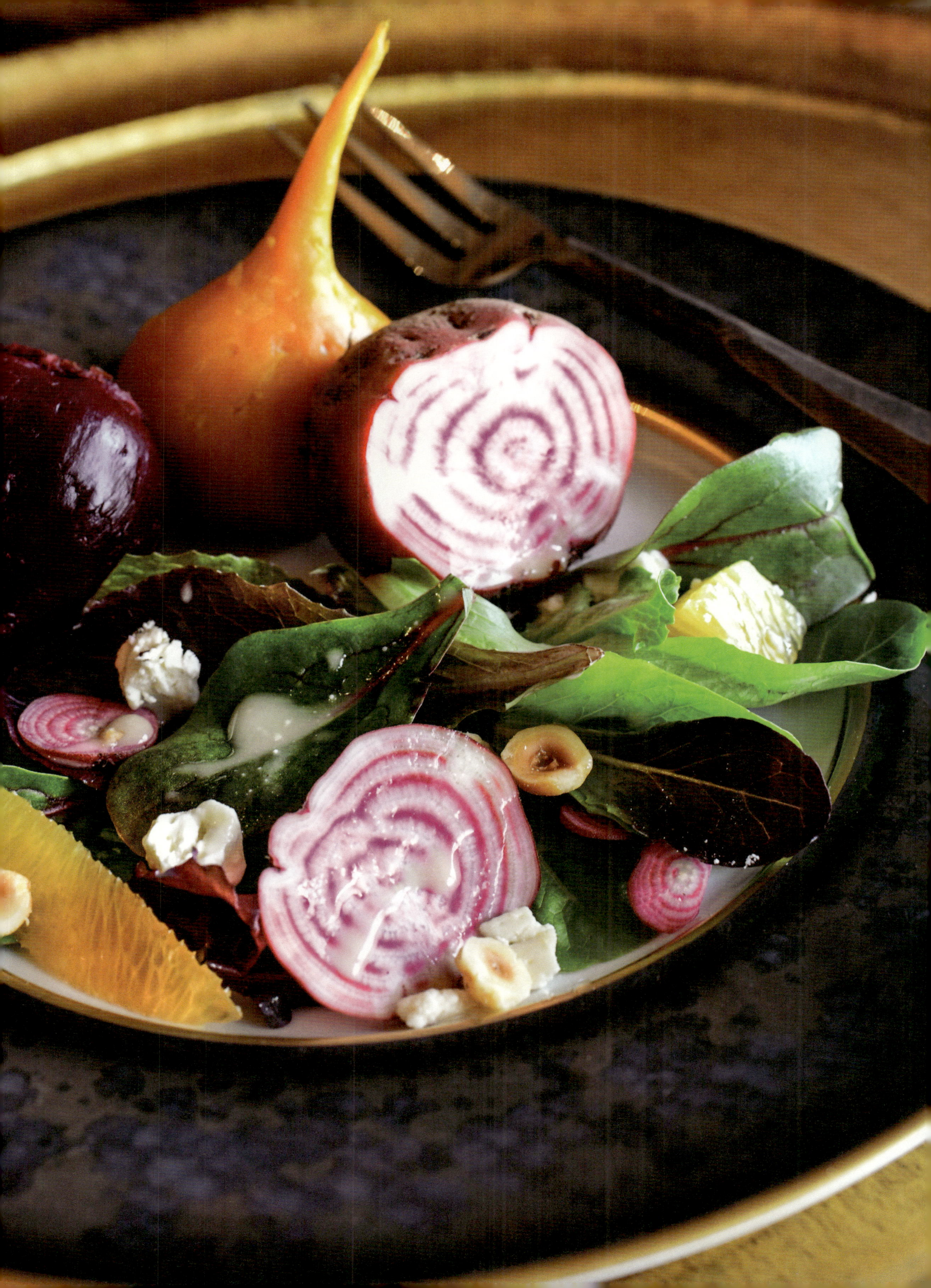

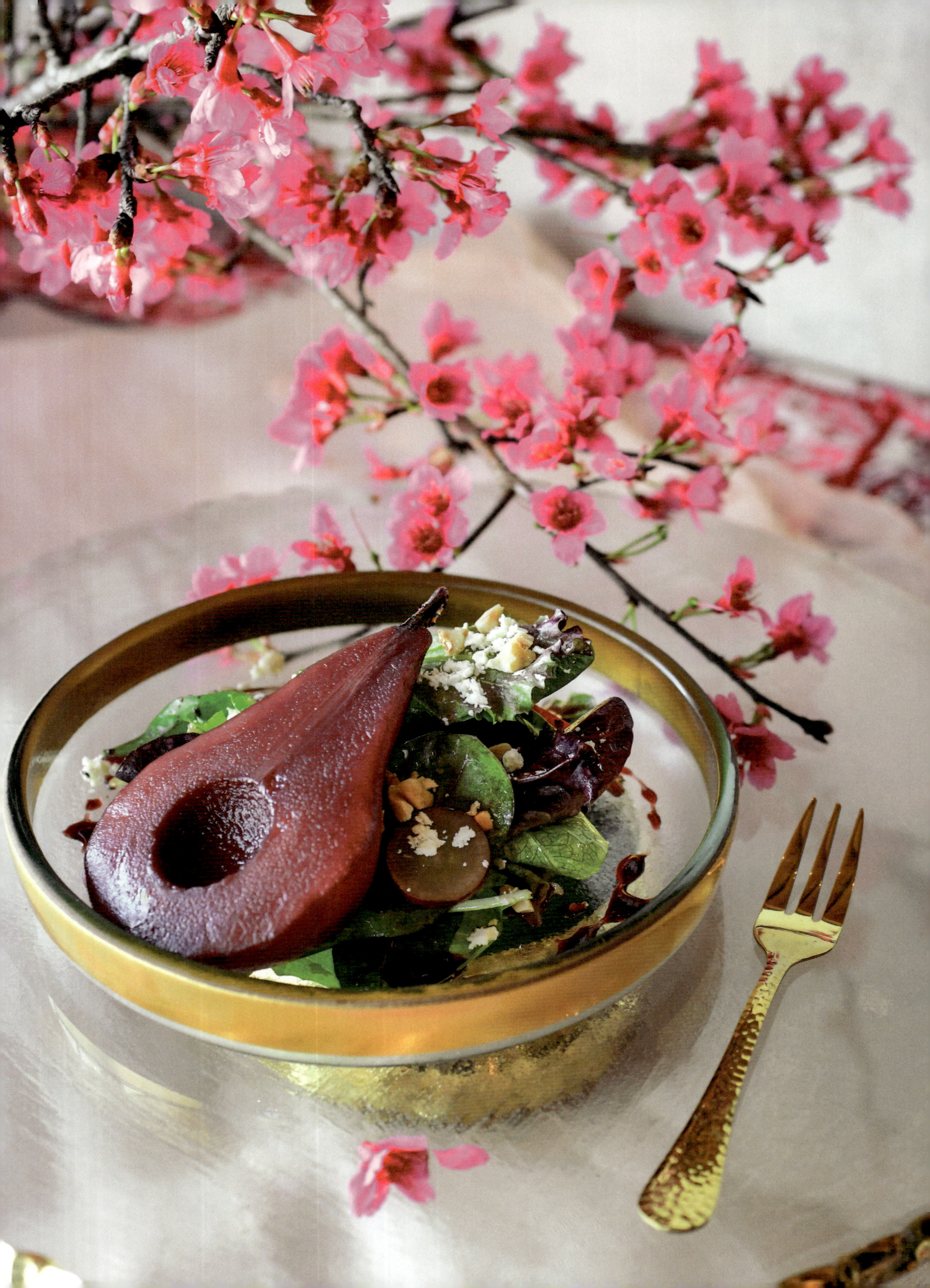

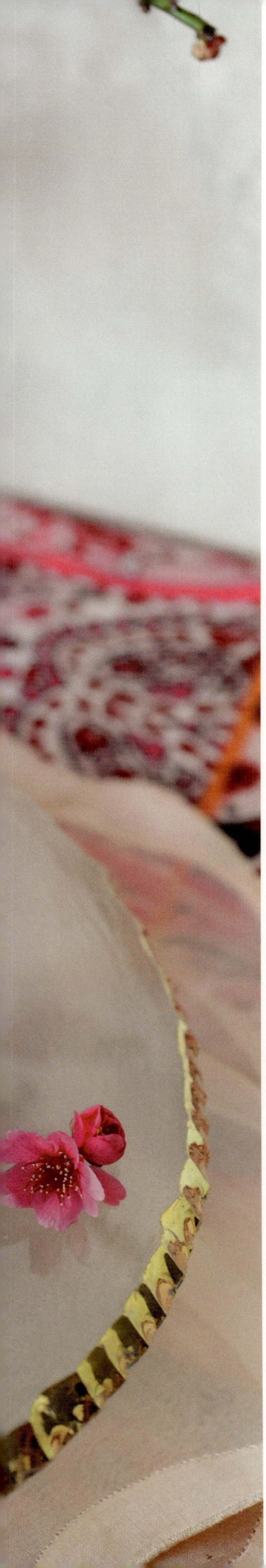

SPICED POACHED PEAR
WITH MIXED GREENS, GRAPES, AND HAZELNUTS

SERVES 8

This poaching technique for pears helps to bring this salad from ordinary to extraordinary. We recommend splurging on a bottle of Banyuls vinegar. It comes from a region in the south of France near the border with Spain; its sweet and nutty flavor pairs well with the pear, grapes, and hazelnuts in our salad.

POACHED BOSC PEARS

3 cups red wine
1 cup water
6 star anise pods
6 black peppercorns
2 cinnamon sticks
8 whole cloves
2 Bosc pears, peeled, halved, and cored

In a large saucepan, bring the wine, water, star anise pods, peppercorns, cinnamon sticks, and cloves to boil. Reduce the heat to a simmer and add the pears. Simmer about 5 minutes or until the pears are soft but not mushy. Gently remove the pears from the poaching liquid with a slotted spoon and let cool.

BANYULS VINAIGRETTE

½ cup Banyuls vinegar
¼ cup water
1 tablespoon honey
1 teaspoon Dijon mustard
1½ cups grapeseed oil
1 teaspoon kosher or sea salt

Combine the vinegar, water, honey, and Dijon mustard in a blender. Slowly add the grapeseed oil until combined. Add the salt. Refrigerate until ready to use.

ASSEMBLY

10 ounces mixed greens
1 cup red seedless grapes, sliced
¼ cup hazelnuts, toasted and chopped
¼ cup crumbled feta cheese
¼ cup Banyuls Vinaigrette
2 Poached Bosc Pears, halved or thinly sliced (¼ pear per person)

In a large bowl, combine all the ingredients except the pears. Toss gently. Place the salad on the plates and top each with a pear per plate. Drizzle with additional Banyuls Vinaigrette.

NUTRITION PER SERVING	Cal	Fat	Protein	Carbs	Sugar	Fiber	Sod
	129	8g	2g	13g	9g	3g	70mg

TEXAS CAVIAR

SERVES 10

Texas Caviar is traditionally served on New Year's Day and is supposed to bring good luck. Folklore says it was first served on New Year's Eve at the Houston Country Club in the 1940s. It's traditionally served with chips, but we've turned it into a healthy salad.

3 cups black-eyed peas, cooked (if using canned, rinsed and drained)
½ cup diced red onion
1 jalapeño, seeded and minced
2 garlic cloves, minced
¼ cup sliced green onions
½ cup diced yellow bell pepper
1 cup diced tomato
2 avocados, peeled, pitted, and chopped
1 tablespoon chopped fresh cilantro
1 tablespoon chopped fresh basil
¼ cup red wine vinegar
½ cup extra-virgin olive oil
2 teaspoons sea salt
1 teaspoon freshly ground black pepper (optional)

In a medium bowl, combine all the ingredients and mix well. Store in an airtight container in the refrigerator until ready to serve.

TIP: When selecting ripe, perfect avocados, go by feel rather than color. A ready-to-eat avocado should feel slightly soft, but not overly soft or mushy.

NUTRITION PER SERVING	Cal	Fat	Protein	Carbs	Sugar	Fiber	Sod
	211	18g	4g	11g	3g	4g	388mg

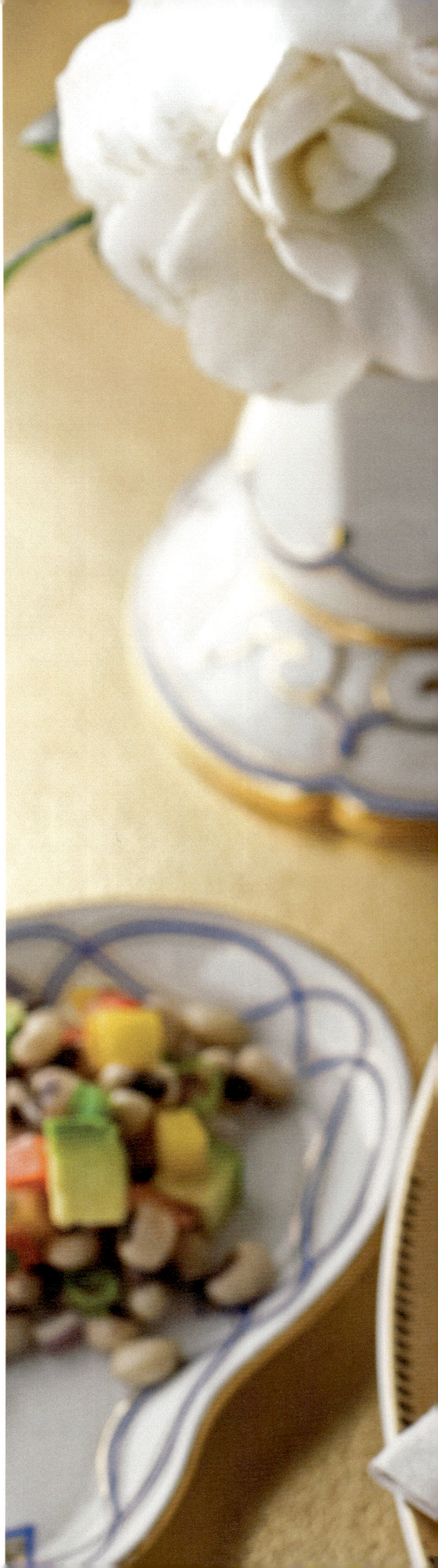

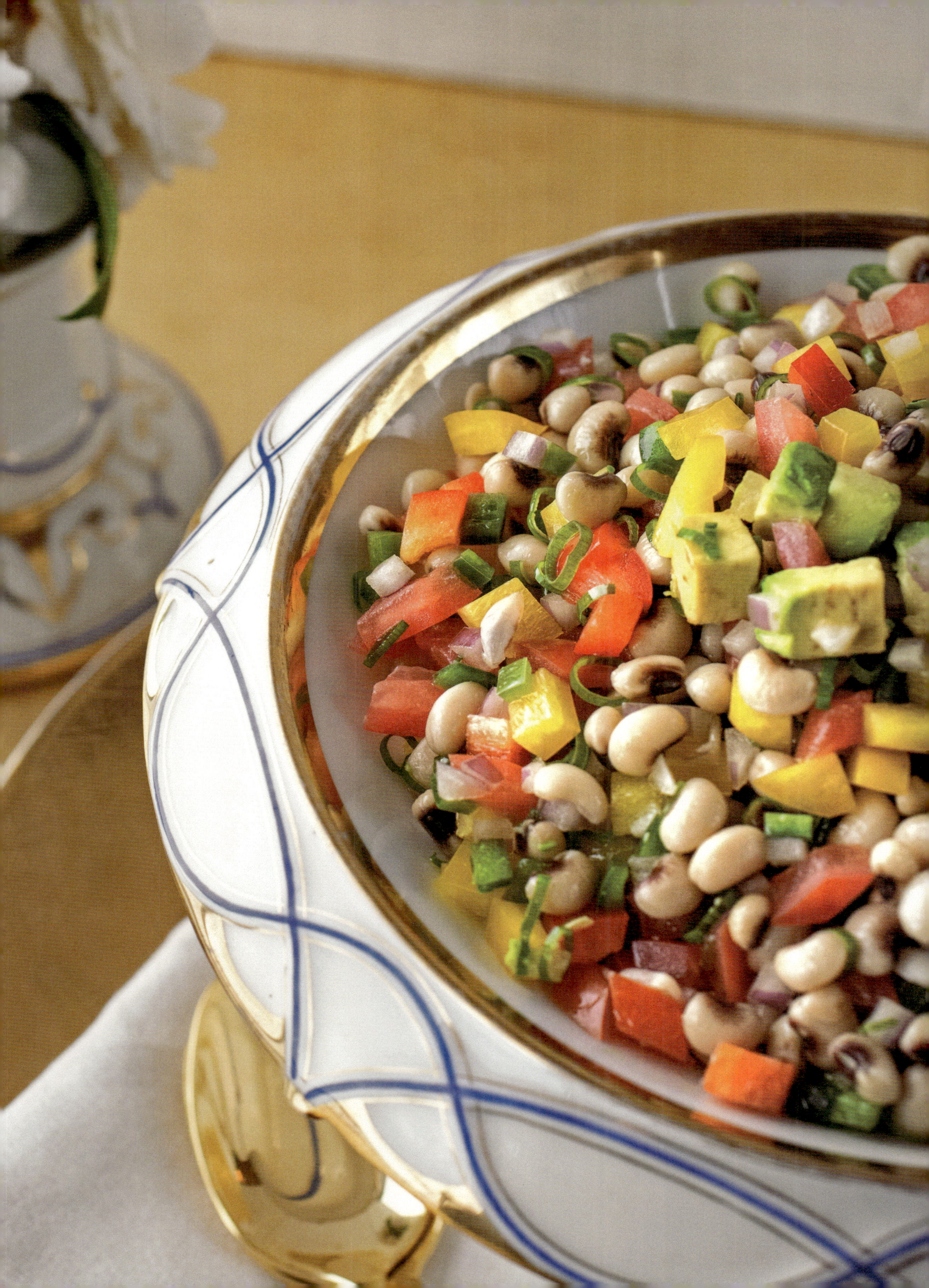

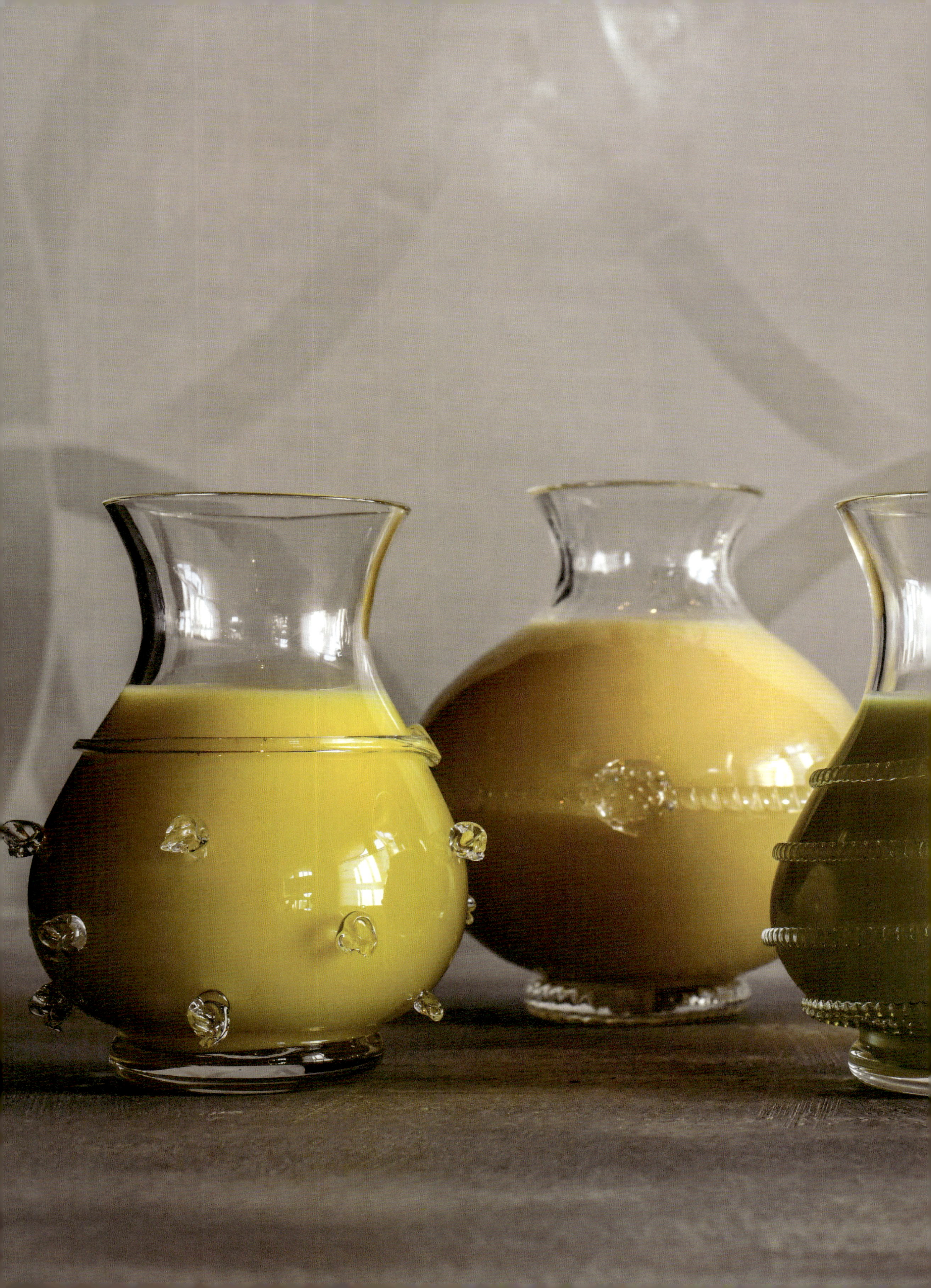

CAL-A-VIE HEALTH SPA VINAIGRETTES

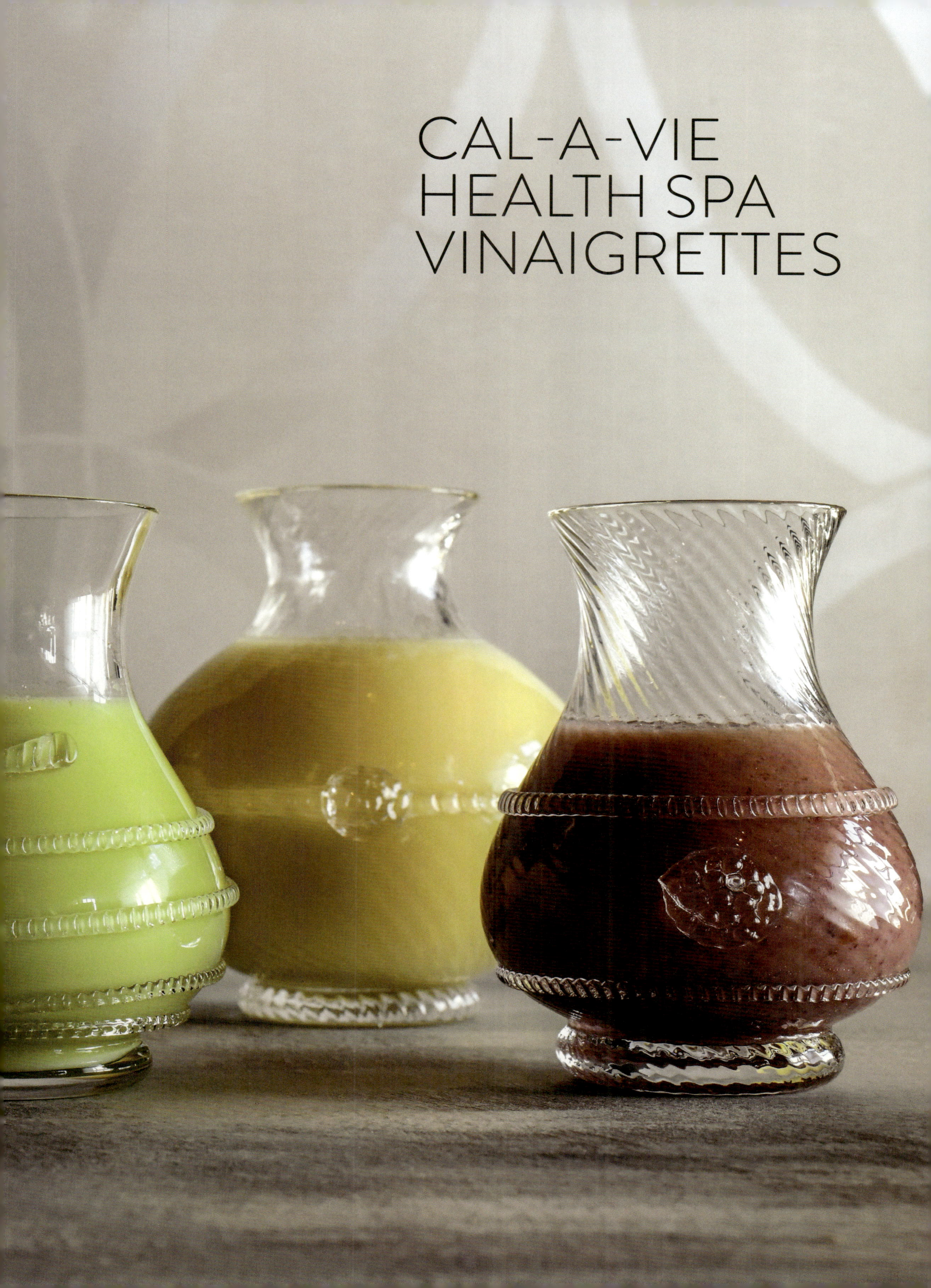

CAL-A-VIE HEALTH SPA VINAIGRETTES

We make our vinaigrettes with grapeseed oil because it's neutral in flavor and does not oxidize easily. Feel free to experiment with other oils for different flavor profiles. Extra-virgin olive oil can be substituted for any of the oils below.

For all of the vinaigrettes below use a blender. Combine the ingredients except the oil and blend on high. Slowly add the oil until completely emulsified. Store in the refrigerator until ready to use, but after two weeks they should be discarded. Consider whisking by hand instead of using the blender as extra-virgin olive oil is much more delicate.

WHITE BALSAMIC VINAIGRETTE (3¼ CUPS = 52 TABLESPOONS)

1 cup white balsamic vinegar
¼ cup honey
2 tablespoons Dijon mustard
1 teaspoon sea salt
½ cup water
1½ cups grapeseed oil

NUTRITION PER SERVING	Cal 65	Fat 6g	Protein 0g	Carbs 2g	Sugar 2g	Fiber 0g	Sod 36mg

GRAPEFRUIT VINAIGRETTE (3¼ CUPS = 52 TABLESPOONS)

1 cup grapefruit juice
2 tablespoons white balsamic vinegar
¼ cup honey
2 tablespoons Dijon mustard
1 teaspoon sea salt
½ cup water
1½ cups grapeseed oil

NUTRITION PER SERVING	Cal 65	Fat 6g	Protein 0g	Carbs 2g	Sugar 2g	Fiber 0g	Sod 36mg

CHAMPAGNE VINAIGRETTE (3¼ CUPS = 52 TABLESPOONS)

1 cup champagne vinegar
¼ cup honey
1 tablespoon Dijon mustard
1 teaspoon sea salt
½ cup water
1½ cups grapeseed oil

NUTRITION PER SERVING	Cal 61	Fat 6g	Protein 0g	Carbs 1g	Sugar 1g	Fiber 0g	Sod 33mg

ORANGE VINAIGRETTE (3¼ CUPS = 52 TABLESPOONS)

¾ cup orange juice
2 tablespoons fresh lemon juice
2 tablespoons white balsamic vinegar
¼ cup honey
2 tablespoons Dijon mustard
½ cup water
1½ cups grapeseed oil

NUTRITION PER SERVING	Cal 63	Fat 6g	Protein 0g	Carbs 2g	Sugar 2g	Fiber 0g	Sod 0mg

JALAPEÑO VINAIGRETTE (2 CUPS = 32 TABLESPOONS)

2 jalapeños, seeded and minced
¾ cup fresh lime juice
6 tablespoons honey
1 tablespoon grated fresh ginger
1 cup grapeseed oil

NUTRITION PER SERVING	Cal 74	Fat 7g	Protein 0g	Carbs 4g	Sugar 3g	Fiber 0g	Sod 0mg

CHILI-LIME VINAIGRETTE (3 CUPS = 48 TABLESPOONS)

2 jalapeños, seeded and minced
1 cup grapeseed oil
¾ cup fresh lime juice
½ cup tamari sauce
6 tablespoons honey
1 tablespoon fish sauce
1 tablespoon grated fresh ginger

In a small bowl, whisk all the ingredients together until fully combined. Set aside in the refrigerator.

NUTRITION PER SERVING	Cal 57	Fat 5g	Protein 0g	Carbs 3g	Sugar 2g	Fiber 0g	Sod 197mg

KALAMATA OLIVE VINAIGRETTE (4 CUPS = 64 TABLESPOONS)

1 cup champagne vinegar
¼ cup honey
1 tablespoon Dijon mustard
1 teaspoon sea salt
1 cup water
1½ cups grapeseed oil
½ cup Kalamata olives, pitted

Add the Kalamata olives at the very end and pulse 10 times.

NUTRITION PER SERVING	Cal 51	Fat 5g	Protein 0g	Carbs 1g	Sugar 1g	Fiber 0g	Sod 35mg

PORK TENDERLOIN
WITH HONEY MUSTARD, PARSNIP MASH, AND SAVOY CABBAGE

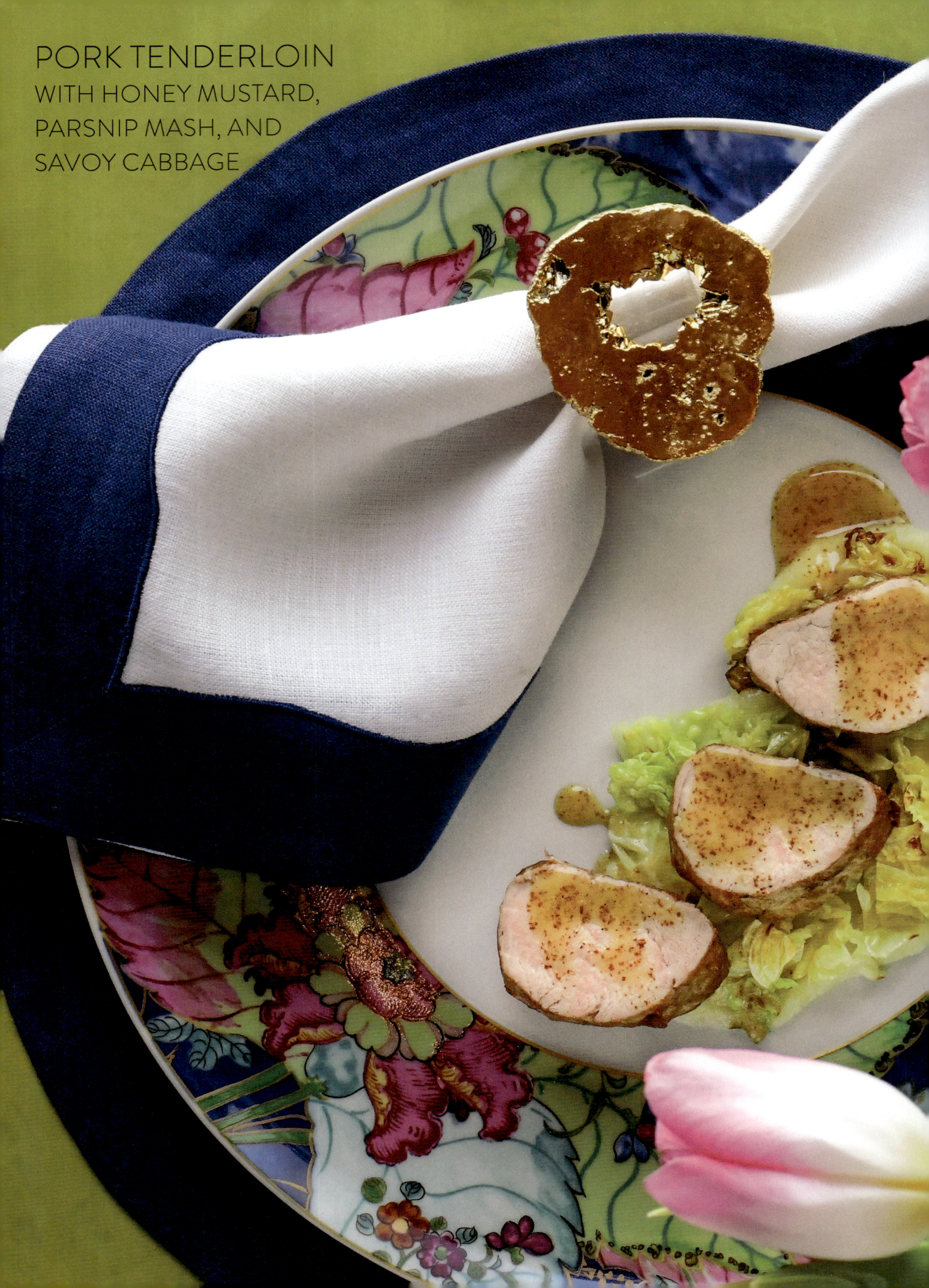

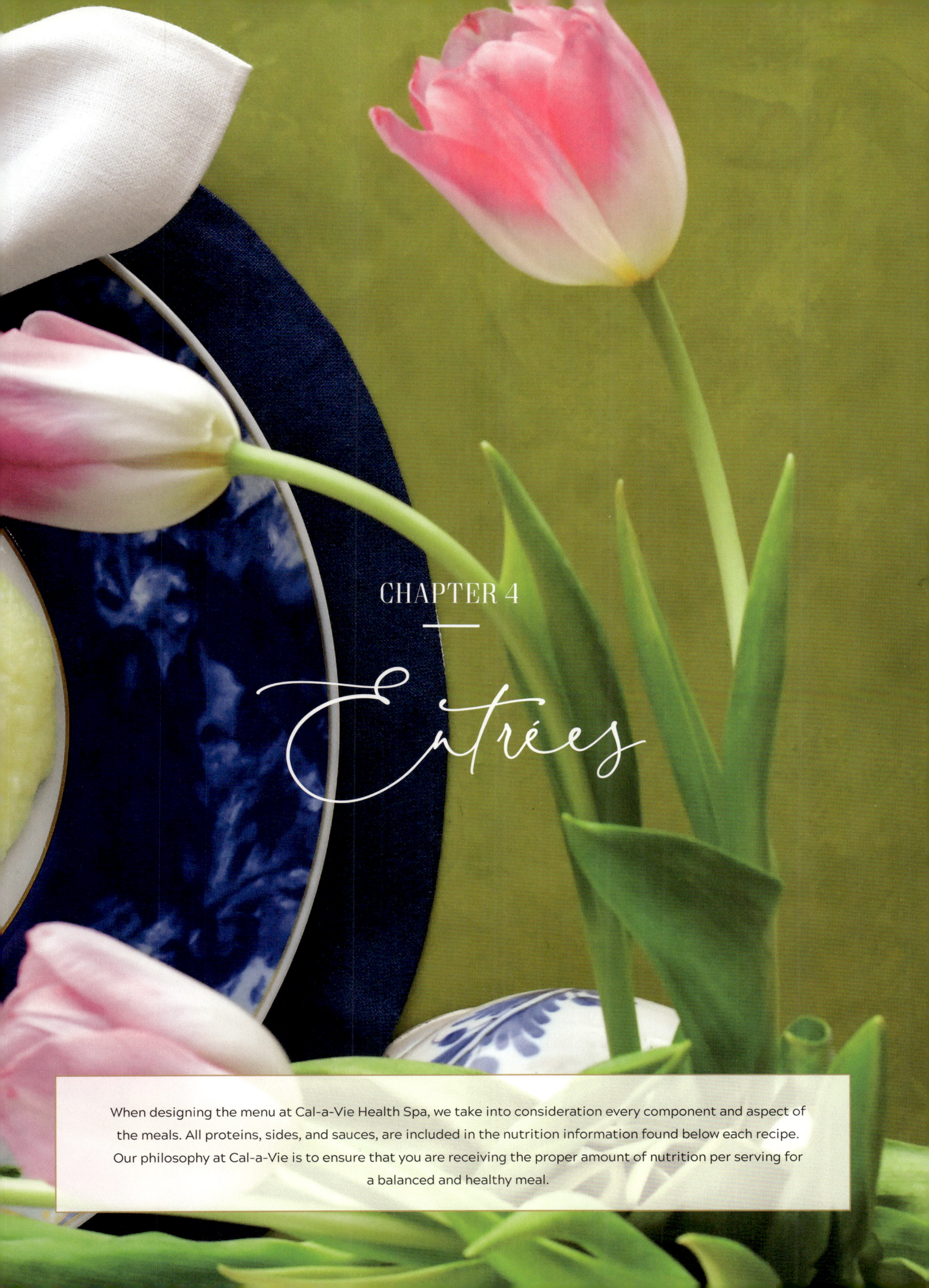

CHAPTER 4

Entrées

When designing the menu at Cal-a-Vie Health Spa, we take into consideration every component and aspect of the meals. All proteins, sides, and sauces, are included in the nutrition information found below each recipe. Our philosophy at Cal-a-Vie is to ensure that you are receiving the proper amount of nutrition per serving for a balanced and healthy meal.

PORK TENDERLOIN

WITH HONEY MUSTARD, PARSNIP MASH, AND SAVOY CABBAGE

SERVES 8

This pork tenderloin is beautifully seared and roasted, making it golden and crispy outside and tender and juicy inside. Containing only 55 calories per half cup, parsnips are a wonderful ingredient to create a nutritious, soul-warming treat.

HONEY MUSTARD

3 tablespoons honey

2 tablespoons whole grain mustard

3 tablespoons Dijon mustard

1 clove garlic

1 teaspoon fresh lemon juice

Combine all the ingredients in a blender and puree until completely smooth. Set aside.

PARSNIP MASH

1 pound parsnips (about 4 medium), peeled, ends trimmed, and cut into large, even-sized pieces

1 herb sachet (5 sprigs fresh thyme and 1 bay leaf wrapped in cheesecloth and tied with butcher's twine)

1¼ teaspoons kosher or sea salt, plus more to taste, divided use

8 cups water (reserving ½ cup after draining)

1½ tablespoons extra-virgin olive oil

In a medium saucepan over high heat, bring the water, parsnips, herb sachet and 1 teaspoon of salt to a boil. Make sure the water covers the parsnips by 2 inches. Boil for 5-7 minutes or until the parsnips are tender enough so you can easily insert a knife. Drain the parsnips, reserving some of the cooking liquid (about ½ cup). Discard the herb sachet. Return the cooked parsnips to the saucepan and heat over medium-low heat until the excess water has evaporated.

Add parsnips to the bowl of a food processor (you'll want to use this instead of a blender to avoid overprocessing). Add ¼ teaspoon salt and olive oil. With food processor running, add in starchy cooking water, 1 tablespoon at a time, until a fluffy, smooth consistency is achieved (about 5 tablespoons total). Taste and season with more salt as needed. Set aside and keep warm.

SAVOY CABBAGE

1 head savoy cabbage

1 tablespoon extra-virgin olive oil

kosher or sea salt

white pepper

Cut the cabbage into quarters. Remove the core from each quarter and slice the cabbage crosswise into ½-inch-thick strips. In a large sauté pan over medium heat, add the olive oil. Add the cabbage and sauté, turning with tongs, to wilt slightly. Season to taste with salt and pepper. Remove from the heat, cover and keep warm.

PORK TENDERLOIN

2 pounds pork tenderloin (keep whole)

kosher or sea salt

freshly ground black pepper

2 tablespoons grapeseed oil

Preheat the oven to 350°F. Season the pork tenderloin with salt and pepper. In a large sauté pan, over medium high heat, add the grapeseed oil. Add the tenderloin and sear on all sides for a deep, rich color. Transfer to a baking sheet and roast in the oven until it reaches an internal temperature of 145°F (medium doneness). Allow the tenderloin to sit for 5 to 7 minutes before slicing it.

ASSEMBLY

Serve each plate with a large spoonful of Parsnip Mash and place two or three slices of Pork Tenderloin on top. Place a serving of Savoy Cabbage on one side. Drizzle the Honey Mustard over the Pork Tenderloin.

NUTRITION PER SERVING	Cal 283	Fat 12g	Protein 25g	Carbs 19g	Sugar 10g	Fiber 4g	Sod 177mg

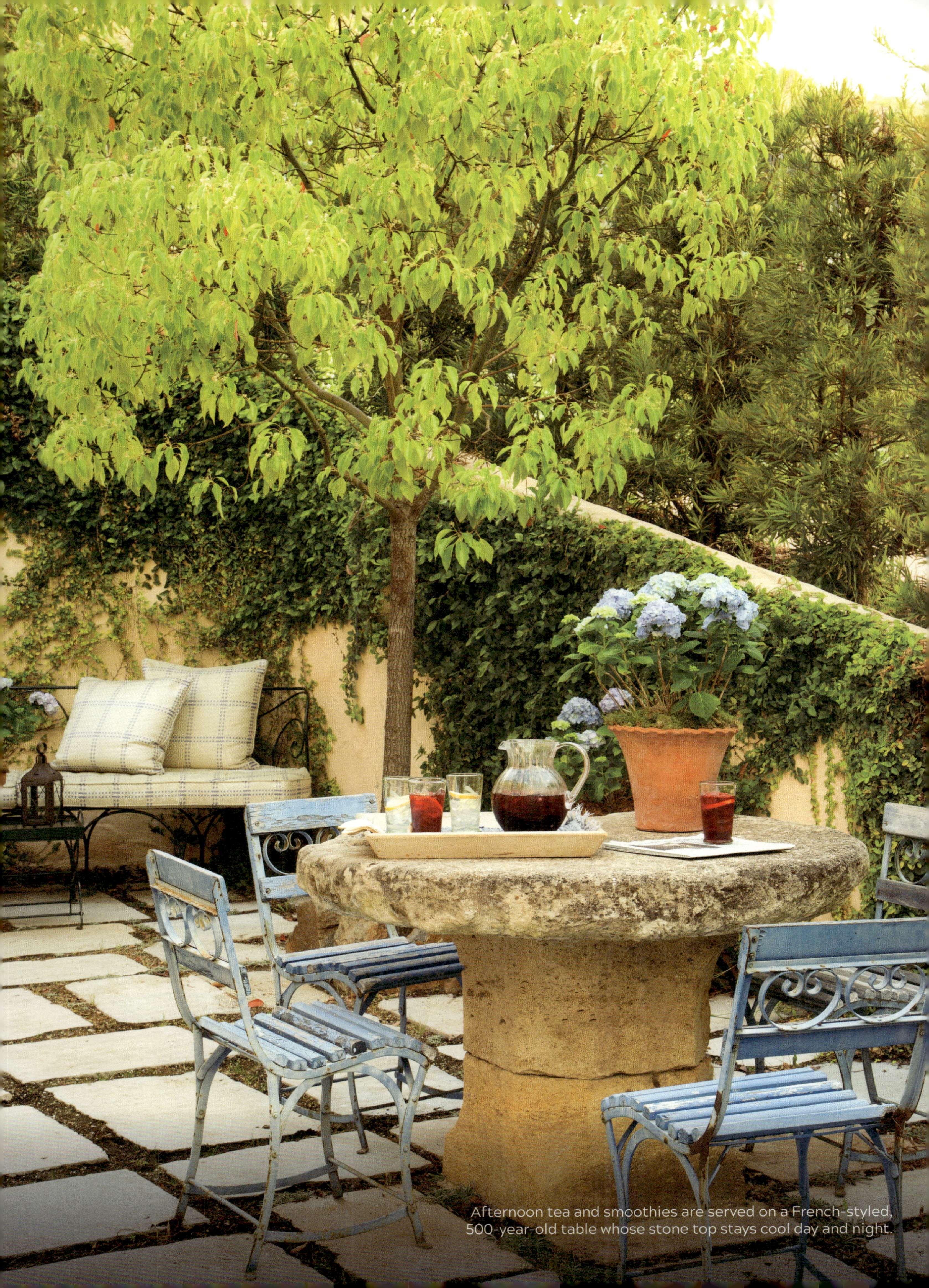

Afternoon tea and smoothies are served on a French-styled, 500-year-old table whose stone top stays cool day and night.

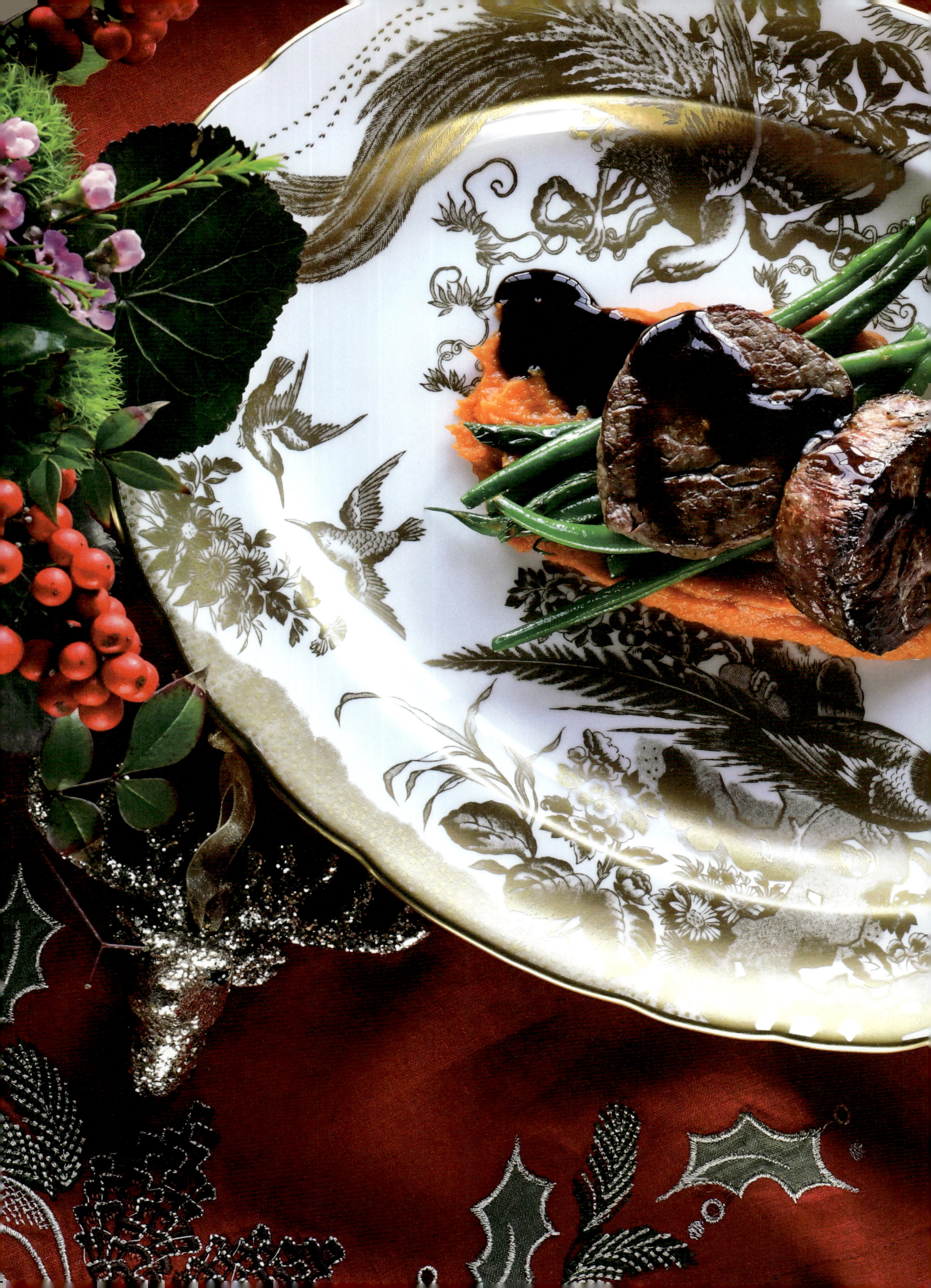

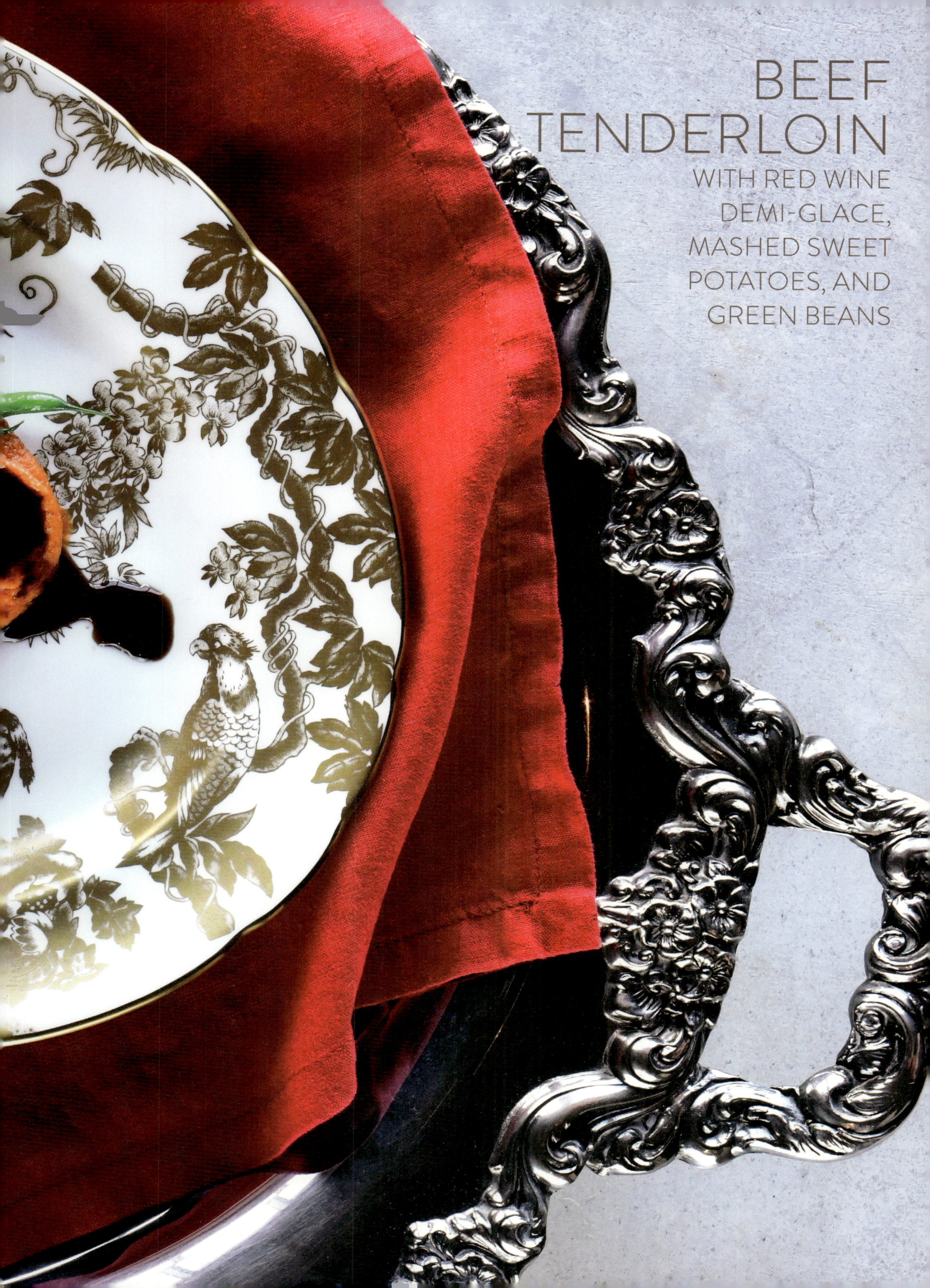

BEEF TENDERLOIN

WITH RED WINE DEMI-GLACE, MASHED SWEET POTATOES, AND GREEN BEANS

BEEF TENDERLOIN

WITH RED WINE DEMI-GLACE, MASHED SWEET POTATOES, AND GREEN BEANS

SERVES 8

Beef is a great source of heme-iron, which is 10 times more absorbable than iron found in plant foods such as spinach. For guests who have low iron or ferritin in their bloodwork, we recommend eating high-quality grass-fed and grass-finished red meat a few times a week, depending on how depleted their levels are. Don't forget to chew your steaks, no matter how tender they are. Chewing helps send signals to the brain to tell your stomach, pancreas, and liver to secrete all the juices necessary to digest meat.

MARINATED BEEF TENDERLOIN

- 1 tablespoon grapeseed oil
- 2 tablespoons chopped fresh parsley
- 2 tablespoons chopped fresh chives
- kosher or sea salt and freshly ground black pepper
- 8 beef tenderloin fillets (4 ounces each), cut 3-inches thick

In a small bowl, combine the oil, parsley, and chives. Salt and pepper the steaks. Rub the marinade over the beef and marinate for 2 hours in the refrigerator.

MASHED SWEET POTATOES

- 1 pound sweet potatoes
- 1 teaspoon smoked paprika
- 1 tablespoon maple syrup
- ½ teaspoon kosher or sea salt
- ¼ cup + 1 tablespoon orange juice

Preheat the oven to 350°F. Thoroughly wash each whole sweet potato to remove any dirt. Place it on a baking sheet and roast for one hour, or until it is soft and tender all the way to the center (pierce with a knife to check).

Peel the sweet potato while still warm, and break it up with a potato masher. Add the paprika, maple syrup, salt, and orange juice and continue mashing until smooth. Set aside and keep warm.

GREEN BEANS

1 tablespoon extra-virgin olive oil
1 pound green beans, trimmed
1 tablespoon water or more
1 teaspoon sea salt

In a large sauté pan over medium heat, add the olive oil and green beans and sauté for about 3 minutes. Add a tablespoon of water and allow the beans to steam. Keep adding additional tablespoons of water until the beans are cooked through. Set aside and keep warm.

RED WINE DEMI-GLACE

2 tablespoons grapeseed oil
1 onion, sliced
2 ribs celery, peeled and sliced
2 carrots, trimmed, peeled and sliced
2 tablespoons tomato paste
2 cups dry red wine
4 cups beef or veal stock
sea salt

In a large saucepan over medium heat, add the oil, onions, celery, and carrots. Sauté for about 10 minutes, stirring often, until the vegetables are caramelized and dark in color. Add the tomato paste and cook until it turns a brick red. Add the red wine, bring to a boil and then reduce the heat to a simmer. When reduced in volume by half, add the beef stock and continue to cook at a simmer until a syrup-like consistency is achieved. Strain the vegetables from the sauce and season with salt to taste. Set aside and keep warm.

TENDERLOIN PREPARATION

Marinated Beef Tenderloins
2 teaspoons grapeseed oil

Preheat the oven to 350°F. Remove the tenderloins from the refrigerator, take out of the marinade and pat dry with paper towels. Let sit for about 30 minutes so they come to room temperature. In a large oven-safe sauté pan over medium-high heat, add the grapeseed oil. Sear the first side of the tenderloins for about a minute, or until they're a golden brown color. Flip the fillets over and sear the other sides. Transfer to the oven and cook for about 5 minutes for a medium finish. Remove from the oven and let rest for 5 minutes.

To serve, place one tenderloin on each plate with Green Beans and Mashed Sweet Potatoes. Top with the Red Wine Demi-Glace sauce.

NUTRITION PER SERVING	Cal 386	Fat 23g	Protein 25g	Carbs 18g	Sugar 6g	Fiber 3g	Sod 200mg

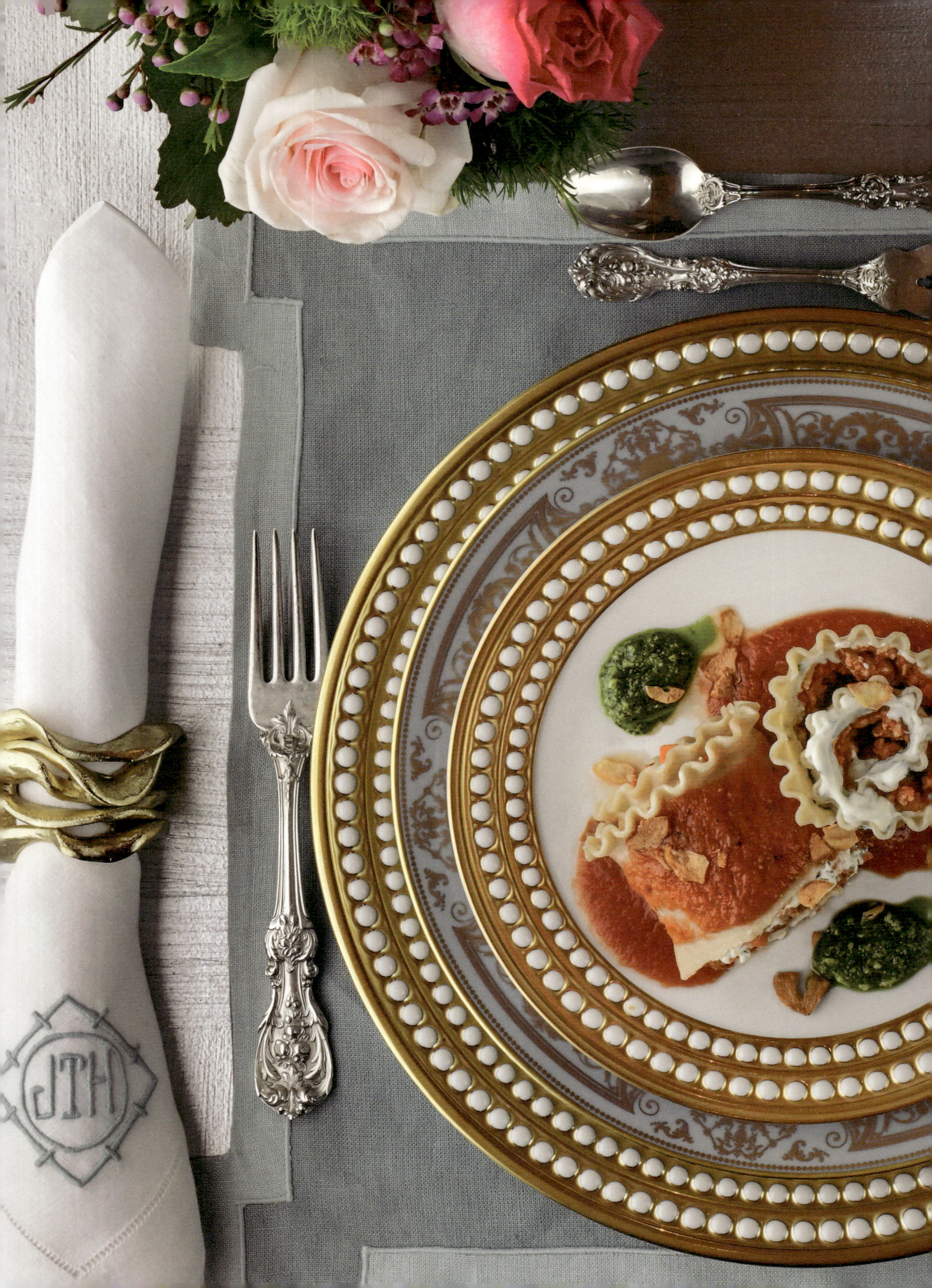
JTH

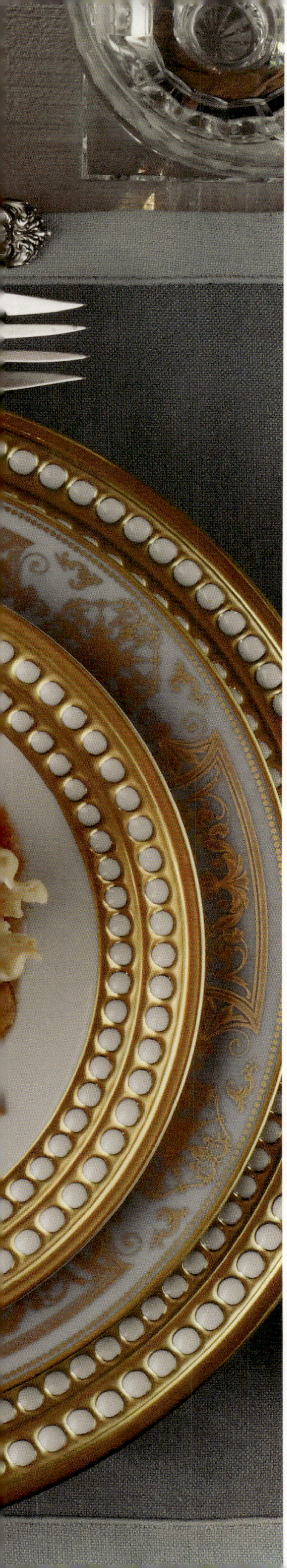

BISON LASAGNA ROLLS
WITH BASIL PESTO AND TOASTED GARLIC

YIELDS 10 LASAGNA ROLLS

This classic Cal-a-Vie entrée has been a favorite for almost a decade, and is always in demand. When it's not on the menu, we hear about it from our guests. But with this recipe, you can make it at home, and still enjoy one of our most requested dishes even if it's not served during your stay with us.

Today, most large grocery stores carry bison, or ask your butcher to source it for you. It's generally more flavorful and contains less fat than beef.

MARINARA SAUCE

- 2 tablespoons extra-virgin olive oil
- 1 cup diced yellow onion
- 3 garlic cloves, minced
- 1 tablespoon tomato paste
- ½ cup dry red wine
- 1 28-ounce can whole tomatoes
- 1 teaspoon fennel seed
- ¼ teaspoon chili flakes
- 2 teaspoons sea salt
- ¼ teaspoon freshly ground black pepper
- 1 cup fresh basil, leaves torn

In a large saucepan over medium heat, add the olive oil. Add the onions and sauté for about 7 minutes. When the onions start to caramelize, turning light brown in color, add the garlic and sauté for 1 minute. Add the tomato paste and stir until it turns brick red in color. Deglaze with the red wine, bring to a boil, then reduce the heat to a simmer and cook until reduced in half. Add the tomatoes, fennel seed, chili flakes, salt, black pepper, and basil. Simmer for about 30 minutes. Transfer the tomato mixture to a blender and puree until completely smooth. Set aside.

BOLOGNESE SAUCE

- 1 tablespoon extra-virgin olive oil
- 1 pound ground bison
- ½ cup diced yellow onion
- ½ cup peeled, diced carrots
- 1 garlic clove, minced
- 1 cup Marinara Sauce (or more if sauce is too dry)

In a medium saucepan over medium heat, add the olive oil. Add the bison and brown. Add the onion, carrots, and garlic and cook for 3 to 5 minutes. Add the Marinara Sauce and simmer for about 15 minutes. Cool and reserve.

BASIL PESTO

- 2 cups fresh basil leaves
- ½ cup pine nuts
- 2 garlic cloves
- ½ cup extra-virgin olive oil
- ½ cup water
- 2 teaspoons kosher or sea salt

In a blender, add all the ingredients and pulse several times until combined. Set aside.

HERB RICOTTA

1 cup ricotta (part skim)

2 tablespoons minced fresh parsley

2 tablespoons minced fresh oregano

1 teaspoon red chili flakes

1 egg

In a small bowl, combine all the ingredients and mix thoroughly. Set aside in the refrigerator.

TOASTED GARLIC FLAKES

12 garlic cloves, sliced extremely thin

Preheat the oven to 200°F. Lay the sliced garlic on a Silpat® silicone-lined baking sheet. Bake in the oven until crispy, about 15 minutes. Set aside.

PASTA PREPARATION

1 box Tinkyada® Brown Rice Pasta Lasagna

1 tablespoon kosher or sea salt

Prepare an ice bath in a bowl, containing 50 percent ice and 50 percent water. In a large pot, bring water to a rolling boil. Add a tablespoon of salt. Working in batches, add 5 lasagna noodles and cook for 9 to 11 minutes or until pliable, but not overcooked. Remove the noodles and immediately plunge into the ice bath to stop the cooking process. Remove from the ice bath and lay flat on a baking sheet covered with parchment or wax paper. Repeat until all pasta sheets are cooked.

TIP: It's important to follow the instructions on the pasta box, as cooking time will vary for different brands of brown rice pasta. Make sure to only cook it 80 percent of the way. If the pasta is overcooked, it will be too soft to roll.

LASAGNA ROLL ASSEMBLY

Preheat the oven to 350°F. Before assembling, let the Bolognese Sauce cool and allow the Herb Ricotta sauce to sit a few minutes out of the refrigerator. This will make assembly easier. Lay 4 noodles at a time next to each other on a flat work surface for maximum efficiency. Evenly spread a heaping tablespoon of the Herb Ricotta from top to bottom of the noodle. Next, spread about ¼ cup of the Bolognese Sauce on top of the ricotta mixture, leaving about 1-inch at the top and keeping it in the middle of the noodle. Starting at the bottom (the opposite end from the 1-inch clearance), gently roll the noodle to create a pinwheel, being careful not to press down. Gently transfer to a casserole dish and top with ¼ cup Marinara Sauce. Repeat this process for the remaining lasagna rolls. Once complete, cover and bake for 8 to 10 minutes to warm the lasagna rolls through. Let rest a few minutes before plating.

TO PLATE

Place one or two warmed lasagna rolls in the center of the plate. After lasagna bakes, it can be tricky to get it to stand up rather than lay down for presentation. Place a few teaspoons of Basil Pesto on the plate and sprinkle with Toasted Garlic Flakes.

NUTRITION PER SERVING	Cal 310	Fat 15g	Protein 15g	Carbs 28g	Sugar 2g	Fiber 2g	Sod 229mg

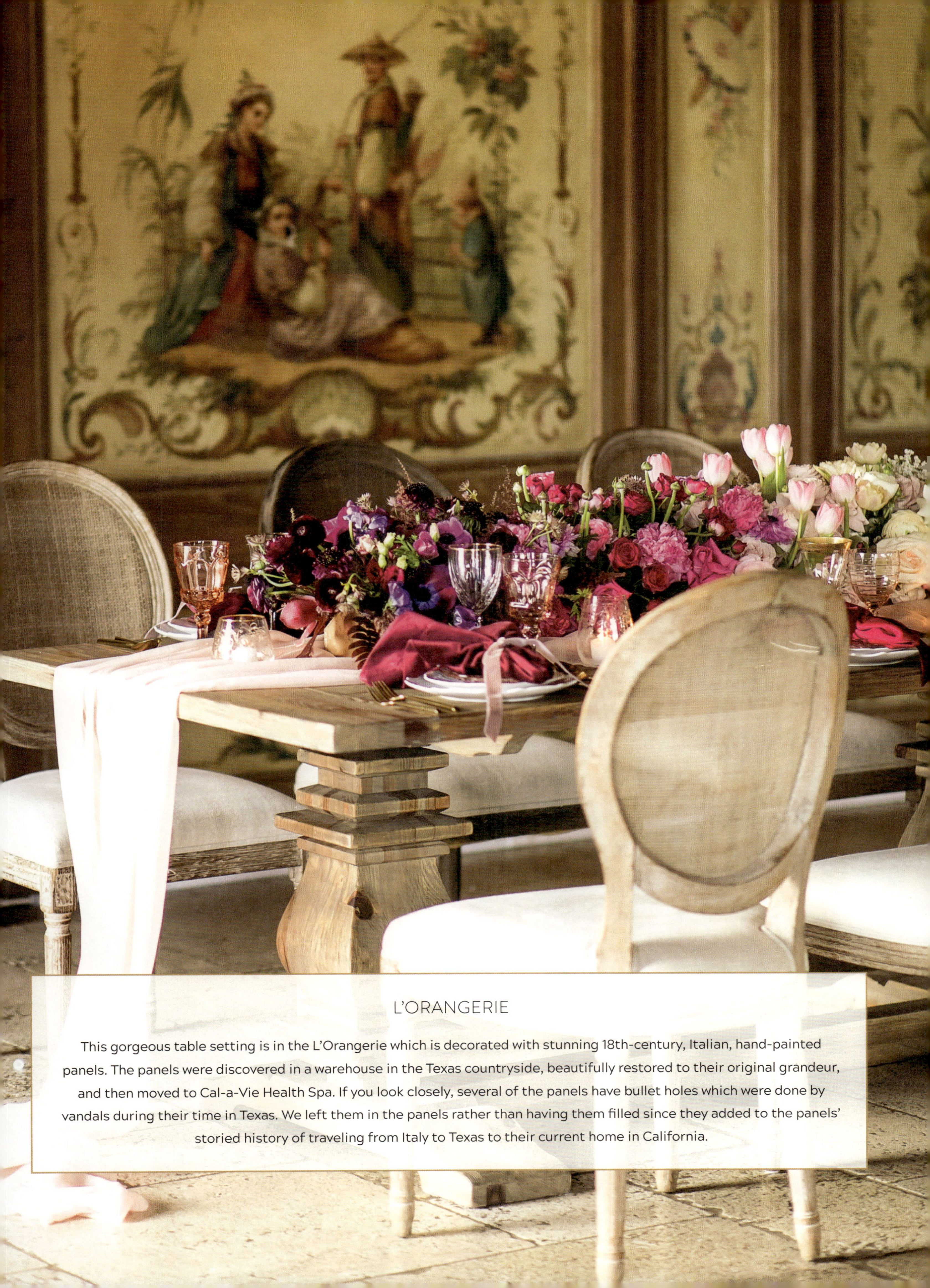

L'ORANGERIE

This gorgeous table setting is in the L'Orangerie which is decorated with stunning 18th-century, Italian, hand-painted panels. The panels were discovered in a warehouse in the Texas countryside, beautifully restored to their original grandeur, and then moved to Cal-a-Vie Health Spa. If you look closely, several of the panels have bullet holes which were done by vandals during their time in Texas. We left them in the panels rather than having them filled since they added to the panels' storied history of traveling from Italy to Texas to their current home in California.

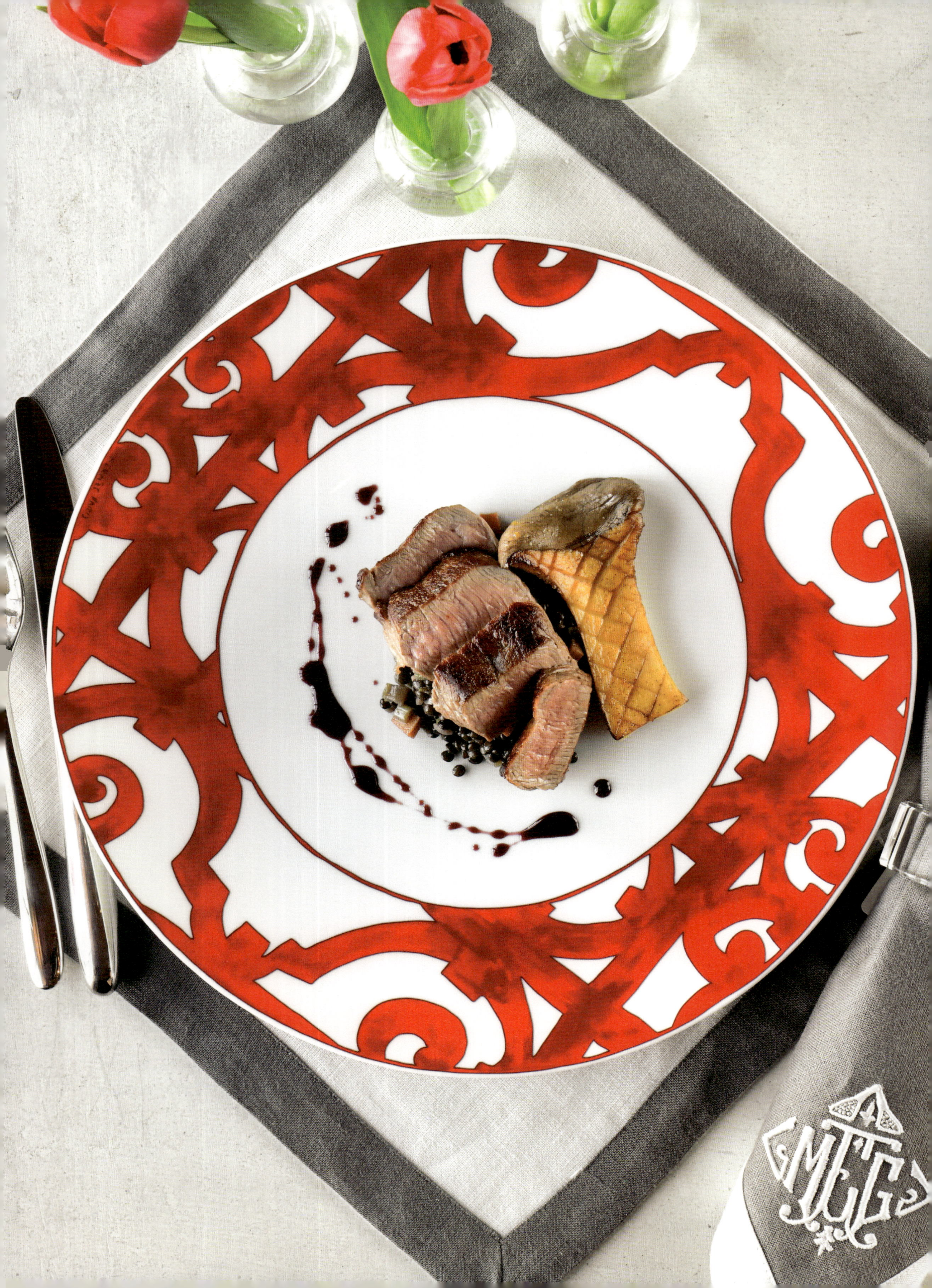

ROASTED LAMB LOIN CHOPS
WITH BELUGA LENTIL RAGU AND KING TRUMPET MUSHROOMS

SERVES 8

Lamb and lentils are the perfect culinary and nutritional duo. They are excellent sources of protein, which can promote healthy muscle growth, and the iron in the lentils delivers oxygen throughout the body that wards off fatigue. Lentils come in many varieties, bringing a diverse array of textures, colors, and flavors to your meals. Beluga lentils in particular resemble small beads of black caviar. They cook quickly but still hold their shape, creating a hearty side dish to accompany the lamb.

PORCINI STOCK AND PORCINI MUSHROOM PASTE

2 quarts water

2 cups dried porcini mushrooms

In a medium saucepan, bring the water to a boil. Remove from the heat and add the dried mushrooms. Allow the mushrooms to steep in the hot water for up to 2 hours. Strain the mushrooms over a large bowl, reserving all the liquid stock. Using a blender, add the reconstituted mushrooms to ¼ cup of the stock. Puree on high to create a mushroom paste. If the paste is too thick, add a tablespoon of stock at a time until you reach the desired consistency. Set aside the Porcini Mushroom Paste and the remaining Porcini Stock.

BELUGA LENTIL RAGU

1 tablespoon grapeseed oil

½ cup diced shallots

½ cup diced celery

½ cup diced carrots

2 garlic cloves, minced

1 tablespoon tomato paste

1 tablespoon Porcini Mushroom Paste

1 cup dry red wine

2 cups beluga lentils (sometimes called black lentils)

4 cups Porcini Stock

2 teaspoons sea salt

In a medium saucepan over medium heat, add the grapeseed oil. Add the shallots, celery, and carrots and sauté for about 3-5 minutes, or until the shallots are translucent. Add the garlic, and sauté for one minute. Add the tomato paste and Porcini Mushroom Paste. Sauté for 1 minute or until the tomato paste turns brick red in color. Add the red wine and bring to a boil, then reduce the heat to simmer and reduce by half. Add the lentils and the Porcini Stock and simmer for about 10 minutes, or until the lentils are just tender. Season with the sea salt. Remove from the heat, cover, and keep warm.

KING TRUMPET MUSHROOMS

1 teaspoon extra-virgin olive oil

1 pound King Trumpet mushrooms
(also known as King Oyster mushrooms), sliced in half

1 garlic clove, minced

1 shallot, minced

¼ cup white wine (we recommend using Chardonnay)

In a large sauté pan over high heat, add the olive oil. Add the mushrooms and sauté for about 2 minutes. Add the garlic and shallots and continue to sauté for another minute. Add the white wine and deglaze until most of the wine has evaporated. Remove from the heat, cover, and keep warm.

RED WINE HONEY SAUCE

2 cups dry red wine

1 cup balsamic vinegar

½ cup honey

In a medium saucepan, add the wine, vinegar, and honey and bring to a simmer. Continue to simmer until a thick, syrupy consistency is achieved. Remove from the heat and set aside. Keep warm.

ROASTED LAMB LOINS

1 2-pound boneless lamb loins

kosher or sea salt

freshly ground black pepper

¼ cup grapeseed oil

Preheat the oven to 375°F. Sprinkle the lamb loins with salt and pepper. In a large skillet over high heat, add the grapeseed oil and sear the loins on all sides for about a minute. Transfer to a baking pan and roast in the oven for 6-8 minutes until cooked. Remove and let rest for about 5 minutes. Slice into 8 pieces.

ASSEMBLY

Place about ½ cup Beluga Lentil Ragu on a plate. Top with 4 ounces Roasted Lamb Loin. Place a large King Trumpet Mushroom and a few teaspoons of the Red Wine Honey Sauce on the plate.

NUTRITION PER SERVING	Cal	Fat	Protein	Carbs	Sugar	Fiber	Sod
	416	27g	24g	14g	5g	2g	204mg

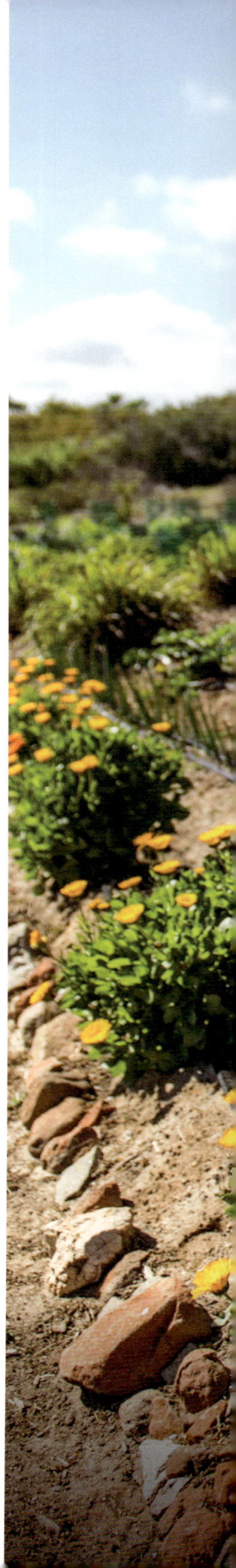

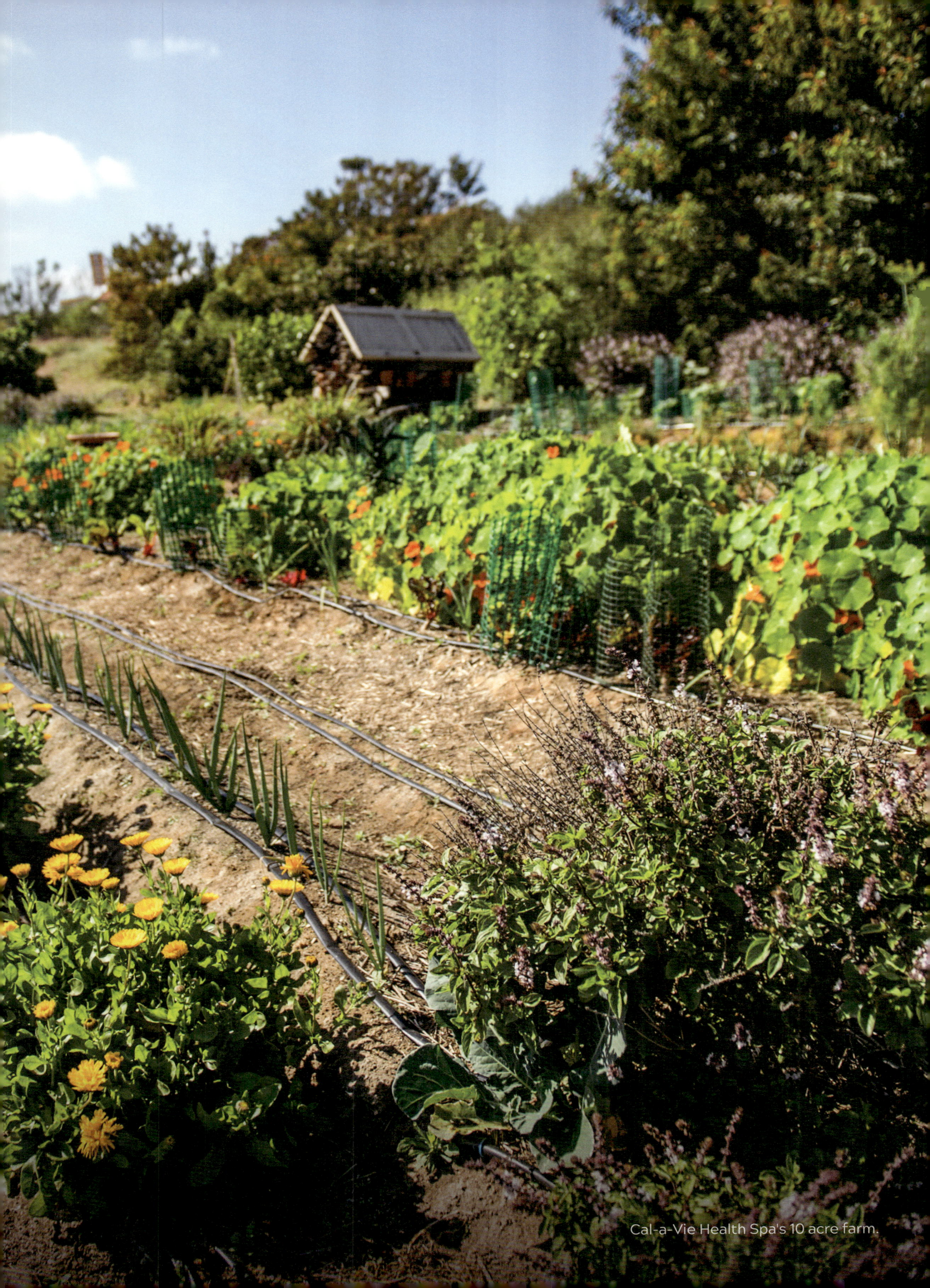

Cal-a-Vie Health Spa's 10 acre farm.

ROASTED RACK OF LAMB
WITH SAUTÉED PEAS AND PIPERADE SAUCE

SERVES 4

The Piment d'Espelette pepper is a key ingredient of the Piperade Sauce that's drizzled over the lamb. Espelette peppers were introduced into France in the 16th century for medicinal uses and later became a culinary delight. At 4,000 units on the Scoville Scale (which measures the "heat" or spiciness of peppers), the Piment d'Espelette powder is much milder than cayenne pepper and adds a subtle warm heat to elevate the flavor of your dish. If you can't find it in your local grocery store, it can be ordered from several online companies.

PIPERADE SAUCE

- ¼ cup extra-virgin olive oil
- 2 yellow onions, diced
- 8 red bell peppers, stems removed, seeded and diced
- 8 garlic cloves
- 12 Roma tomatoes, peeled and diced
- 2 teaspoons kosher or sea salt
- 1 tablespoon sugar
- 1 tablespoon Piment d'Espelette powder (you can substitute a smaller amount of cayenne pepper)

In a medium sauté pan over medium heat, add the olive oil. Add the onion and peppers and sauté for about 10 minutes. Add the garlic, tomatoes, salt, sugar, and Piment d'Espelette powder and continue to cook for an additional 15 minutes. Using a stick blender, pulse the sauce until all the vegetables are broken up into a chunky sauce. Set aside and keep warm.

SAUTÉED PEAS

- 2 cups English peas
- 2 cups snap peas
- 2 tablespoons extra-virgin olive oil
- 1 cup sliced spring onions or scallions
- ½ cup diced fennel
- 2 garlic cloves, sliced

Prepare an ice bath in a large bowl with 50 percent ice and 50 percent water. In a large saucepan over high heat, boil the English peas and snap peas for about 2 minutes. Immediately remove and place in the ice bath so they will retain their color and texture. Drain and set aside.

In a large sauté pan over medium heat, add the olive oil. Add the onions and fennel. Slowly sauté the vegetables until they become translucent. Add the garlic and continue to sauté for about a minute. Add the English peas and snap peas and warm through. Set aside and keep warm.

ROASTED RACK OF LAMB LOINS

- 4 2-bone in racks of lamb loins (about 2 pounds)
- kosher or sea salt
- freshly ground black pepper
- 2 tablespoons grapeseed oil, divided use

Preheat the oven to 350°F. Sprinkle the lamb loin chops with salt and pepper. In a large sauté pan over high heat, add 1 tablespoon of grapeseed oil to coat the bottom of the pan. Add only 2 lamb racks to the pan. Sear each side for about a minute. Transfer to a baking sheet. Repeat with the other 2 lamb racks. Roast the racks in the oven for about 7 minutes. Remove and let rest before slicing each lamb rack in two.

Serve the Lamb Loins plated with the Piperade Sauce and Sautéed Peas.

NUTRITION PER SERVING	Cal 409	Fat 34g	Protein 17g	Carbs 10g	Sugar 4g	Fiber 3g	Sod 444mg

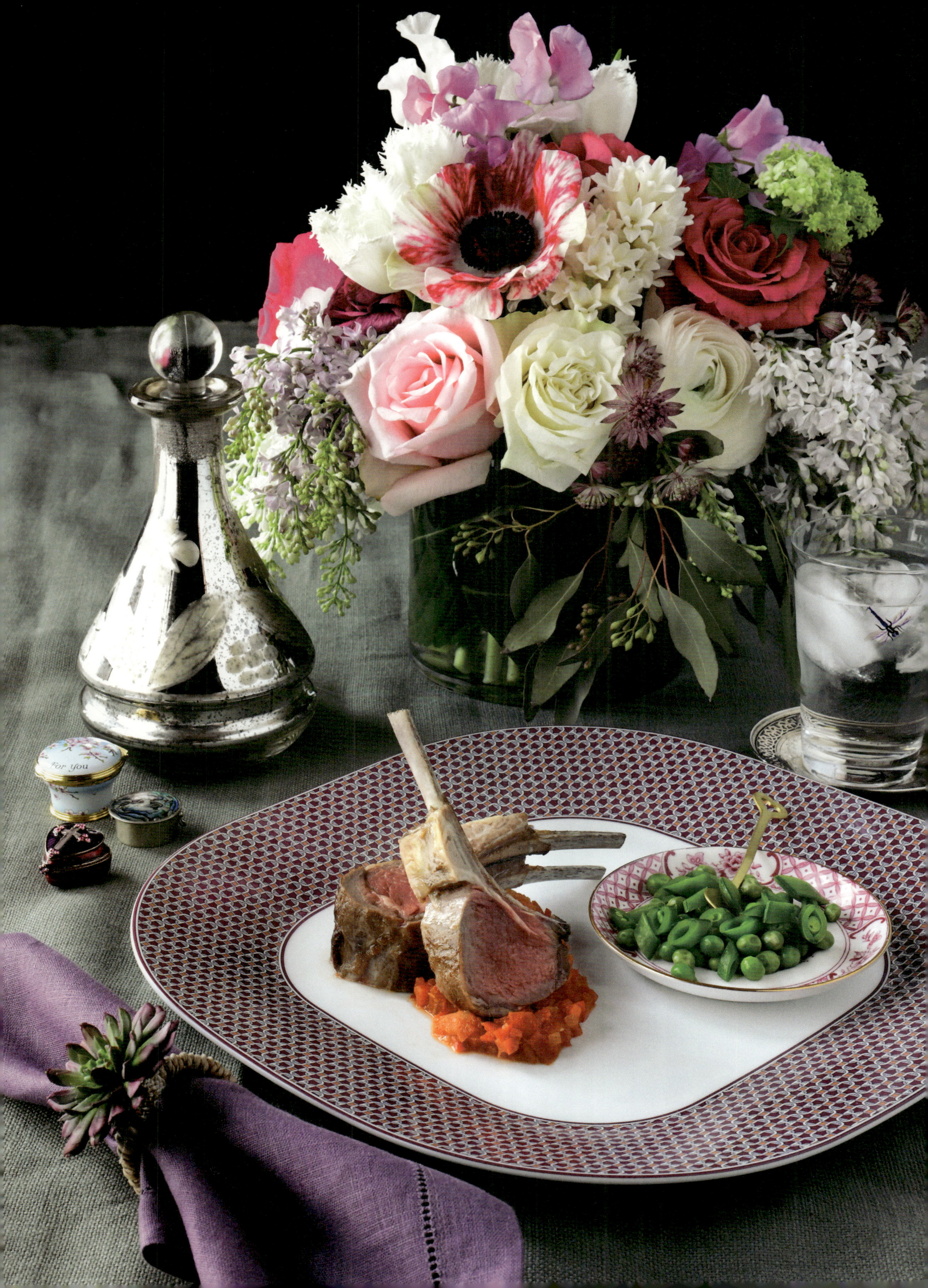
For you

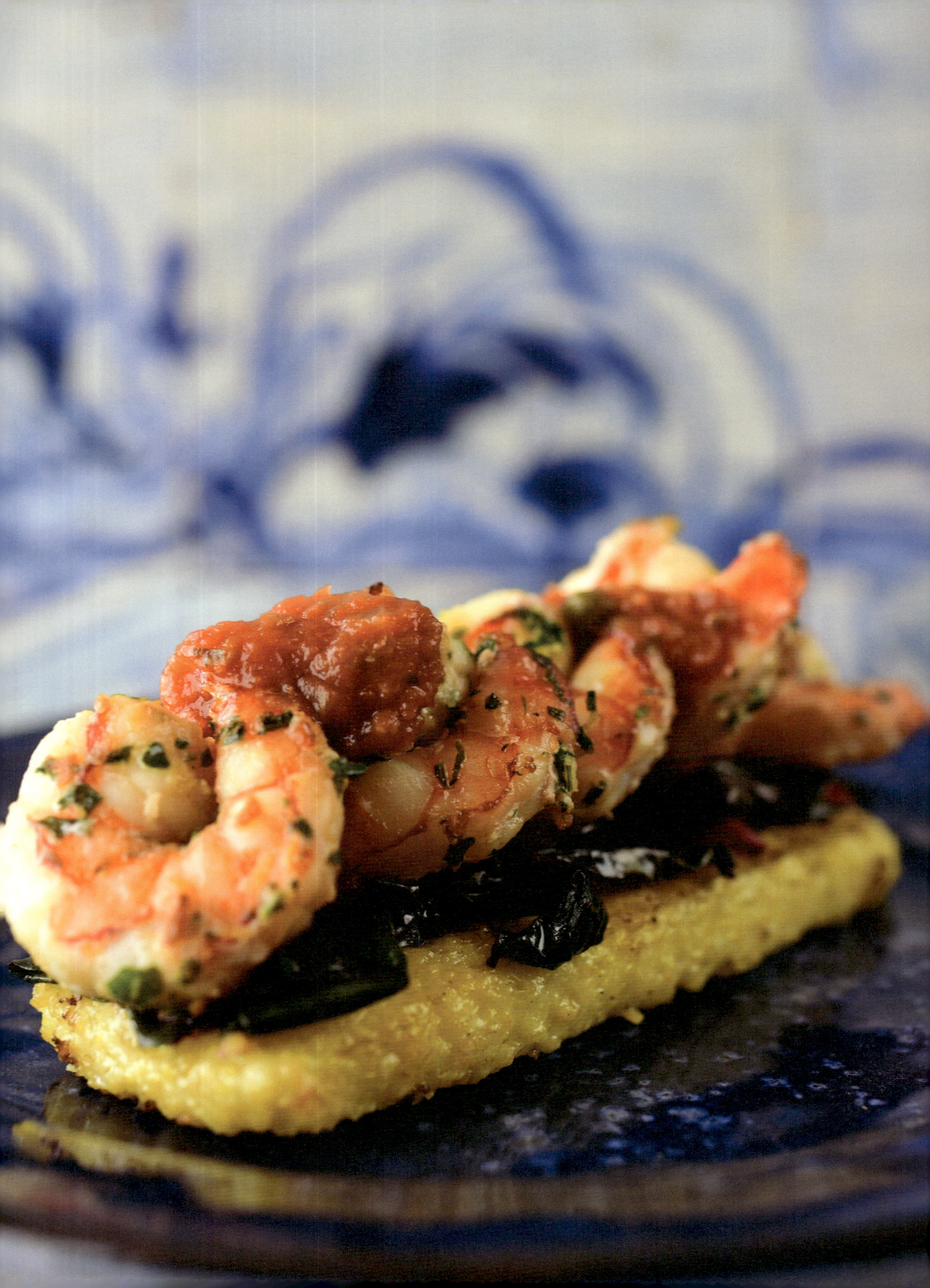

HERB SHRIMP

WITH PUTTANESCA SAUCE, PARMESAN POLENTA, AND SWISS CHARD

SERVES 4

The Puttanesca Sauce in this dish brings the whole meal together with a crescendo of flavor. While the capers and anchovies contain sodium, proper amounts of salt help to heighten flavors and mineralize your meals. A far bigger concern is how much hidden sodium is in restaurant and packaged foods. But when you can cook like this at home, who needs to eat out anyway?

PARMESAN POLENTA

4 cups chicken stock
1 cup coarse ground polenta
1 cup grated Parmesan cheese
1 teaspoon sea salt

In a medium saucepan, add the chicken stock and bring to a boil. Slowly whisk in the polenta. Turn the heat down to low and continue to cook the polenta, whisking frequently, for about 20 minutes, or until the polenta is soft to the bite. Add the Parmesan and salt. Remove from the stove, spread the polenta on a baking sheet into a ½-inch-thick rectangle and let cool. Once it's slightly cooled, cut into 6-inch by 3-inch rectangle pieces. Cover and keep warm.

PUTTANESCA SAUCE

2 tablespoons extra-virgin olive oil
½ yellow onion, diced
3 garlic cloves, minced
10 Roma tomatoes, chopped
1 tablespoon anchovy paste
1 teaspoon honey
2 tablespoons capers, drained and rinsed
2 tablespoons finely chopped fresh basil
2 tablespoons finely chopped fresh parsley

In a medium saucepan over medium-high heat, add the olive oil. Add the onions and sauté until golden brown, about 5-6 minutes. Add the garlic and continue to sauté for 1 minute. Add the chopped tomatoes, anchovy paste, honey, capers, basil, and parsley. Simmer for about 10-12 minutes. Transfer to a food processor and blend. Cover and keep warm.

SWISS CHARD

1 pound Swiss chard (2 bunches)
1 teaspoon extra-virgin olive oil
2 garlic cloves, minced
½ teaspoon sea salt

Rinse the Swiss chard leaves and pat dry. Tear away the leaves from the thick stalks. Chop the leaves into 1-inch-wide pieces, then chop the stalks into smaller pieces and keep separate. In a large sauté pan over medium heat, add the olive oil. Sauté the Swiss chard stems for 2 minutes. Add the garlic and continue to sauté for another minute. Add the Swiss chard leaves and sauté together for about 3-4 minutes. Season with salt. Remove from the stove, cover, and keep warm.

HERB SHRIMP

16 large shrimp, peeled and deveined
1 tablespoon finely chopped fresh oregano
1 tablespoon finely chopped fresh parsley
1 tablespoon finely chopped fresh basil
1 teaspoon sea salt
1 tablespoon grapeseed oil

In a medium bowl, toss the shrimp with the herbs and salt. In a large sauté pan, add the grapeseed oil and heat to almost smoking. Add the shrimp to the pan and sauté for about 5 minutes, or until completely cooked. Remove from the stove, cover, and keep warm.

To assemble, place a polenta rectangle on each plate, top with Swiss Chard, 4 Herb Shrimp, and then the Puttanesca Sauce.

NUTRITION PER SERVING	Cal 210	Fat 8g	Protein 23g	Carbs 12g	Sugar 3g	Fiber 3g	Sod 792mg

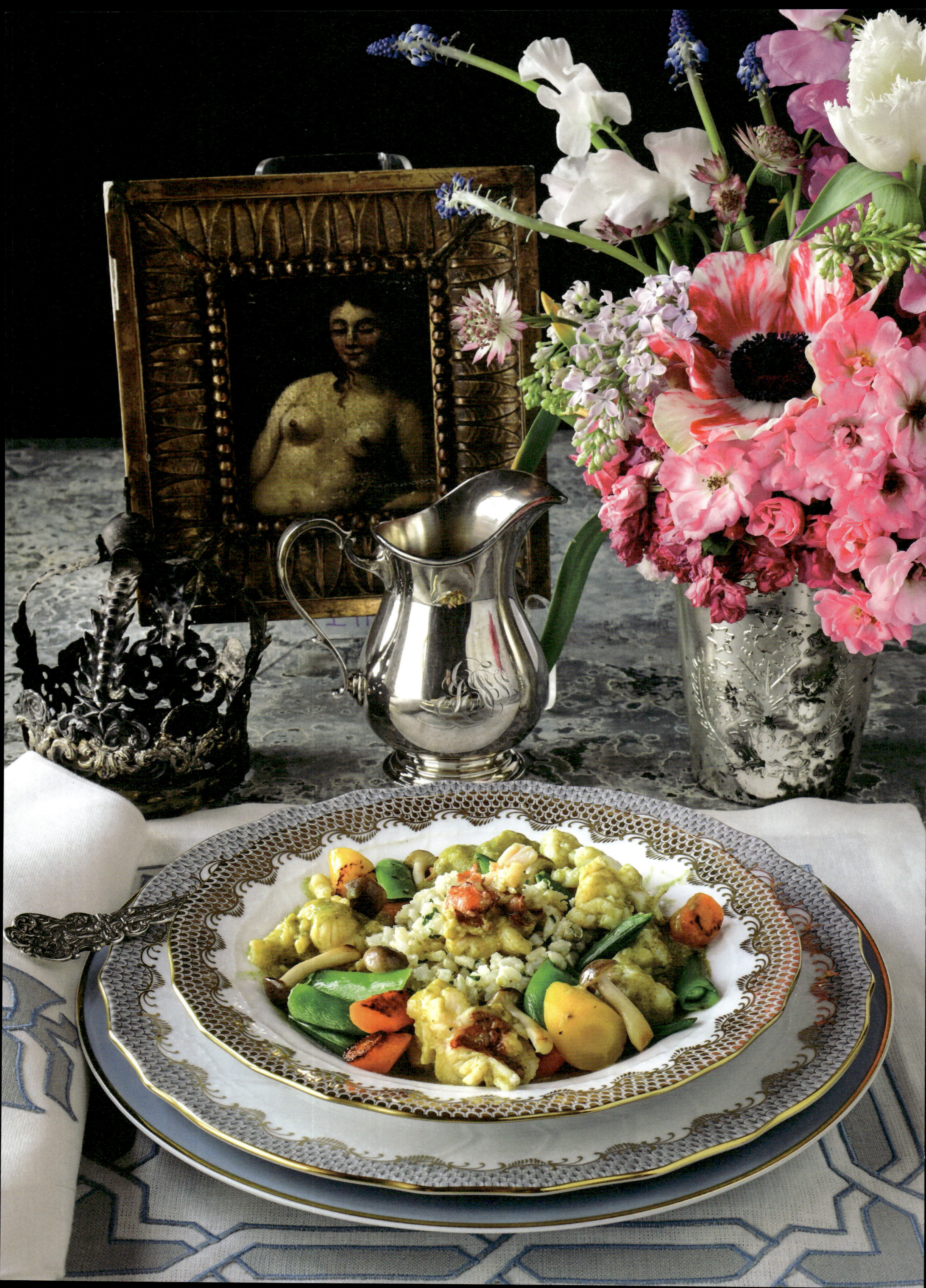

LOBSTER CURRY

WITH BABY CARROTS, BEECH MUSHROOMS, SNAP PEAS, AND COCONUT CILANTRO RICE

SERVES 6

You won't believe how easy this curry is to make after you've sourced and prepped all the ingredients. One of the main lessons guests learn during the hands-on cooking demonstrations with our executive chef is the importance of "mise en place"—everything in its place. If you can plan ahead and make the Green Curry Paste the night before, you'll be able to serve this for lunch or dinner within an hour.

GREEN CURRY PASTE

2 bunches fresh cilantro

½ cup fresh chopped basil

2 bunches fresh flat-leaf parsley

1 tablespoon fresh minced ginger

1 garlic clove

2 teaspoons black peppercorns

1 shallot, minced

½ teaspoon cumin

¼ teaspoon coriander

2 teaspoons tamari

½ teaspoon fish sauce

¼ cup chopped lemongrass, white parts only

⅓ cup grapeseed oil

2 limes, zest and juice

½ cup chicken stock

In a blender, combine all the ingredients and blend until completely smooth. Set aside in the refrigerator in an airtight container.

COCONUT CILANTRO RICE

1 cup short-grain brown rice

2½ cups water

1 teaspoon grated fresh ginger

2 tablespoons honey

2 tablespoons chopped fresh cilantro

2 teaspoons chopped fresh mint

1 tablespoon chopped fresh green onion

3 tablespoons coconut milk

In a medium saucepan over high heat, bring the water to a boil. Add the brown rice. Lower the heat to medium, cover the pan, and simmer for about 20 minutes, or until the rice has absorbed all the liquid and is tender. Spread the cooked rice on a baking sheet and chill in the refrigerator until cool. In a medium-sized bowl, whisk together the ginger, honey, cilantro, mint, green onion, and coconut milk. Fold in the cooled brown rice and set aside.

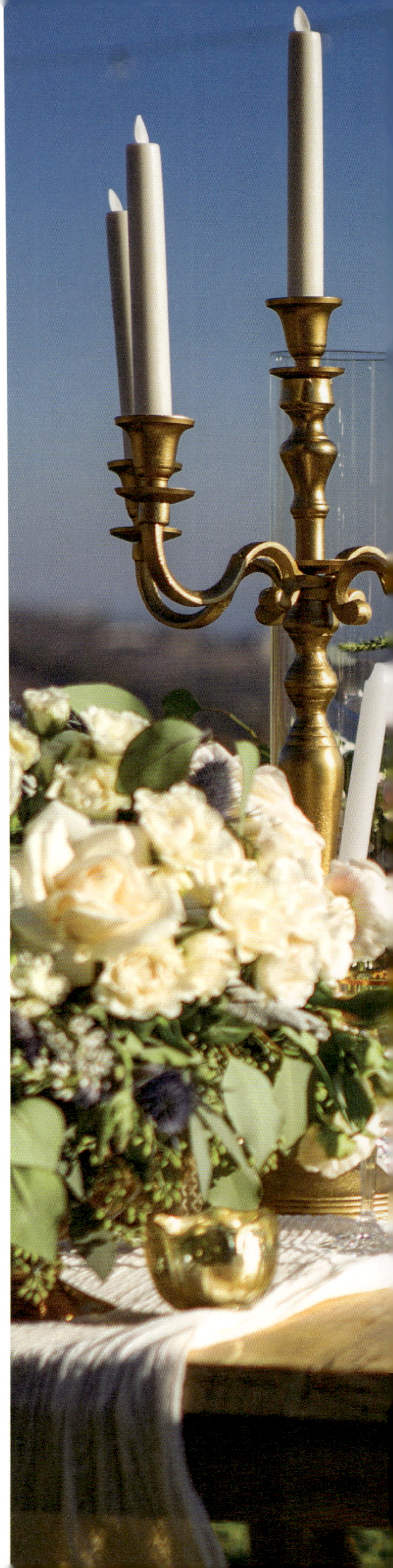

BLANCHED CARROTS AND PEAS

2 cups baby carrots, trimmed and peeled

2 cups baby snap peas

In a large pot, fill with water and bring to a boil. Prepare an ice bath with 60 percent ice and 40 percent water. Working in small batches, add one cup of the carrots to the boiling water. Cook them for about 3 minutes, or until just tender. Remove them from the boiling water and immediately plunge them into the ice bath. Leave in the bath until the carrots are completely chilled. Repeat this process for the rest of the carrots and the snap peas. When cooled, cut into bite-sized pieces. Set aside.

LOBSTER CURRY AND ASSEMBLY

2 tablespoons cornstarch

1½ pounds lobster tail, cut into large pieces

1 tablespoon grapeseed oil

½ cup Green Curry Paste

½ cup chicken stock

½ cup coconut milk

1 tablespoon grapeseed oil

Blanched Carrots and Peas

2 cups beech mushrooms, cleaned and trimmed

3 cups Coconut Cilantro Rice

In a medium bowl, toss the lobster in the cornstarch. In a large skillet over medium-high heat, add the grapeseed oil. When hot, add the lobster and sauté for about 2 minutes. Add the Green Curry Paste and toss with the lobster for another minute. Add the chicken stock and the coconut milk and simmer for about 4 minutes, or until the lobster is cooked through and the sauce is thickened. Keep warm.

In a large skillet over medium-high heat, add the grapeseed oil. When hot, add the Blanched Carrots and Peas and the mushrooms. Sauté for about 3 minutes. Remove from the heat and combine with lobster mixture.

Remove the Coconut Cilantro Rice from the refrigerator. Warm it in a small saucepan over low heat.

To plate, place ½ cup of Coconut-Cilantro Rice in the center of each of 6 large soup bowls. Gently add the Lobster Curry around the rice so it's evenly presented.

NUTRITION PER SERVING	Cal	Fat	Protein	Carbs	Sugar	Fiber	Sod
	392	15g	25g	42g	10g	4g	992mg

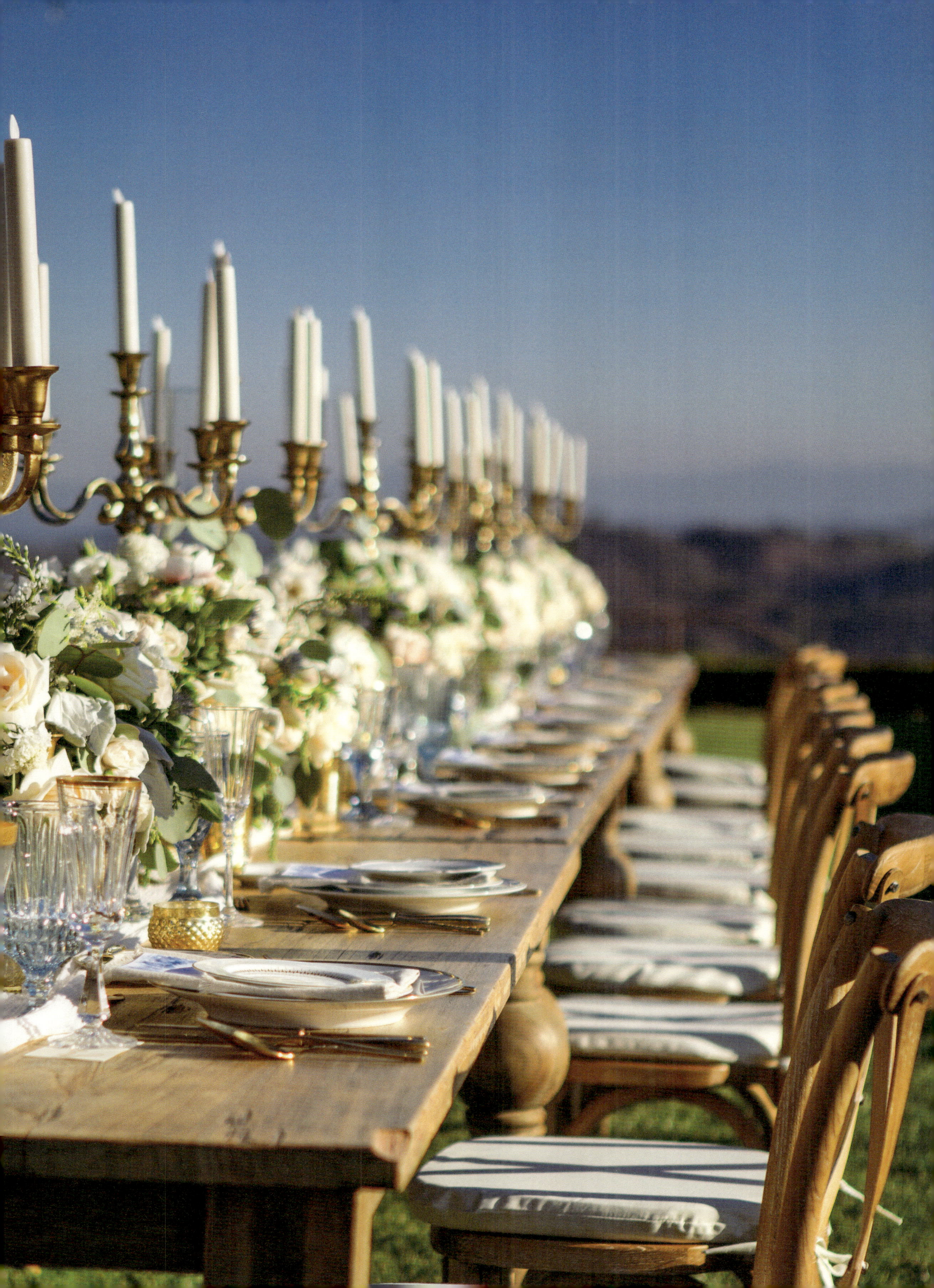

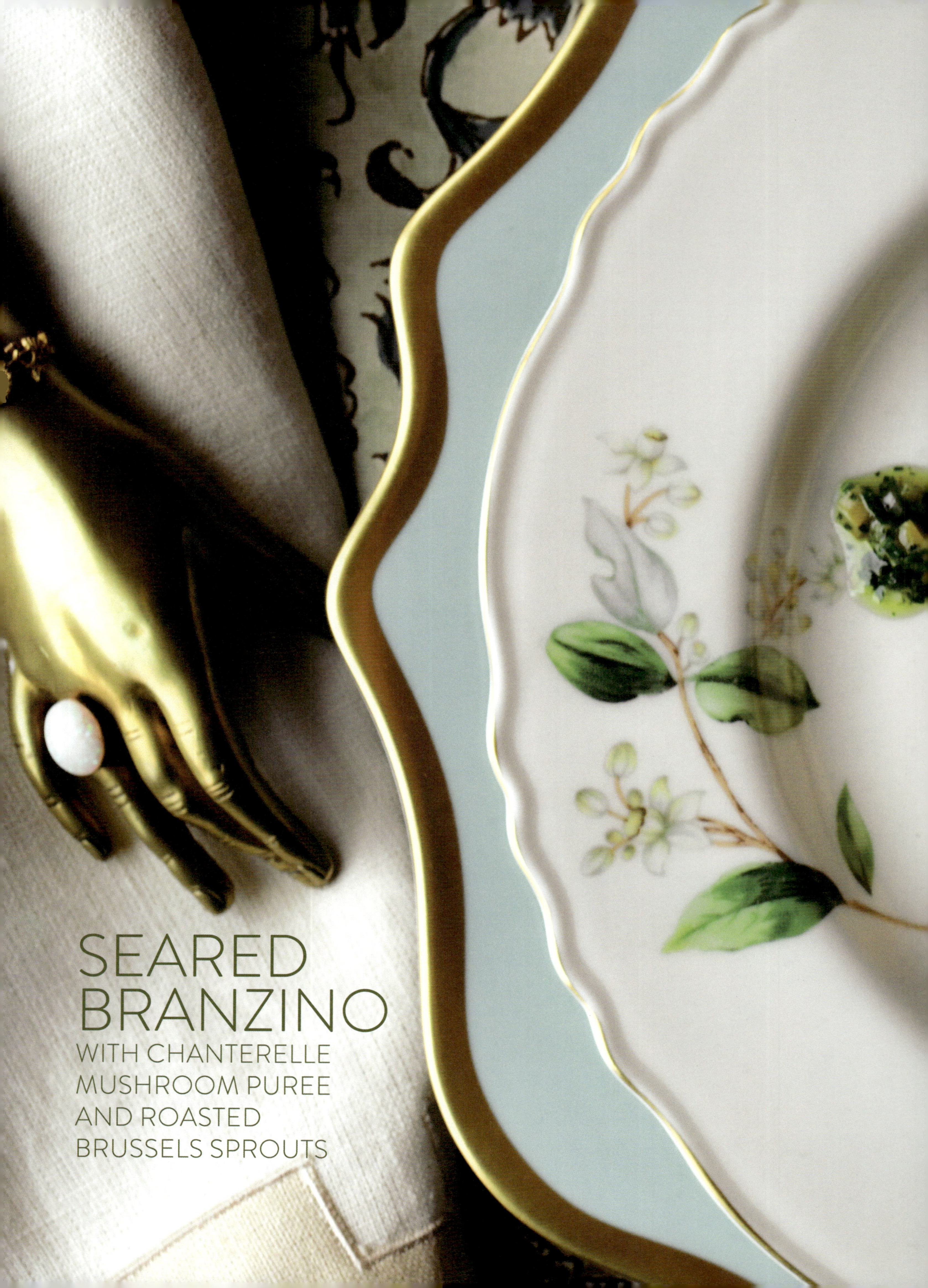

SEARED BRANZINO

WITH CHANTERELLE MUSHROOM PUREE AND ROASTED BRUSSELS SPROUTS

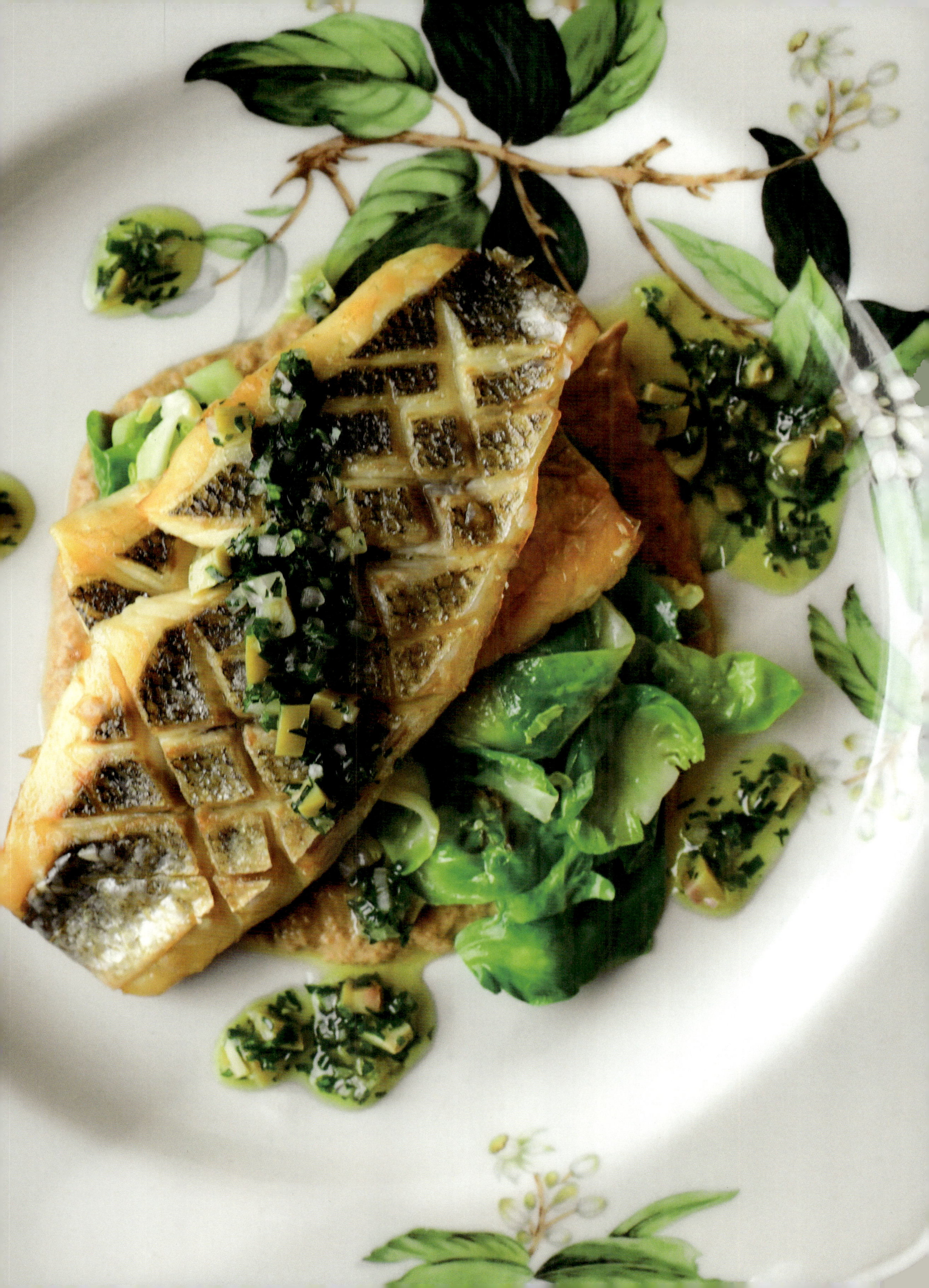

SEARED BRANZINO WITH CHANTERELLE MUSHROOM PUREE AND ROASTED BRUSSELS SPROUTS

SERVES 4

Branzino is a sustainable fish, native to the Mediterranean Sea. It is also called Loup de Mer, or European Sea Bass, and is one of the ocean's most delicious, tender, white-flesh fish. Small trout can be used in place of branzino if you have difficulty sourcing it. When buying fish, remember to look for the signs of freshness: taut skin, clear eyes, and bright red gills. Brussels sprouts are high in glucosinolates and offer additional benefits especially for people who genetically need extra liver detox or glutathione support.

SALSA VERDE

¼ cup minced fresh parsley

2 tablespoons minced fresh chives

2 tablespoons minced fresh tarragon

1 tablespoon minced shallots

2 tablespoons finely chopped green olives

¼ cup extra-virgin olive oil

juice of 1 lemon

In a small bowl, mix all the ingredients until combined. Set aside.

CHANTERELLE MUSHROOM PUREE

2 tablespoons grapeseed oil

2½ cups chanterelle mushrooms, cleaned

2 tablespoons minced shallots

2 tablespoons sherry wine

½ teaspoon sea salt

1 cup vegetable stock

In a large sauté pan over high heat, add the grapeseed oil. Add the mushrooms and sauté until crisp and golden brown. Add the shallots and continue to sauté for 1 minute. Deglaze with the sherry wine. Season with salt. While the mushrooms are still hot, puree in a blender with the vegetable stock. Keep warm and set aside.

SAUTÉED BRUSSELS SPROUT LEAVES

1 pound Brussels sprouts, trimmed and halved

¼ cup extra-virgin olive oil

kosher or sea salt

freshly ground black pepper

Remove the leaves from the Brussels sprouts. In a large pan over medium heat, add the olive oil. When warm, add the leaves and sauté until tender, about 4 minutes. Add salt and pepper to taste. Set aside and keep warm.

BRANZINO PREPARATION

4 Branzino fillets, skin on one side (6 ounces each)

kosher or sea salt

rice flour for dusting

2 tablespoons grapeseed oil

Score the skin side of the fillets with cross marks and season with salt. In a small, wide bowl, gently dust both sides of the fillets with rice flour to keep the skin dry. In a large skillet over medium heat, add the grapeseed oil. When the oil is hot, place the fillet skin side down and cook for about 3 minutes, then turn over and cook the skinless side until slightly crispy and fish is cooked through, about 1 minute. To plate, place about ½ cup of the mushroom puree in the middle and top with the Brussels sprout leaves and one fish fillet. Drizzle several teaspoons of Salsa Verde over the fish.

NUTRITION PER SERVING	Cal 429	Fat 32g	Protein 25g	Carbs 13g	Sugar 3g	Fiber 5g	Sod 255mg

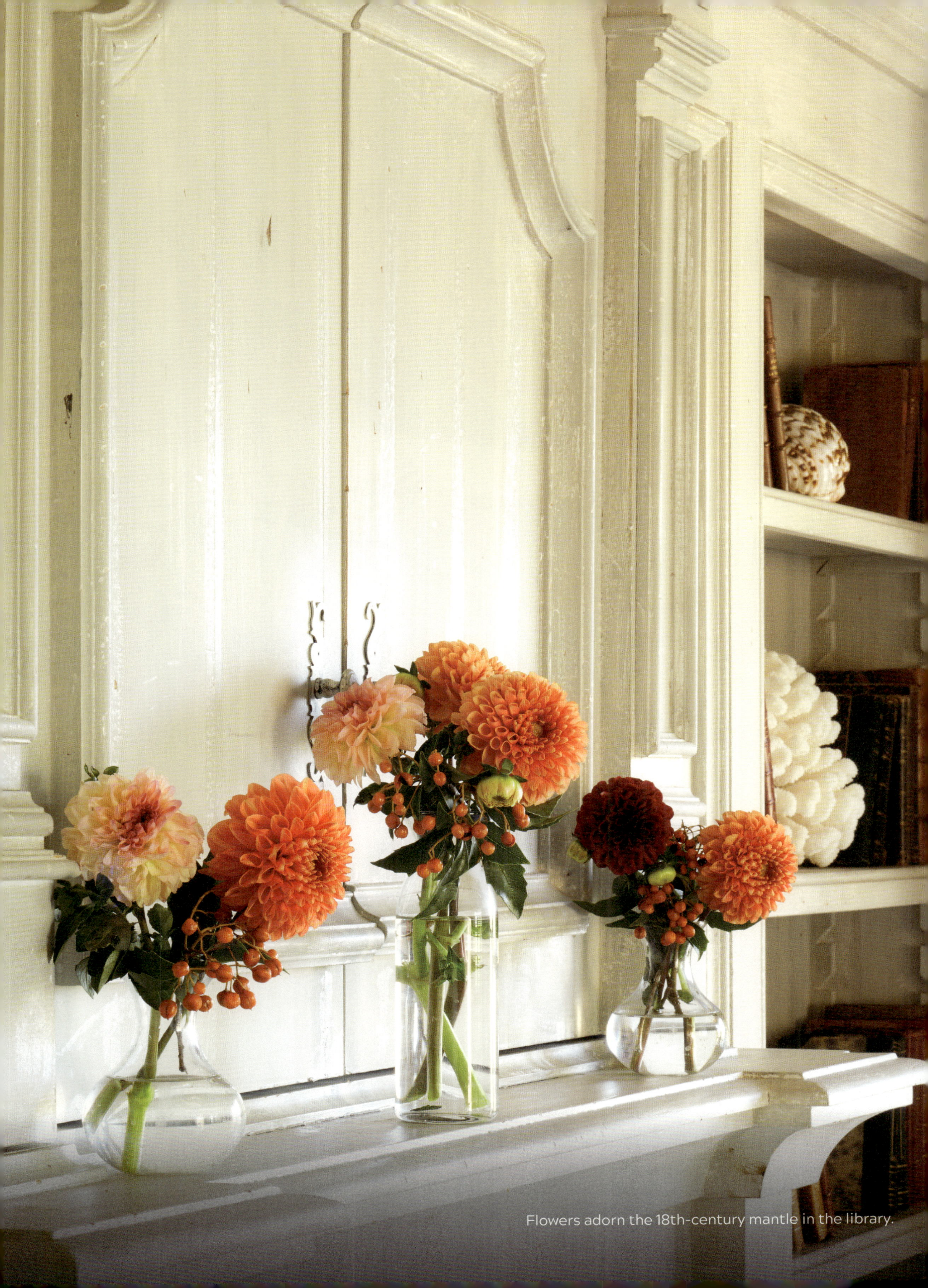

Flowers adorn the 18th-century mantle in the library.

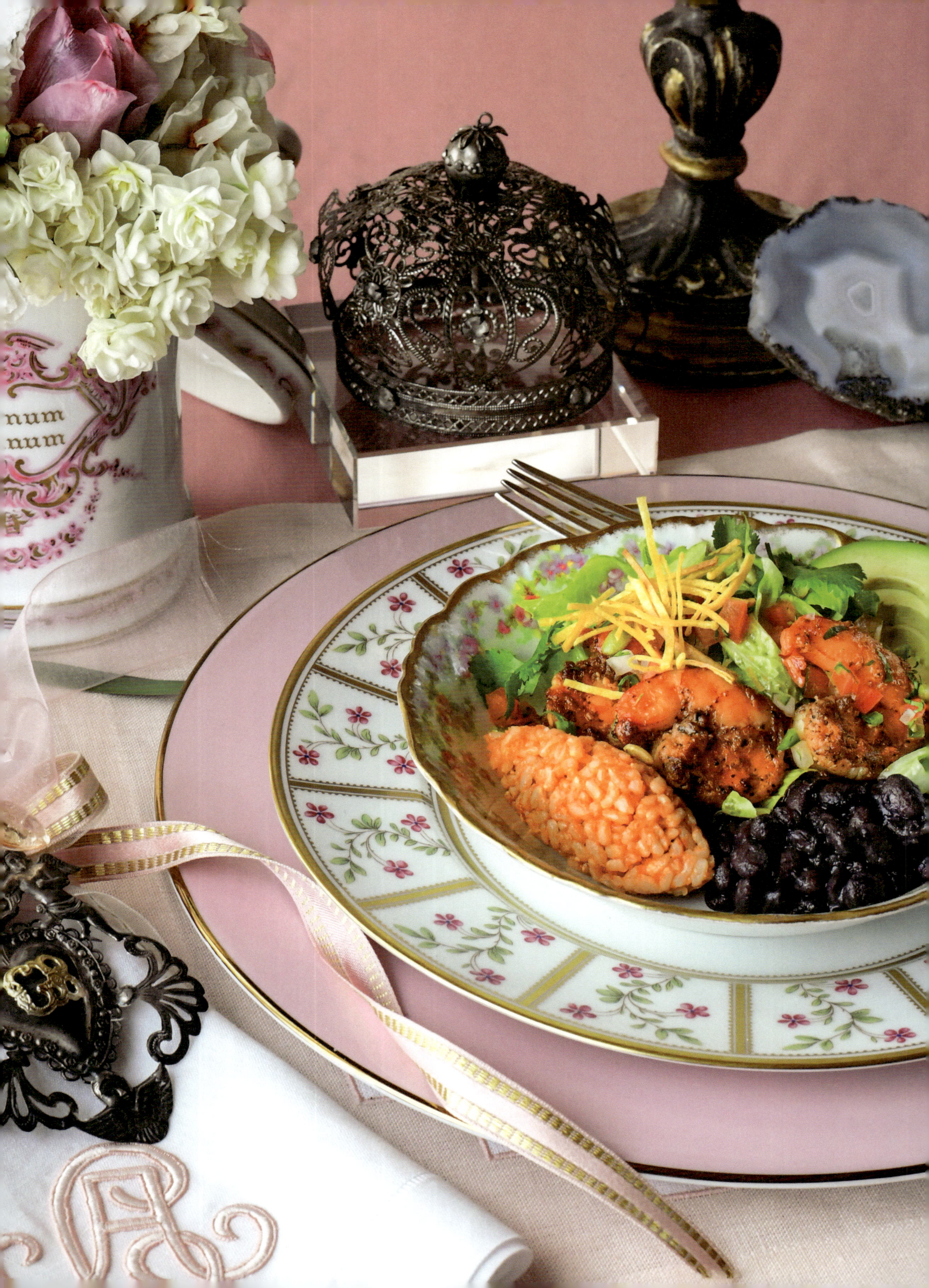
num
num

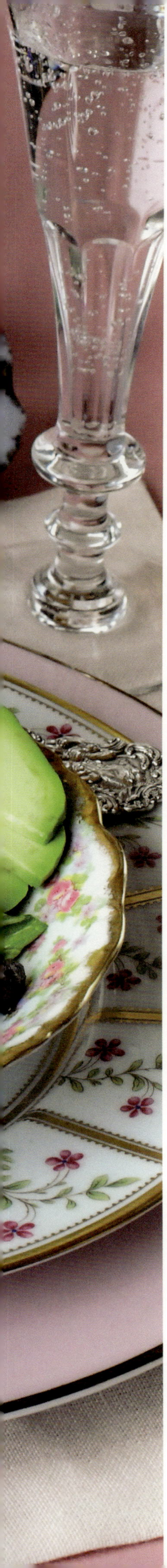

SHRIMP TACO BOWL

SERVES 8

This is our healthy take on the popular taco bowls that you find at local Southern California restaurants. You won't miss traditional deep-fried corn chips when you have the crunch from roasted pepitas and a sprinkle of your own homemade crisp tortillas strips.

TACO SPICE

2 tablespoons finely ground black peppercorns

2 tablespoons finely ground cumin seeds

½ tablespoon sea salt

2 tablespoons garlic powder

1 teaspoon smoked paprika

In a small bowl, combine all the spices and stir until completely incorporated. Store in a small glass jar.

PICO DE GALLO

1 cup diced tomato

½ cup diced red onion

¼ cup minced jalapeño, seeds and veins removed

2 tablespoons finely chopped fresh cilantro

juice of 1-2 limes

1 teaspoon kosher salt

In a medium bowl, combine the tomato, onion, jalapeño, and cilantro. Mix thoroughly. Season with lime juice and salt to taste. Set aside in the refrigerator.

LEMON-LIME VINAIGRETTE

¼ cup fresh lemon juice

¼ cup fresh lime juice

2 tablespoons honey

½ teaspoon kosher or sea salt

1 tablespoon Dijon mustard

¼ cup water

¾ cup grapeseed oil

In a blender, add all of the ingredients except the grapeseed oil and pulse. With the blender running, slowly add the grapeseed oil until incorporated. Set aside in the refrigerator.

CRISPY TORTILLAS

4-5 corn tortillas (we recommend using 6-inch size Mission® gluten free)

cooking spray

Preheat the oven to 350°F. Stack the tortillas and slice into very thin strips. Place strips on a baking sheet and spray with cooking spray. Bake for 7 minutes until crispy. Remove and set aside.

BLACK BEANS

- 1 cup black beans, soaked overnight
- 4 cups water
- 1 teaspoon kosher or sea salt

In a medium saucepan, add the black beans and bring to a boil. Turn down to a simmer and cook until the black beans are tender (about 30-45 minutes). Stir in the salt. Drain the black beans to serve them whole, or using a stick blender, roughly puree them. Cover, keep warm, and set aside.

SPANISH RICE

- ¼ cup diced onion
- 1 garlic clove
- 1 tablespoon tomato paste
- 3 Roma tomatoes, rough chopped
- 4 cups vegetable stock (or chicken stock)
- 2 cups brown rice
- 1 teaspoon kosher or sea salt
- 1 tablespoon grapeseed oil

In a blender, combine the onion, garlic, tomato paste, Roma tomatoes, and vegetable stock. Puree until completely smooth. Reserve. In a medium pot over medium heat, add the grapeseed oil. Add the brown rice and continuously stir for about 2 minutes, to toast the rice. Add the pureed mixture and bring to a simmer. Cover the pot and cook for about 20 minutes or until the rice is tender. Keep warm and set aside.

SAUTÉED OR GRILLED SHRIMP

- 24 shrimp (U10) peeled, tails removed, and deveined
- 2 tablespoons Taco Spice
- 2 tablespoons extra-virgin olive oil

Preheat the grill to medium high. In a medium bowl, toss the shrimp with olive oil, making sure to evenly coat each shrimp. Evenly sprinkle the Taco Spice over the shrimp and toss to coat. Place the shrimp on the grill and cook for about 1-2 minutes per side. Remove and keep warm.

TIP: We use U10 shrimp which means Extra Colossal or about 10 shrimps per pound.

BOWL ASSEMBLY

- 2 cups Black Beans
- 2 cups Spanish Rice
- 4 cups Romaine lettuce
- 24 Grilled Shrimp
- 1 cup Pico de Gallo
- ½ cup toasted pepitas (pumpkin seeds)
- 2 avocados, quartered and sliced
- ½ cup Crispy Tortillas
- ½ cup Lemon Lime Vinaigrette

In each bowl, place ½ cup of Black Beans and ½ cup of Spanish Rice on one side. Add the lettuce to the other half and top with 6 shrimp, a large spoonful of Pico de Gallo, a tablespoon of pepitas, sliced avocado, and Crispy Tortillas. Drizzle with the Lemon-Lime Vinaigrette.

NUTRITION PER SERVING	Cal 329	Fat 17g	Protein 12g	Carbs 36g	Sugar 5g	Fiber 9g	Sod 452mg

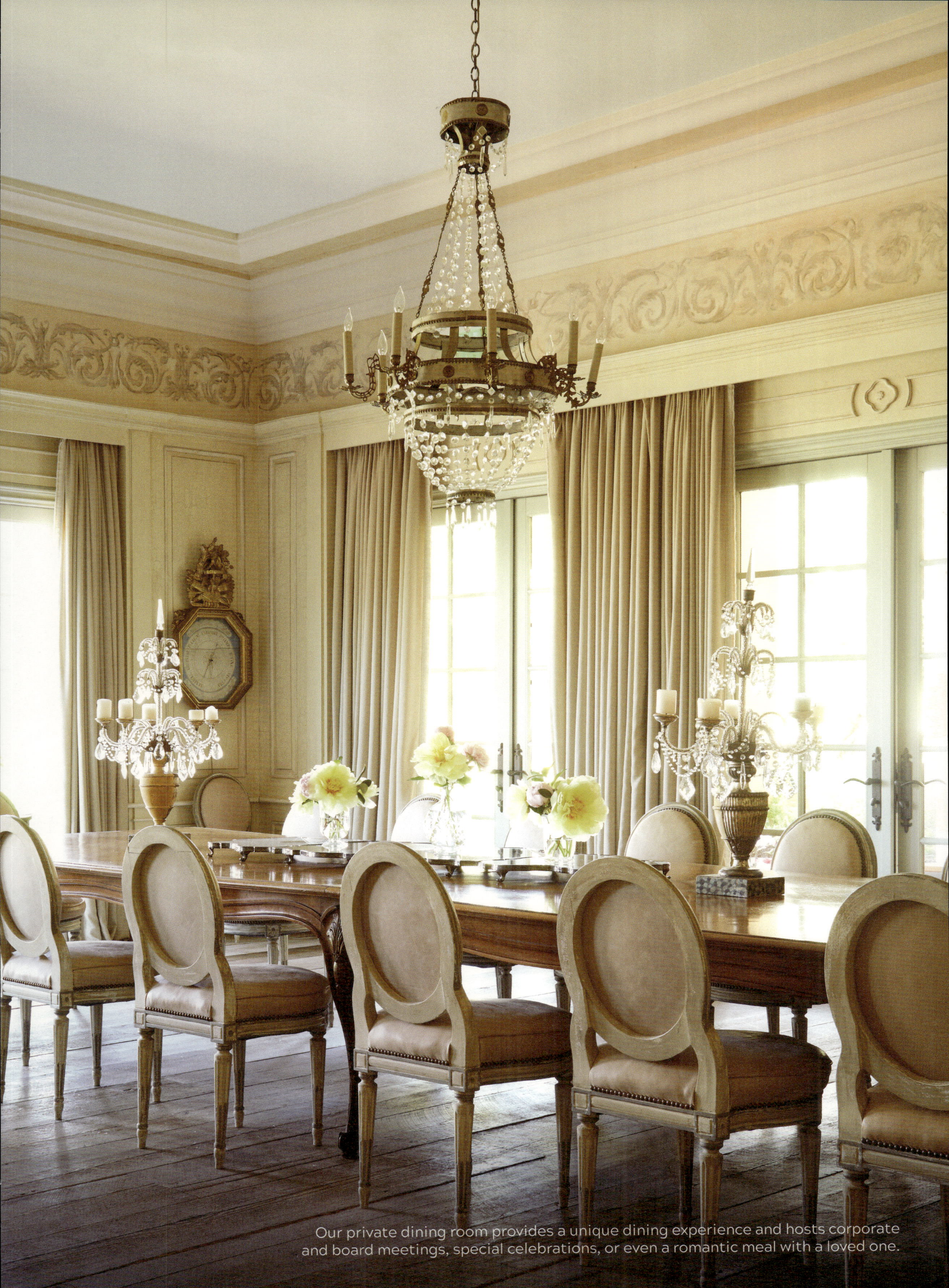

Our private dining room provides a unique dining experience and hosts corporate and board meetings, special celebrations, or even a romantic meal with a loved one.

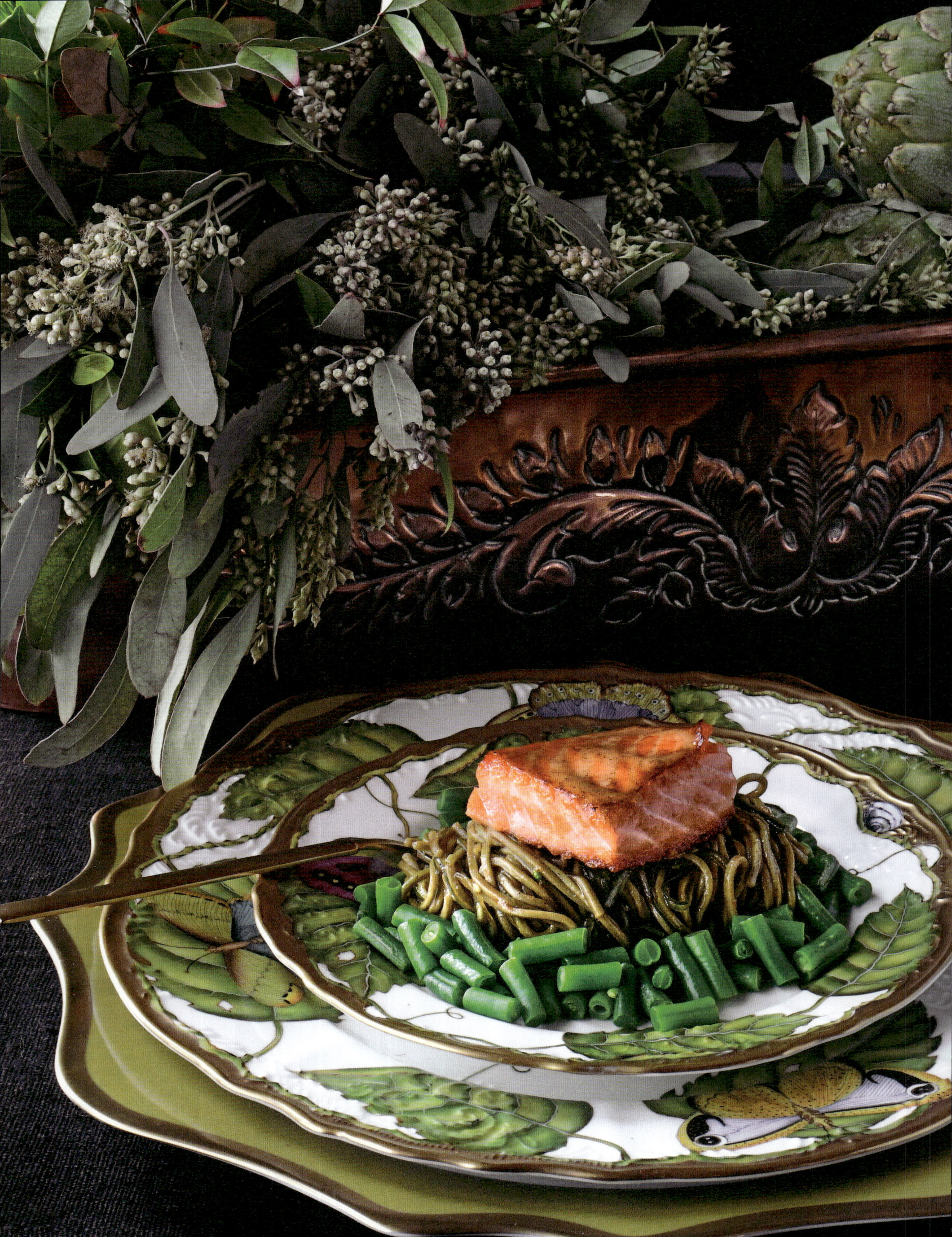

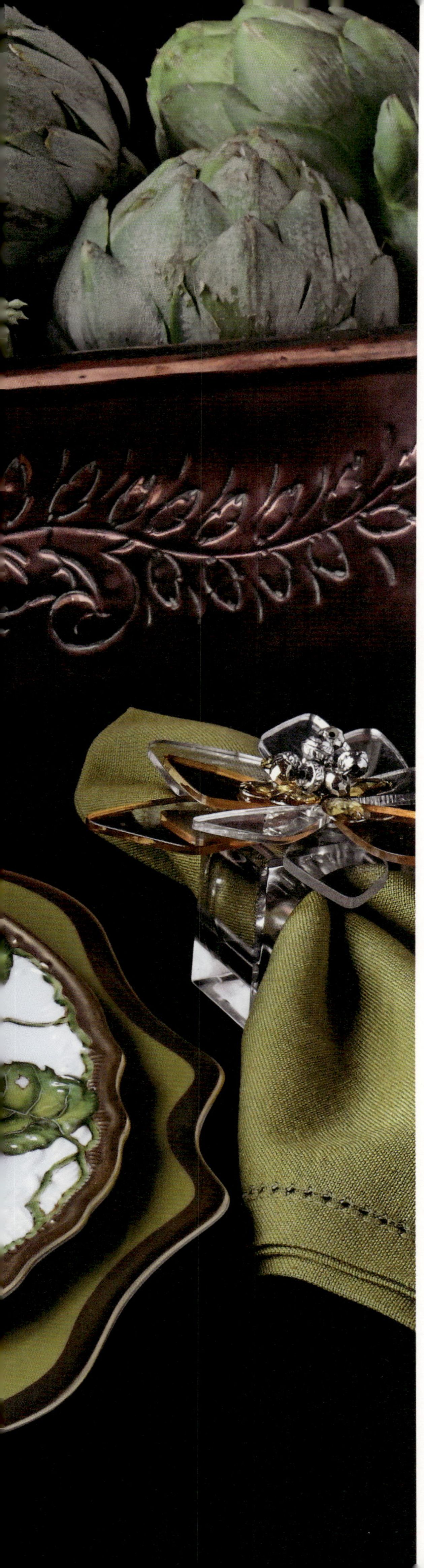

KING SALMON
WITH HONEY SESAME GLAZE, SOBA NOODLES, AND GREEN BEANS

SERVES 6

This is an extremely popular lunch for guests who frequent Cal-a-Vie. The high omega-3 content of salmon paired with the Asian-inspired soba noodles and lightly blanched green beans make for a satisfying recovery meal after a good morning workout. We source our salmon from the North Atlantic Shetland Islands and Wild Isles, a salmon farm that follows global GAPs (Good Aquaculture Practices) and approved sustainable farming methods.

SWEET AND SOUR SAUCE

1 cup tamari sauce
¾ cup rice wine vinegar
½ cup ketchup
½ cup sugar
¼ cup mirin (Japanese sweet rice wine)
1 tablespoon sambal sauce

In a small bowl, combine all the ingredients and stir until thoroughly incorporated. Set aside.

GREEN BEANS

1 pound fresh green beans, snapped and cut into 1-inch pieces
kosher or sea salt to taste

In a large stock pot, bring 2 quarts of water to a rolling boil. In a large bowl, prepare an ice bath with 60 percent ice and 40 percent water. Add the green beans to the boiling water and cook for about 4 minutes, or until tender to the bite. Remove the beans from the boiling water and immediately plunge into the ice bath to stop the cooking and preserve the color. Drain and set aside.

HONEY SESAME GLAZE

6 tablespoons honey
¼ cup whole grain mustard
2 tablespoons sesame oil
2 tablespoons Dijon mustard
2 tablespoons tamari sauce
1 tablespoon mirin
1 teaspoon sambal sauce
1 tablespoon wasabi powder or wasabi paste
1½ cups water
1 teaspoon minced garlic
1½ teaspoons xanthan gum

In a blender, combine all the ingredients. Blend on high for 2 minutes. Set aside.

SOBA NOODLES

1 pound green-tea, buckwheat, soba noodles, cooked (follow the instructions on the package)
1 tablespoon sesame oil
¼ cup Sweet and Sour Sauce
1 tablespoon grated fresh ginger
1 teaspoon sambal or sriracha sauce
½ cup tamari sauce

Combine all of the ingredients and mix thoroughly. Cover, keep warm, and set aside.

KING SALMON

6 king salmon fillets (3 ounces each), skinless
1 teaspoon sea salt
1 tablespoon grapeseed oil
1 cup Honey Sesame Glaze

Preheat the oven to 350°F. Season the salmon with salt. In a 10-inch non-stick oven-safe pan over medium-high heat, add the grapeseed oil. Add the salmon fillets and sear for 1-2 minutes. Flip the salmon over and sear again. Remove from the heat and brush both sides with the Honey Sesame Glaze. Place the pan in the oven for 5-7 minutes, depending on the thickness of the salmon fillets.

While the salmon is in the oven, reheat the green beans in a medium saucepan.

To plate, using a fork, spin about a cup of the noodles to make a circle. Place in the middle of the plate, surround with green beans, and top the noodles with a salmon fillet.

TIP: Don't let the extra Honey Sesame Glaze and Sweet and Sour Sauce go to waste. They can be stored in tightly covered containers for about a week in the refrigerator. Try them on all sorts of vegetables and proteins.

NUTRITION PER SERVING	Cal 495	Fat 15g	Protein 30g	Carbs 65g	Sugar 6g	Fiber 2g	Sod 914mg

WINE-TASTING

Guests can enjoy wine tastings at the Presbitaire, which was built around 1715 and imported to Cal-A-Vie from Dijon, in the heart of Burgundy country. They feature our own estate wines that are produced from organic grapes grown under ideal conditions and cultivated from our hillside vineyards. The selections include both reds and whites, all of which are perfectly balanced and a treat for even the most discriminating palate.

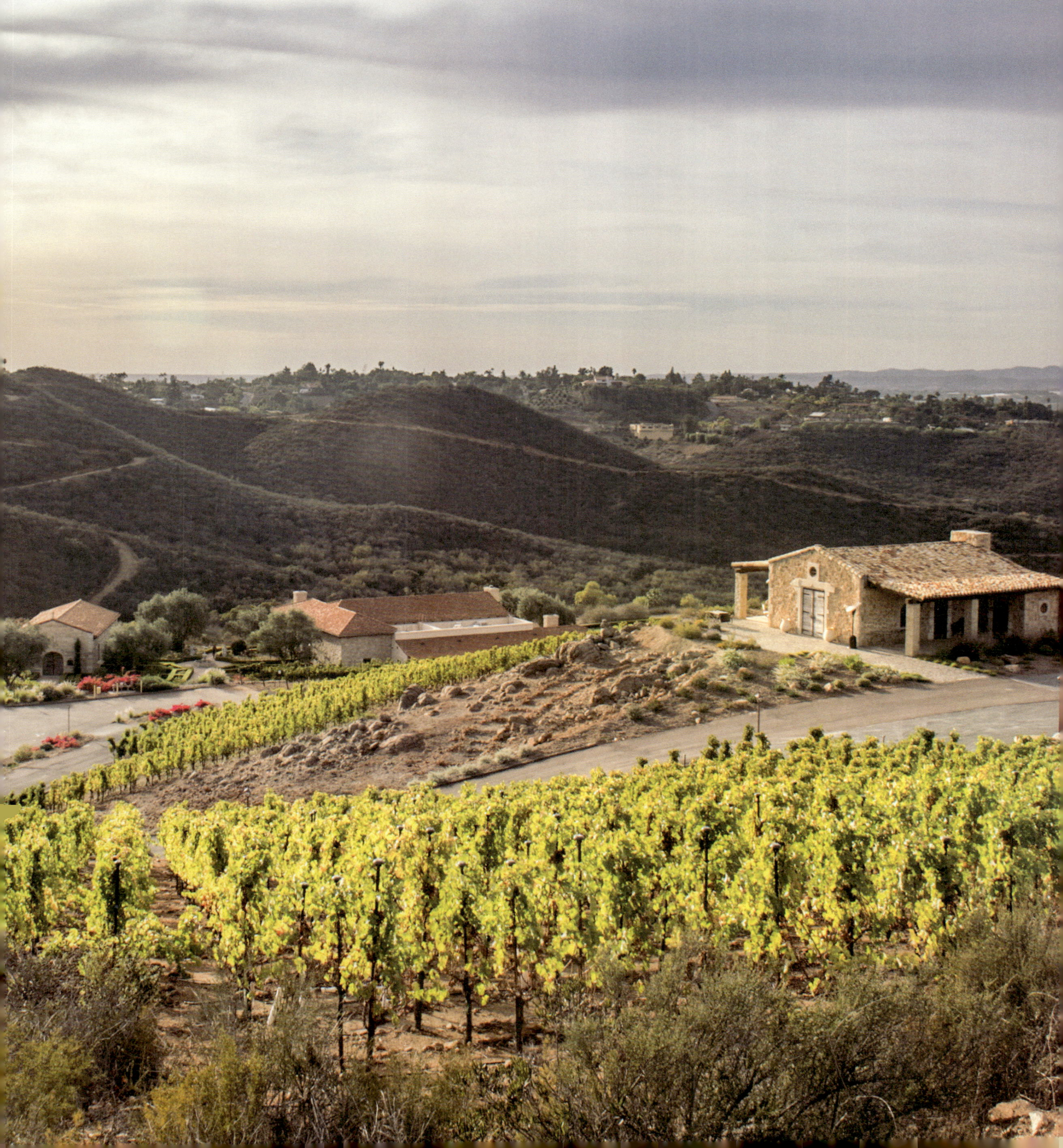

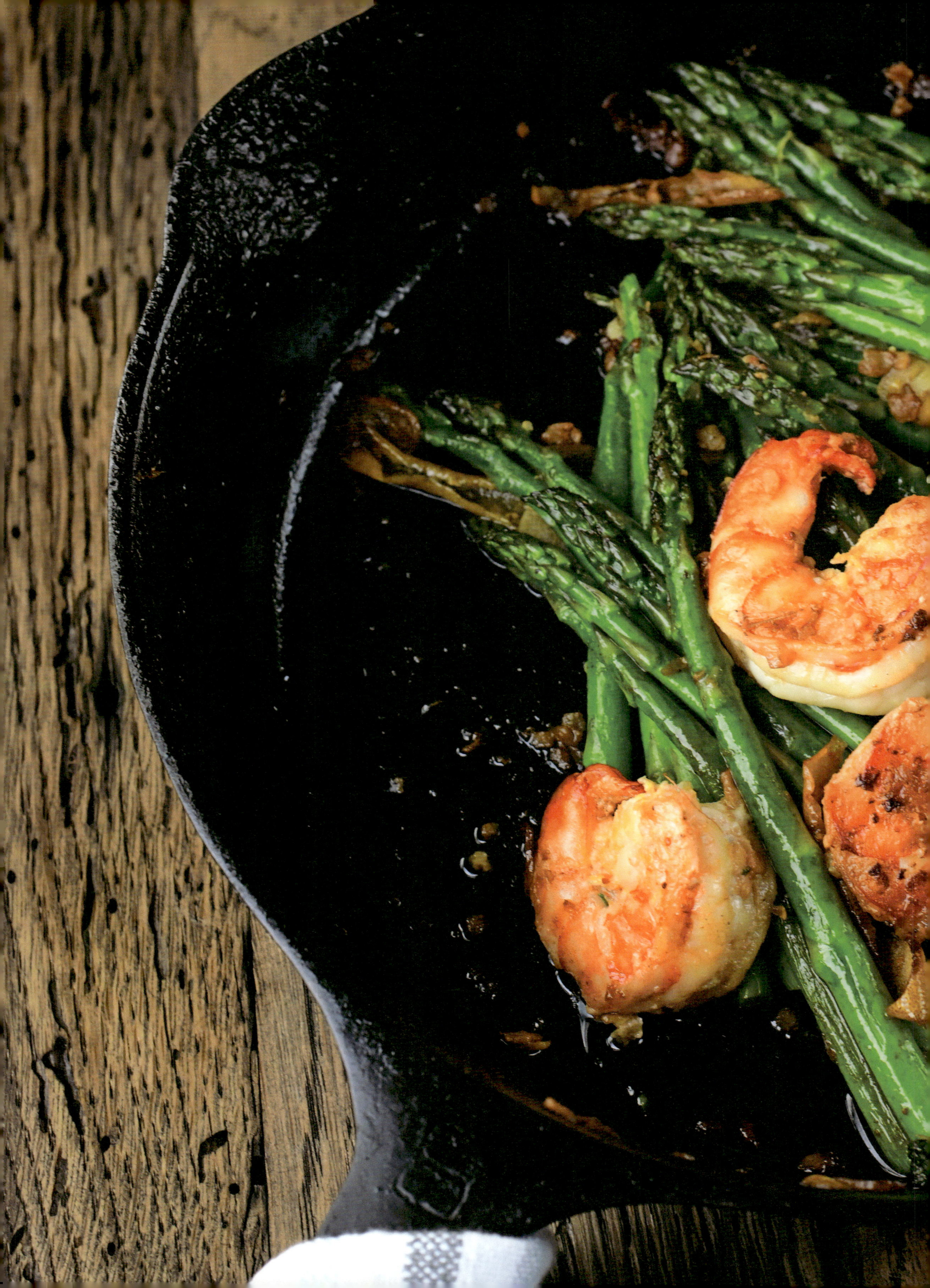

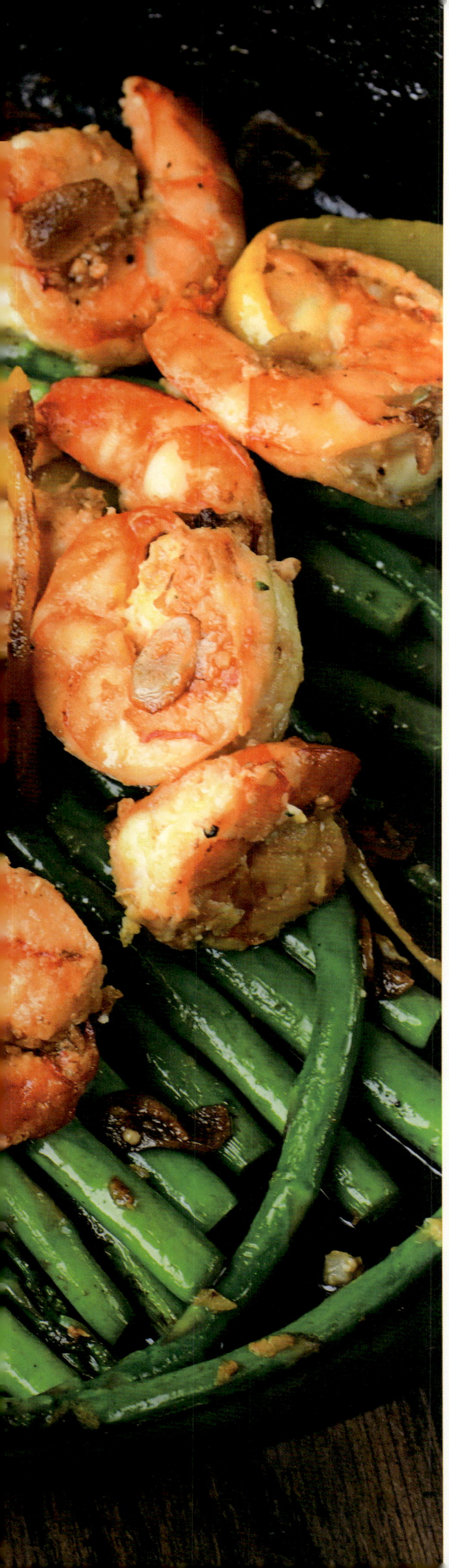

LEMON-GARLIC SHRIMP
WITH SAUTÉED ASPARAGUS

SERVES 4

We serve our Lemon-Garlic Shrimp with Sautéed Asparagus, but they can easily be thrown over any salad for a tasty lunch or paired with any other cooked vegetable for a satisfying dinner. Make sure to source your shrimp from reputable seafood providers. Shrimp is a great lean protein that offers a healthy dose of selenium, iodine, and vitamin B12.

- ¼ cup extra-virgin olive oil
- 3 garlic cloves, minced
- 1 lemon, zested into thin strips of peel and juiced (keep zest and juice separate as they will be used in different steps)
- 1¼ teaspoons kosher or sea salt, divided
- 1 pound extra-large shrimp (U10), peeled and deveined
- 1 tablespoon grapeseed oil
- 1 pound thin asparagus spears, trimmed

Add olive oil, garlic, lemon zest and 1 teaspoon salt to a medium bowl and whisk to combine. Add the shrimp and toss to fully coat each shrimp in marinade. Cover and refrigerate for about an hour. Remove from refrigerator and add the lemon juice. Toss to coat and allow shrimp to marinate for an additional 15 minutes.

In a large skillet over medium-high heat, add the grapeseed oil. Drain off the excess marinade from the shrimp, keeping the lemon zest strips, and add shrimp to the hot pan. Allow to cook for about 2 minutes, then turn them over. At this point you can move the shrimp to one side of the pan, add the asparagus spears and toss in the pan. Cook for another 3-5 minutes until the asparagus are soft but not overcooked. When adequately cooked, shrimp should take on the shape of the letter "c." Remove from the heat and serve immediately.

TIP: Shrimp is often sold by the number of shrimp per pound, but you will see it labeled many different ways in the grocery store. For this recipe, we use U10 Shrimp, which means Extra Colossal or 10 shrimps per pound, but you might also see these labeled as extra-large shrimp at your neighborhood seafood counter.

NUTRITION PER SERVING	Cal	Fat	Protein	Carbs	Sugar	Fiber	Sod
	260	18g	20g	6g	3g	4g	430mg

LOUP DE MER
WITH THAI CHILI-GLAZE VINAIGRETTE AND ROASTED BROCCOLI

SERVES 4

Loup de Mer is also known as branzino, bronzini, or Mediterranean Sea Bass. The acid from the Thai Chili-Glaze Vinaigrette awakens digestive juices while the heat from the chilis tantalizes the mouth. It's a perfect pairing to make your evening protein satisfying with every bite! This makes a beautiful presentation served in the pan.

THAI CHILI-GLAZE VINAIGRETTE

1-3 dried Thai chili peppers, minced or crumbled (amount to use varies with personal preference, depending on how much heat you like)

1 tablespoon minced garlic

2 tablespoons honey

2 limes, juiced and zested (about ⅓ cup)

½ cup extra-virgin olive oil

1 tablespoon minced fresh chives

1 shallot, minced

In a medium bowl, whisk all the ingredients together thoroughly. Set aside in the refrigerator.

TIP: We use Saladmaster© cooking and baking pans since they can go from stove to oven and maintain their even cooking temperature. Cooking times will vary depending on the kind of ovenproof skillet you use.

ROASTED BROCCOLI AND GARLIC

1 broccoli head,
trimmed into large pieces (1 pound)

4 garlic cloves, paper skin left on

2 tablespoons extra-virgin olive oil

kosher or sea salt, to taste

Preheat the oven to 375°F. Toss the broccoli pieces and garlic cloves in olive oil and lightly salt. Roast on a baking sheet in the oven for about 10 minutes. Do not let the broccoli heads get too brown. Remove from the oven, set aside, and keep warm.

LOUP DE MER PREPARATION

1 whole Loup de Mer (about 1½ pounds); ask your neighborhood fishmonger to remove the bones, butterflied

1 lemon, thinly sliced

1 cup fresh parsley sprigs

2 tablespoons grapeseed oil

1 teaspoon kosher or sea salt

3-4 tablespoons Thai Chili Glaze Vinaigrette

Preheat the oven to 400°F. Pat the fish very dry with paper towels. Score the fish on both sides about 3 times with a very sharp knife so the fish cooks evenly. Stuff the inside of the fish with sliced lemons and parsley. Drizzle with oil and season with salt on both sides and on the inside. Place the fish in a pan and roast it in the oven for about 15-20 minutes. The fish does not need to be turned. Once the fish is cooked, remove from the oven, place the Roasted Broccoli and Garlic around the fish, and drizzle with Thai Chili-Glaze Vinaigrette. Serve immediately.

NUTRITION PER SERVING	Cal 355	Fat 19g	Protein 35g	Carbs 12g	Sugar 4g	Fiber 4g	Sod 698mg

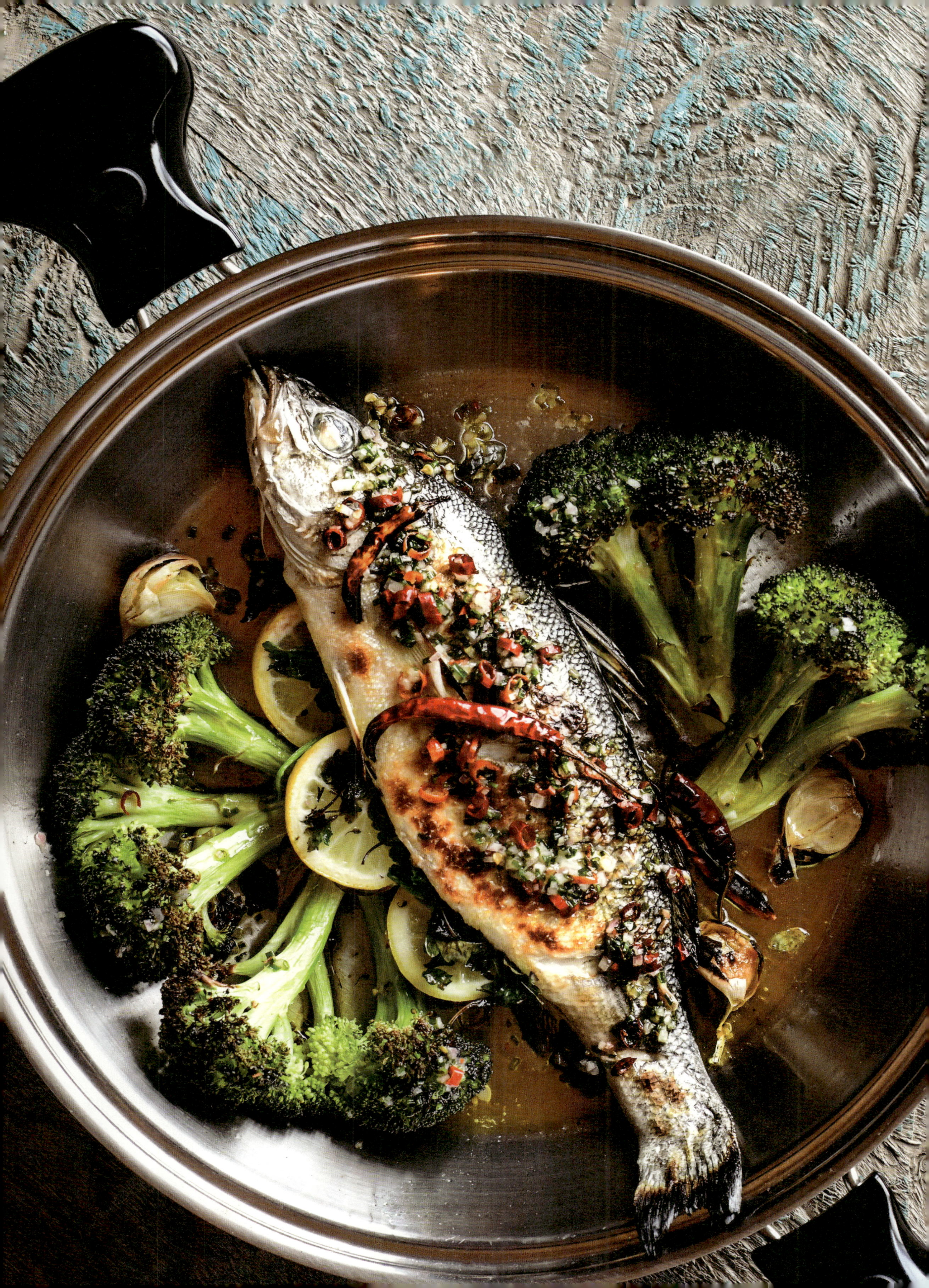

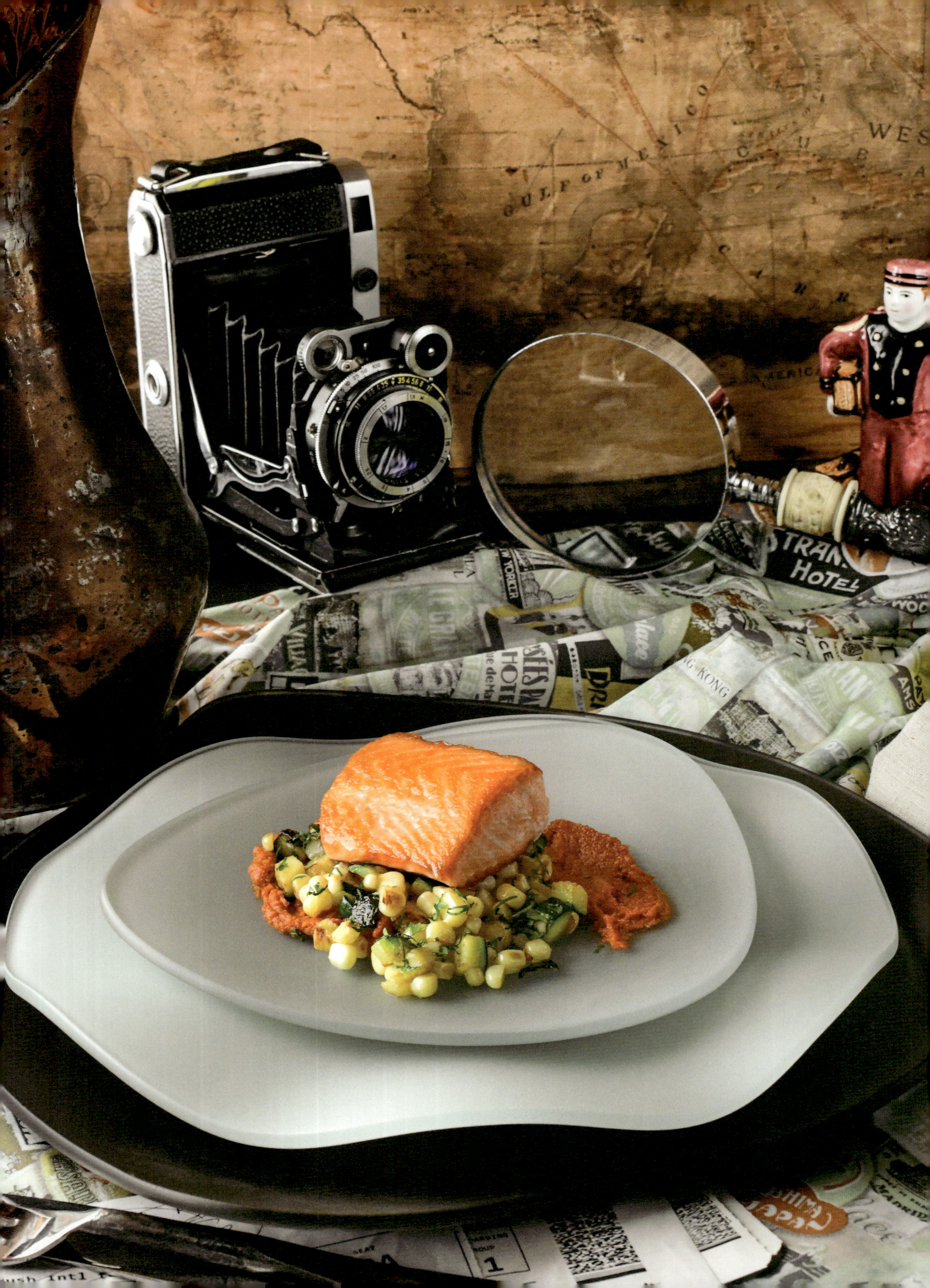
GULF OF MEXICO
HOTEL

ROASTED ŌRA KING SALMON
WITH ROMESCO SAUCE, SKILLET ZUCCHINI, AND CORN

SERVES 4

Ōra King salmon is considered by many experts as the finest of the salmon breeds. It is the largest species of Pacific salmon, and is now considered by many environmentalists to be endangered and overfished. In our efforts to support sustainably farmed seafood, we source our Ōra King salmon from New Zealand, where they are raised in clean, environmentally friendly ways. It is flown in fresh every day. Ōra has a unique, delicious buttery texture and is prized for its high fat content and abundant omega-3's. Romesco Sauce is a traditional Spanish dish that has a rich, earthy flavor.

ROMESCO SAUCE
(YIELDS ABOUT 2 CUPS)

3 medium tomatoes, cored and the skin on the bottom scored in an X

3 medium red bell peppers

8 garlic cloves, peeled and wrapped in foil with a teaspoon of extra-virgin olive oil

3 dried ancho chili peppers

½ cup slivered almonds

2 tablespoons sherry vinegar

⅓ cup extra-virgin olive oil

1 teaspoon smoked paprika

2 teaspoons sea salt

1 slice whole wheat bread, toasted and cubed (about 1 cup)

Preheat the oven to 350°F. Place tomatoes, bell peppers, and garlic on a baking sheet. Roast in the oven for 15-20 minutes. Remove the tomatoes and garlic and continue roasting the bell peppers another 10 minutes or so until the skin becomes blistered. Remove from the oven and allow to cool. Once cool enough to handle, remove the core and seeds from the bell peppers. Using your hands, remove the skins from the tomatoes and the peppers. Set aside.

While vegetables are roasting, bring two cups of water to a boil and add the ancho chili peppers. Remove from the heat and let the peppers sit for 15 minutes or until soft. Once softened and cooled, remove the seeds and stem. Set aside.

Place the almonds on a baking sheet and roast for 5-6 minutes or until golden brown.

Place all the ingredients except the bread in a food processor. Blend until smooth. Slowly pulse in the bread cubes so the sauce takes on a thick texture. Cover to keep warm.

SKILLET ZUCCHINI AND CORN

2 tablespoons extra-virgin olive oil

1 shallot, minced

1 garlic, minced

2 cups corn, cut from the cob

2 cups diced zucchini

3 tablespoons minced fresh cilantro

In a large skillet over medium heat, heat the oil. Add the shallots and garlic and sauté until translucent. Add the corn and zucchini and cook 3-5 minutes until softened. Fold in the cilantro and set aside. Keep warm.

SALMON PREPARATION

1 tablespoon grapeseed oil

kosher or sea salt and freshly ground black pepper

4 salmon fillets (4 ounces each), skinless

Preheat the oven to 350°F. Lightly salt and pepper the salmon fillets. In a 10-inch non-stick pan over medium-high heat, add the grapeseed oil. Add the salmon fillets and sear for 1-2 minutes. Flip the salmon over and place into the oven for 3-5 minutes, depending on the thickness of the salmon fillet.

To plate, place 2 tablespoons of Romesco Sauce in the middle of the plate. Lay the Skillet Zucchini and Corn across the sauce in a linear fashion and place the salmon on top.

TIP: Save the extra Romesco Sauce in the refrigerator. It will keep for a week or so. A very versatile sauce, it's perfect served with roasted chicken, pork, or fresh vegetables.

NUTRITION PER SERVING	Cal 410	Fat 27g	Protein 27g	Carbs 16g	Sugar 6g	Fiber 3g	Sod 146mg

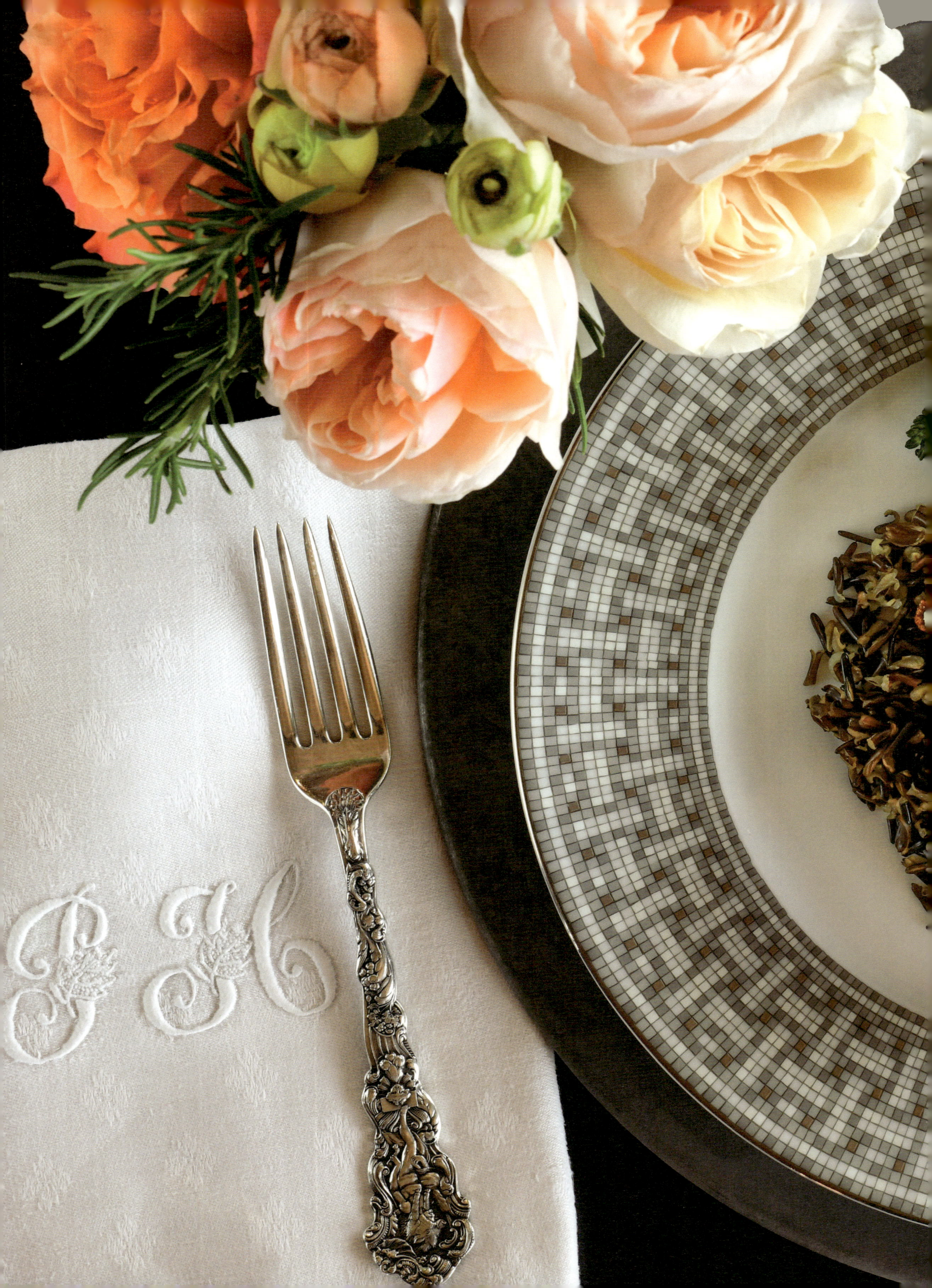

SEA BASS VERACRUZ
WITH WILD RICE AND BROCCOLINI

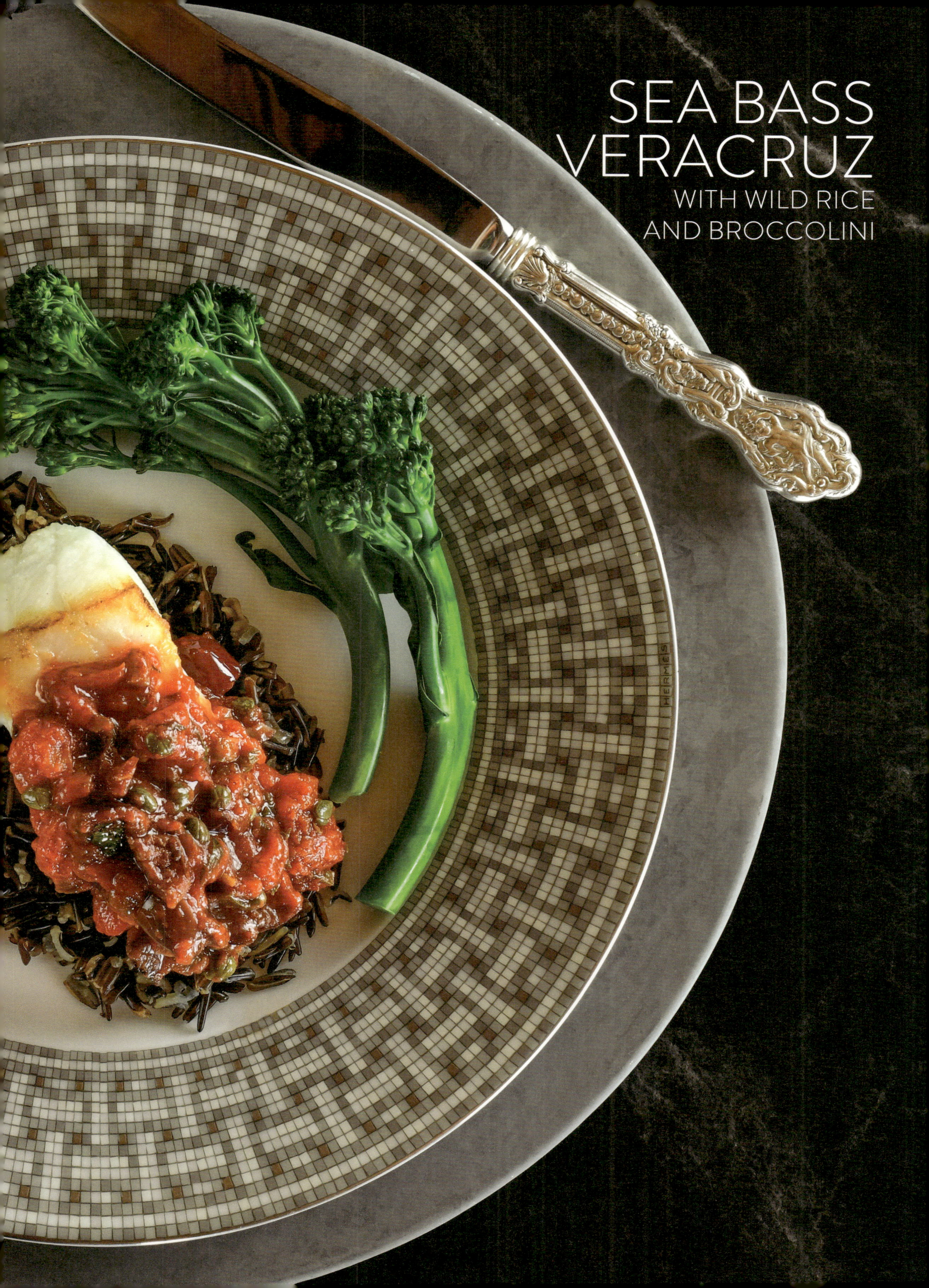

SEA BASS VERACRUZ
WITH WILD RICE AND BROCCOLINI

SERVES 4

Wild rice is actually a grass, so this meal fits the bill for guests trying out a grain-free diet. And sea bass is a great source of omega-3's, the healthy fat that has anti-inflammatory effects in your body. It's important to eat a variety of fish, usually in low-to-moderate mercury categories. (See "Mercury in Fish" on page 280.) Since sea bass contains a moderate amount of the metal, we recommend eating fewer than three servings per month. Keep in mind, too, that the 4-ounce portions the recipe calls for are about the size of a deck of cards.

VERACRUZ SAUCE

½ tablespoon extra-virgin olive oil
½ onion, thinly sliced
2 garlic cloves, minced
1 jalapeño pepper, seeded, diced
1 28-ounce can diced tomatoes, drained
1 fresh bay leaf
1 tablespoon chopped fresh oregano
1 tablespoon chopped fresh parsley
¾ cup sliced Kalamata olives
1 tablespoon capers, drained, rinsed

In a medium sauté pan over medium heat, add the olive oil. Add the onions, garlic, and jalapeños and slowly sauté until the vegetables are caramelized (about 10 minutes). Add the tomatoes, bay leaf, oregano, parsley, olives, and capers. Turn the heat down to a simmer and continue to cook for about 20 minutes. Remove from the heat, cover, and keep warm.

WILD RICE

2 cups vegetable stock
1 teaspoon kosher or sea salt
1 cup wild rice
¼ cup toasted almonds

In a medium saucepan over high heat, bring the vegetable stock to a boil. Add the salt and wild rice and turn down to a simmer. Cover with a lid and cook for 15 minutes or until the rice absorbs the liquid. Fold in the toasted almonds. Cover and keep warm.

BROCCOLINI

1 tablespoon extra-virgin olive oil
2 cups broccolini, the bottom third trimmed
1 tablespoon chopped fresh parsley

In a large sauté pan over medium heat, add the olive oil. Add the broccolini and sauté for about 2 minutes. Add 2 tablespoons of water and steam. Toss in the parsley. Remove from the heat and keep warm.

SEA BASS

1 pound sea bass (4 4-ounce portions), cleaned, skin on
kosher or sea salt
1 tablespoon grapeseed oil

Preheat the oven to 350°F. Lightly salt the sea bass. In a non-stick, oven-safe, sauté pan over medium-high heat, add the grapeseed oil. Sear the sea bass for about 1 minute on each side, or until you achieve a golden brown color. Place in the oven skin side down for about 7 minutes. Remove from the oven.

To assemble, place the Wild Rice in the middle of the plate with the Broccolini surrounding it and the Sea Bass on top, covered with the Veracruz Sauce.

NUTRITION PER SERVING	Cal 364	Fat 18g	Protein 28g	Carbs 26g	Sugar 3g	Fiber 5g	Sod 374mg

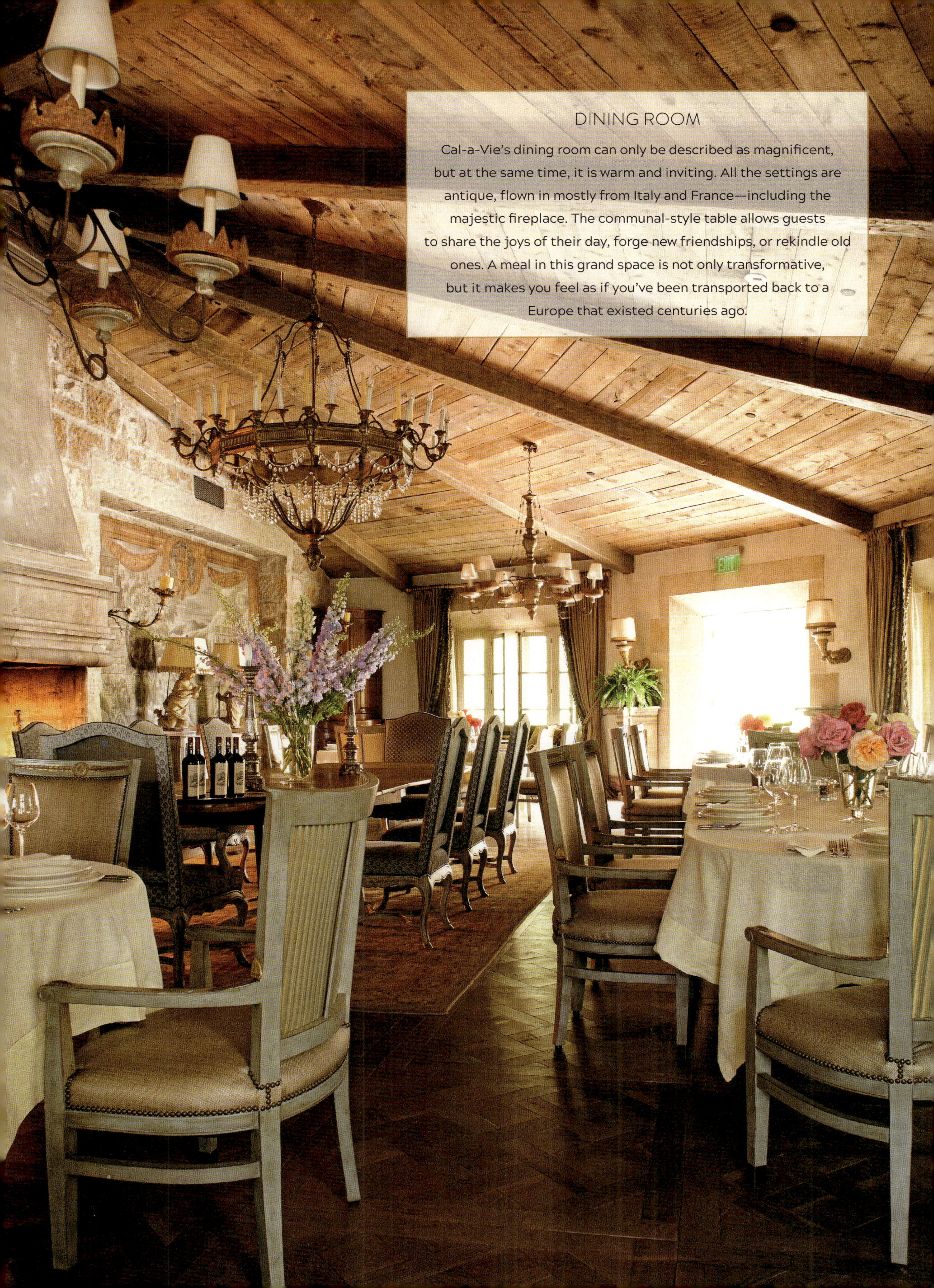

DINING ROOM

Cal-a-Vie's dining room can only be described as magnificent, but at the same time, it is warm and inviting. All the settings are antique, flown in mostly from Italy and France—including the majestic fireplace. The communal-style table allows guests to share the joys of their day, forge new friendships, or rekindle old ones. A meal in this grand space is not only transformative, but it makes you feel as if you've been transported back to a Europe that existed centuries ago.

HERB CHICKEN

WITH HEIRLOOM TOMATO PROVENÇAL, ZUCCHINI NOODLES, AND CALYPSO BEANS

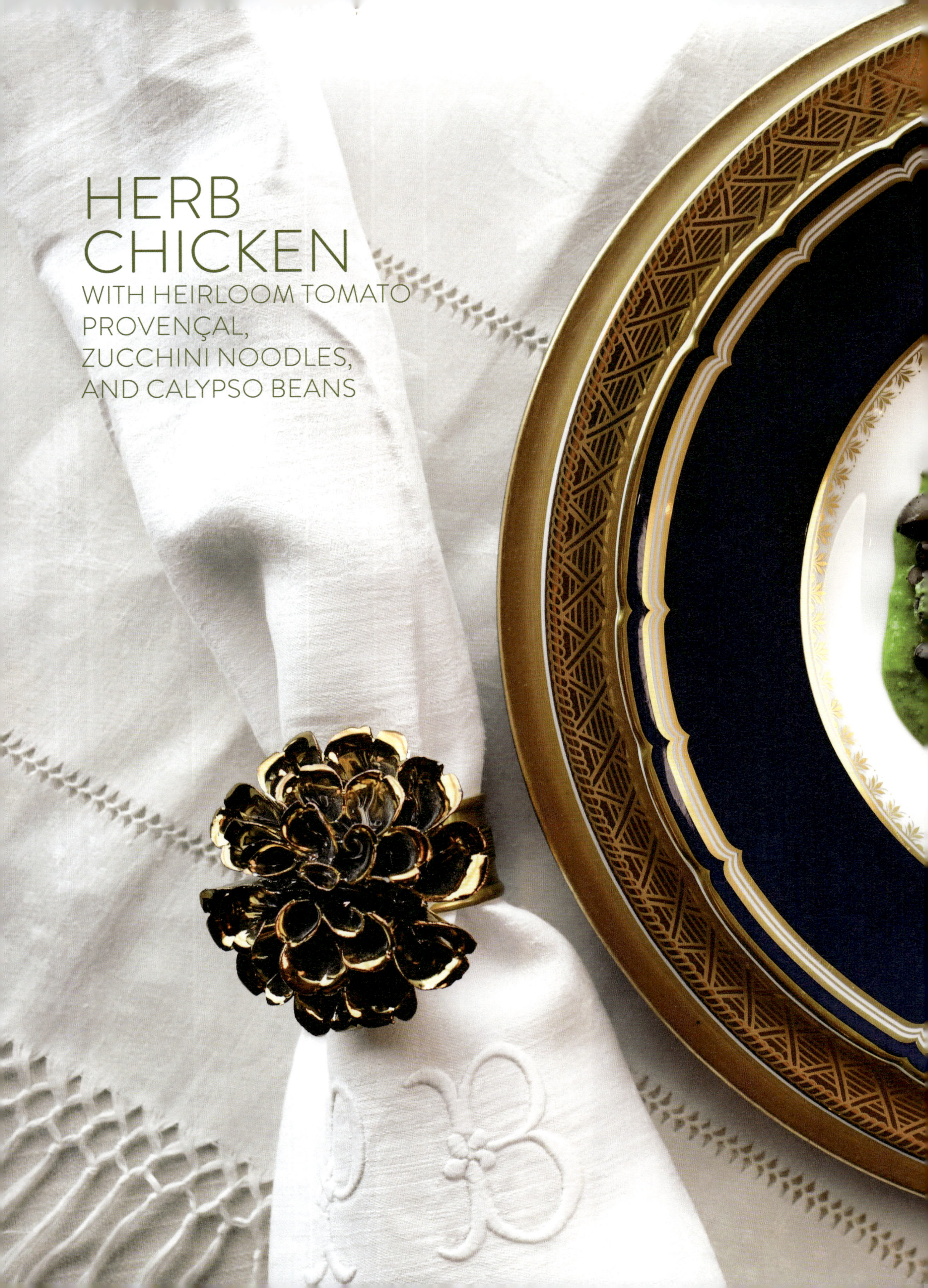

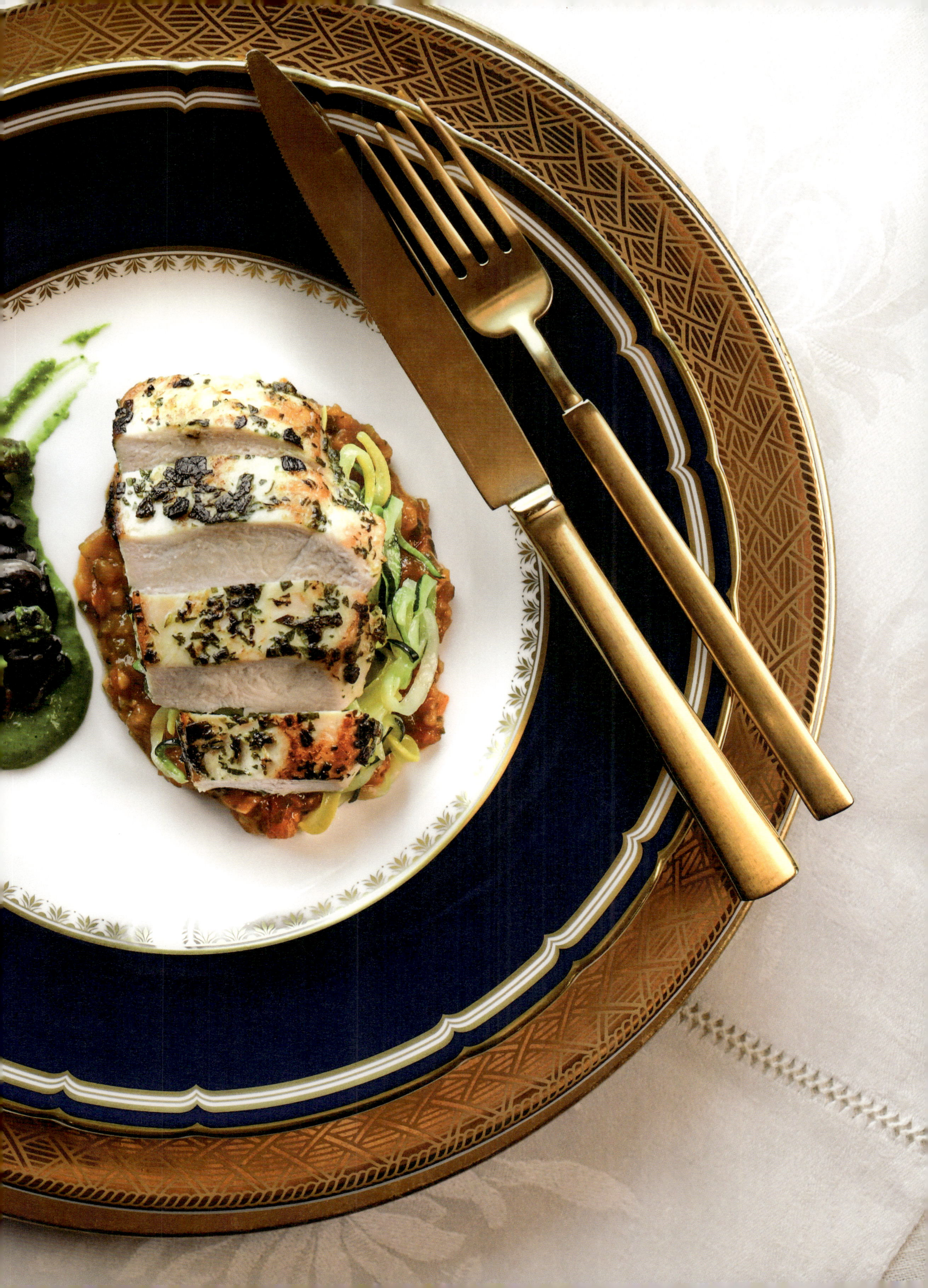

HERB CHICKEN
WITH HEIRLOOM TOMATO PROVENÇAL, ZUCCHINI NOODLES, AND CALYPSO BEANS

SERVES 4

This delicious meal features flavors from the South of France. Don't be intimidated by the four components of this dish; each is easy to make, and the final product is sure to wow your friends and family. The beans in this dish are a low-glycemic carbohydrate paired with soluble fiber and protein—so a little goes a long way toward keeping your blood sugar stable and making sure you're sated right up until bedtime.

BASIL PESTO

- 2 cups fresh basil leaves
- ½ cup pine nuts
- 3 teaspoons minced garlic
- ½ cup extra-virgin olive oil
- ½ cup water
- 2 teaspoons kosher or sea salt

In a blender, add all the ingredients and puree on high until very smooth. Set aside.

CALYPSO BEANS

- 2 cups Calypso beans
- 1 carrot, peeled and cut into large pieces
- 1 celery stalk, cut into large pieces
- ½ yellow onion, cut into large pieces
- 2 quarts water
- 2 tablespoons extra-virgin olive oil
- ½ cup Basil Pesto (more if necessary)

In a medium saucepan, bring the beans, carrots, celery, onion, and water to a boil. Reduce the heat to a simmer and cook the beans until you can easily crush one with your tongue on the roof of your mouth (about an hour). Strain the beans, discard the carrot, celery, and onion pieces, and let cool. In a medium sauté pan over high heat, add the olive oil. Once the oil is heated, add the beans and sauté until their exterior is crispy. Toss with the Basil Pesto. Set aside, cover, and keep warm.

HEIRLOOM TOMATO PROVENÇAL

- 1 tablespoon extra-virgin olive oil
- ¼ cup minced shallots
- 2 garlic cloves, minced
- ½ cup dry white wine (we recommend using Chardonnay)
- 2 cups baby heirloom tomatoes, halved
- 1 tablespoon finely chopped fresh basil
- 1 tablespoon finely chopped fresh oregano
- 1 tablespoon finely chopped fresh parsley
- 1 teaspoon sea salt

In a medium saucepan over medium-high heat, add the olive oil. When oil is heated, add the shallots and garlic and sauté for 1-2 minutes. Add the white wine and deglaze the pan. Simmer until reduced in half. Add the tomatoes, reduce heat to low, and simmer for about 20 minutes. Add the herbs and season with salt. Remove from the stove. Keep warm and set aside.

ZUCCHINI NOODLES

1 large zucchini, ends trimmed (packaged zucchini noodles are usually available in the grocery produce section)

1 teaspoon extra-virgin olive oil

1 garlic clove, minced

Using a turning slicer, slice the zucchini into long noodles. In a large skillet, heat the olive oil. Add the zucchini and garlic and sauté for about 4 minutes. Set aside, cover, and keep warm.

HERB CHICKEN

2 skinless, boneless chicken breasts (6 ounces each), sliced, 3 ounces per portion

1 tablespoon finely chopped fresh chives

1 tablespoon finely chopped fresh parsley

1 tablespoon finely chopped fresh tarragon

1 teaspoon sea salt

1 tablespoon grapeseed oil

Preheat the oven to 350°F. In a medium bowl, toss the chicken with the herbs and salt. In a large sauté pan over medium heat, add the grapeseed oil. Add the chicken and sauté on each side for 2-3 minutes to develop a nice golden brown color. Transfer the chicken breasts to a baking sheet and place in the oven for 4-6 minutes until they reach 165°F on a meat thermometer.

Remove from the oven and add to the Heirloom Tomato Provençal. Put a spoonful of Calypso Beans on one side of the plate and Zucchini Noodles on the other. Add the Herb Chicken with Tomato Provençal to the middle.

TIP: Kidney beans can be used if calypso beans are unavailable, though you can order calypso beans online. Our favorite specialty store for beans and other dry goods is the Chieftain Wild Rice Company in Wisconsin at www.chieftainwildrice.com.

NUTRITION PER SERVING	Cal 290	Fat 15g	Protein 27g	Carbs 10g	Sugar 3g	Fiber 4g	Sod 232mg

CORNISH GAME HENS
WITH GRILLED ZUCCHINI, ROASTED TOMATOES, AND CHIMICHURRI

SERVES 8 PEOPLE (½ BIRD EACH)

Cornish game hens are featured in fine dining restaurants for their attractive presentation possibilities, yet are easy for the home chef to prepare—and our Chimichurri adds bright and bold flavors to this juicy bird. While the hens are cooking, prepare the Chimichurri sauce, the Grilled Zucchini, and Roasted Tomatoes to make this meal in less than an hour. You'll impress your family and friends with kitchen skills that would make a five-star restaurant proud.

CORNISH GAME HENS

4 Cornish game hens (if frozen, make sure to properly defrost)

1 orange, quartered

1 lemon, quartered

4 garlic cloves

8 sprigs fresh thyme

kosher or sea salt

Preheat the oven to 350°F. Stuff each hen with ¼ orange, ¼ lemon, 1 garlic clove, and 2 sprigs of thyme. Truss the bird using butcher's twine and place in a roasting tray with a drip pan. Season the skin with salt.

Roast in the oven for about 45 minutes until the temperature inside reaches 165°F, making sure to measure the thickest part of the bird but not puncturing through to the cavity with the thermometer. Remove from the oven and allow to rest before slicing each hen in half, cutting around the backbone.

CHIMICHURRI SAUCE

1 cup fresh cilantro leaves

½ cup fresh oregano leaves

½ cup fresh mint leaves

2 tablespoons red wine vinegar

¼ cup extra-virgin olive oil

2 tablespoons water

½ teaspoon sea salt

1 garlic clove

In a blender, add all of the ingredients and puree until smooth. Set aside.

ROASTED TOMATOES

40 cherry tomatoes (mixed varieties are always good)

2 tablespoons extra-virgin olive oil

8 sprigs fresh thyme

kosher or sea salt

Preheat the oven to 350°F. In a large bowl, toss the tomatoes with the oil, thyme, and salt. Evenly spread out on a baking sheet. Place in the oven for about 8-10 minutes. The tomatoes should be lightly roasted, still retaining their shape. Remove and set aside.

GRILLED ZUCCHINI

2 large zucchinis, cut in half, lengthwise

2 teaspoons extra-virgin olive oil

1 teaspoon kosher or sea salt

4 tablespoons Chimichurri Sauce

Brush the front and back of the zucchini strips with olive oil. Heat the grill or use a grill pan, and cook the zucchinis for 2-3 minutes on each side, turning them 45 degrees once to get nice grill marks. Remove and slice into half-moon shapes. In a large bowl, mix with Roasted Tomatoes and Chimichurri Sauce.

Serve with Cornish Game Hens.

NUTRITION PER SERVING	Cal 439	Fat 33g	Protein 30g	Carbs 4g	Sugar 2g	Fiber 1g	Sod 204mg

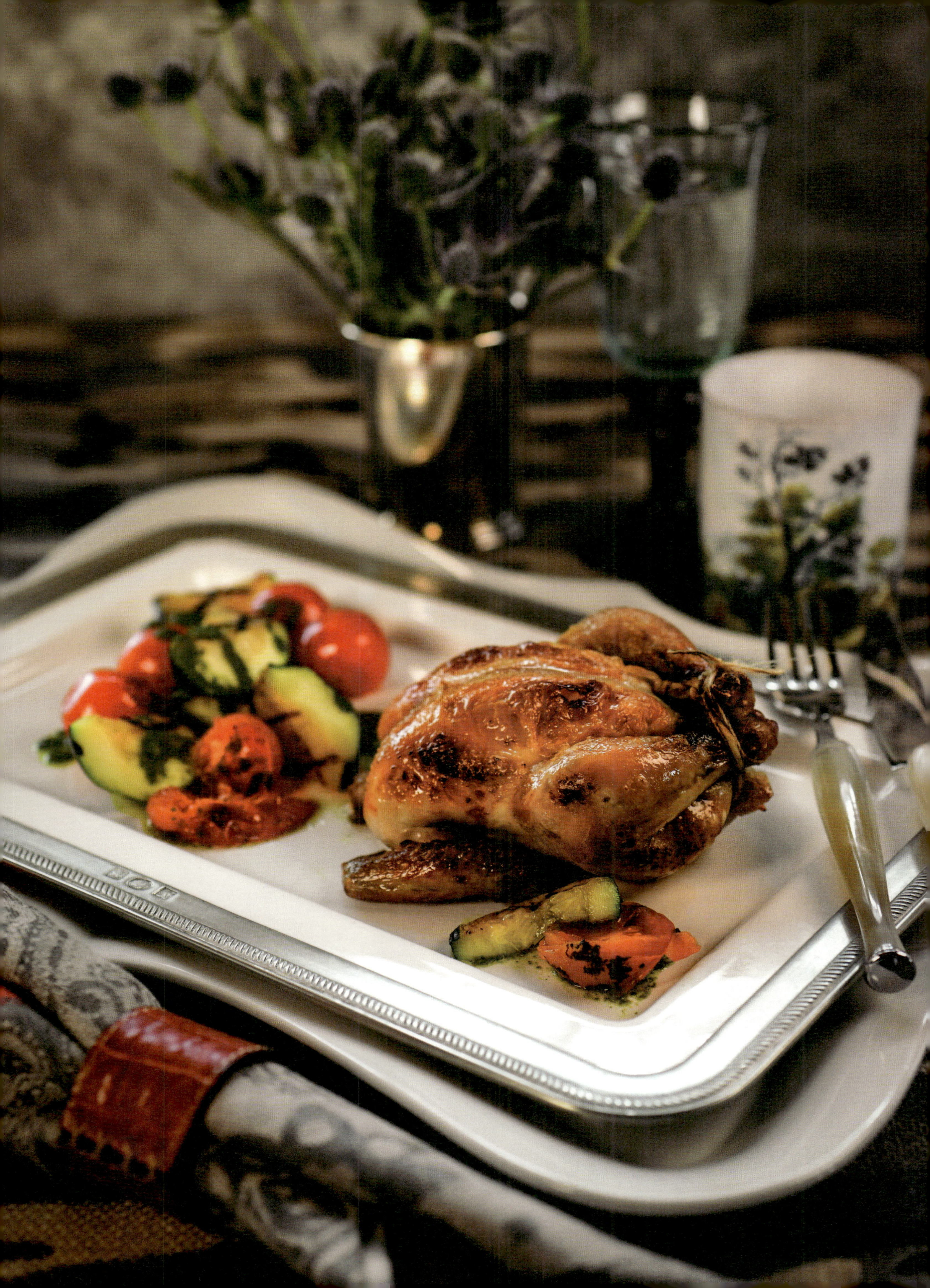

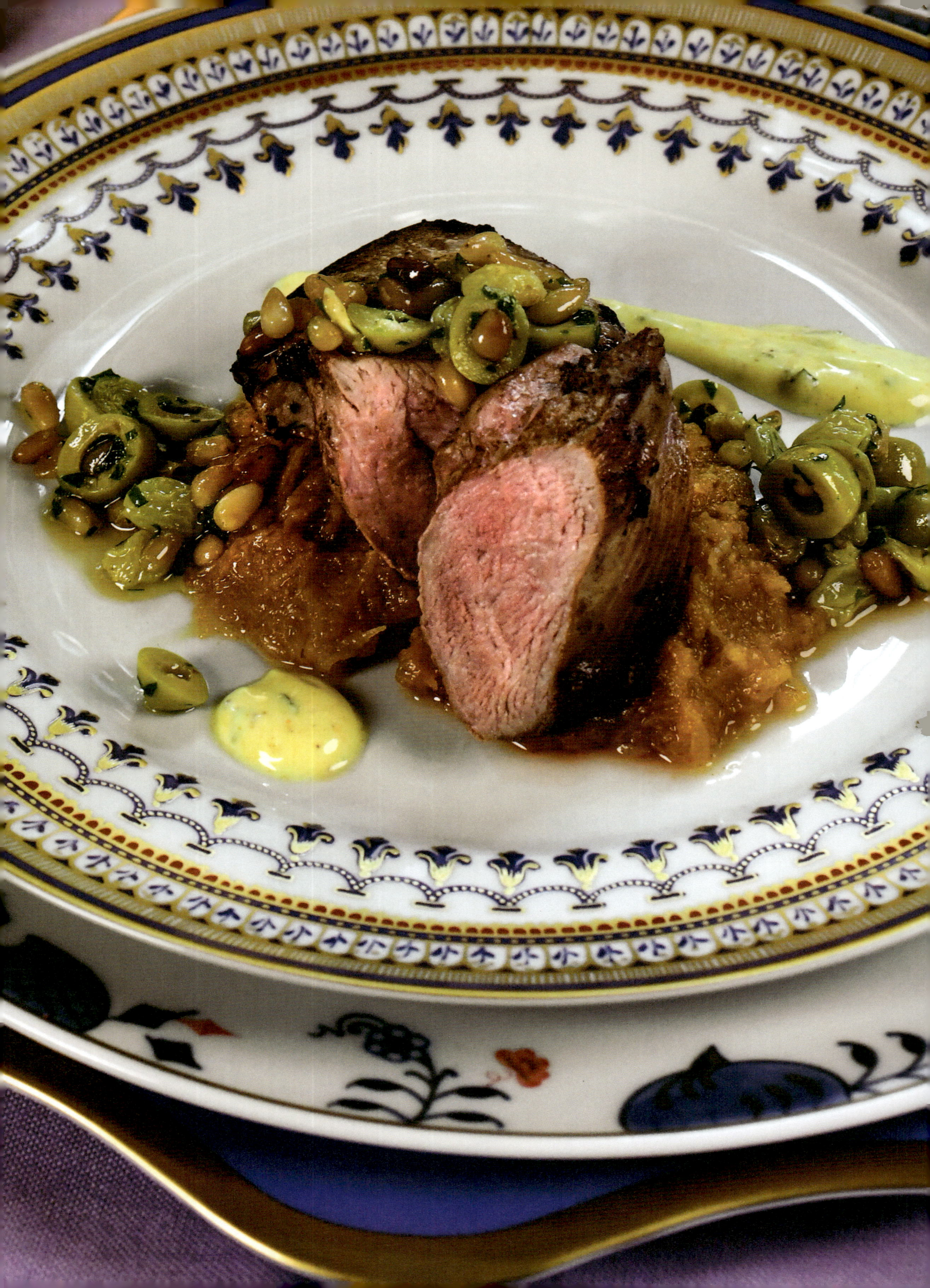

DUCK BREAST

WITH SPAGHETTI SQUASH, OLIVE GOLDEN-RAISIN RELISH, AND SPICED YOGURT

SERVES 4

People often keep duck out of their recipe repertoire because they don't know how to cook the breasts or would rather not take on roasting a whole duck. But our chef walks you through how to easily prepare succulent duck breasts with our unique olive relish, creating a heavenly meal and an unforgettable experience.

SPICED YOGURT

½ cup plain yogurt
1 teaspoon chopped fresh mint
¼ teaspoon turmeric
¼ teaspoon sumac

In a small bowl, whisk all the ingredients together. Set aside in the refrigerator.

OLIVE GOLDEN-RAISIN RELISH

½ cup golden raisins
½ cup pine nuts
½ cup pitted and quartered green olives
¼ cup extra-virgin olive oil
1 tablespoon chopped fresh chives
1 tablespoon chopped fresh parsley

In a small bowl, add the golden raisins and cover with hot water. Allow them to sit for 15 minutes to plump up. Drain the raisins and set aside. In a small sauté pan over medium heat, add the pine nuts and toast for 3-5 minutes, constantly moving the pan to avoid burning the nuts.

In a small bowl, combine the raisins, pine nuts, olives, olive oil, chives, and parsley. Mix thoroughly and set aside.

CHILI PASTE

3 garlic cloves
3 tablespoons + ½ teaspoon extra-virgin olive oil, divided use
1 teaspoon whole coriander seeds
1 teaspoon whole cumin seeds
1 teaspoon whole caraway seeds
5 dried pasilla chilis
1 dried aji amarillo chili
3 tablespoons water
kosher or sea salt

Preheat the oven to 350°F. In a small bowl, mix the garlic cloves with ½ teaspoon olive oil. Wrap the cloves in aluminum foil and place on a baking sheet. Roast for 12 minutes or until the garlic is soft, and set aside. In a small skillet over medium heat, mix the coriander, cumin, and caraway seeds. Stir for 2 minutes until the seeds are lightly toasted. Set aside.

In a small saucepan, bring 2 quarts of water to a boil. Add the dried chilis, turn off the heat, and allow the chilis to soak for 15 minutes. Take the chilis out of the pan and remove the stems and seeds. In a food processor, add the softened chilis, roasted garlic, toasted spices, 3 tablespoons olive oil, and 3 tablespoons water. Puree until completely smooth. Season with salt to taste. Set aside.

SPAGHETTI SQUASH

1 tablespoon extra-virgin olive oil

1 spaghetti squash, halved

¼ cup + 1 teaspoon Chili Paste

kosher or sea salt

Preheat oven to 350°F. Coat a sheet tray with olive oil. Using a spoon, remove the seeds from inside the spaghetti squash and discard. Coat each cut side of the squash with ¼ cup of Chili Paste (about 2 tablespoons per half). Carefully place the squash halves cut-side down on the oiled sheet tray. Place in the oven and roast until the skin has darkened, and a knife can easily be inserted into the flesh of the squash, about 40 minutes.

Remove the squash from oven. Using a fork, scrape the thin strands of squash from the outer skin and place in a large bowl. Fold in the remaining teaspoon of chili paste and season with salt to taste. Keep warm.

DUCK BREAST PREPARATION

4 duck breasts (6 ounces each), skin removed

kosher or sea salt

freshly ground black pepper, to taste

2 tablespoons grapeseed oil

Preheat the oven to 350°F. Season the duck breasts with salt and black pepper. In a large, oven-safe, sauté pan over medium heat, add the grapeseed oil. Add the duck breasts and sauté for about 3 minutes to give them a nice golden brown color. Flip the duck breasts and continue to cook for 1 minute. Transfer the breasts to the oven and roast until they're medium done, 4 minutes. Allow the breasts to rest for 3 minutes before slicing.

To plate, place ½ cup of the Spaghetti Squash in the middle of the plate. Spoon a tablespoon or two of Spiced Yogurt around the outside of the squash. Place the sliced duck breast on top of the squash. Spoon ¼ cup of Olive Golden-Raisin Relish on top of the duck, allowing it to spill over the breast.

NUTRITION PER SERVING	Cal	Fat	Protein	Carbs	Sugar	Fiber	Sod
	257	17g	18g	8g	5g	1g	116mg

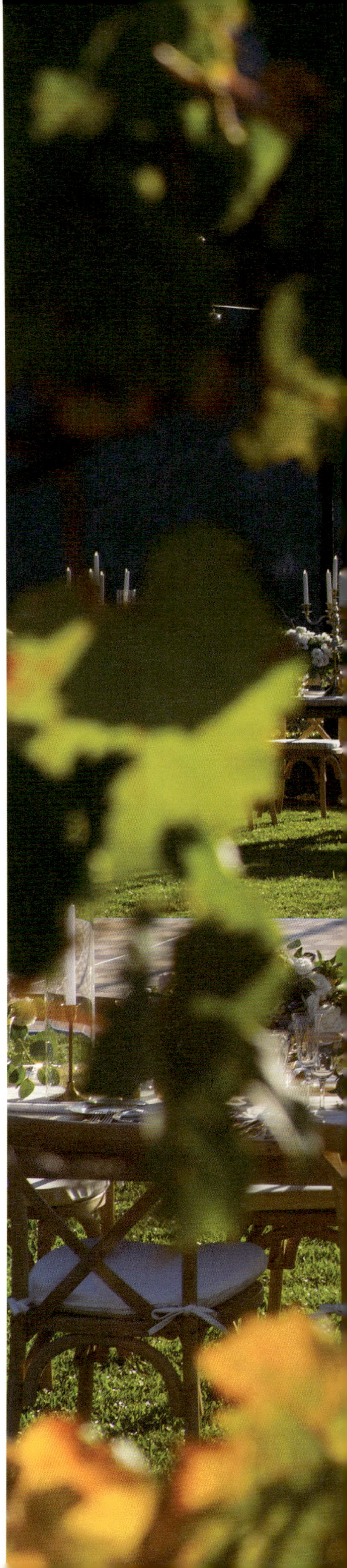

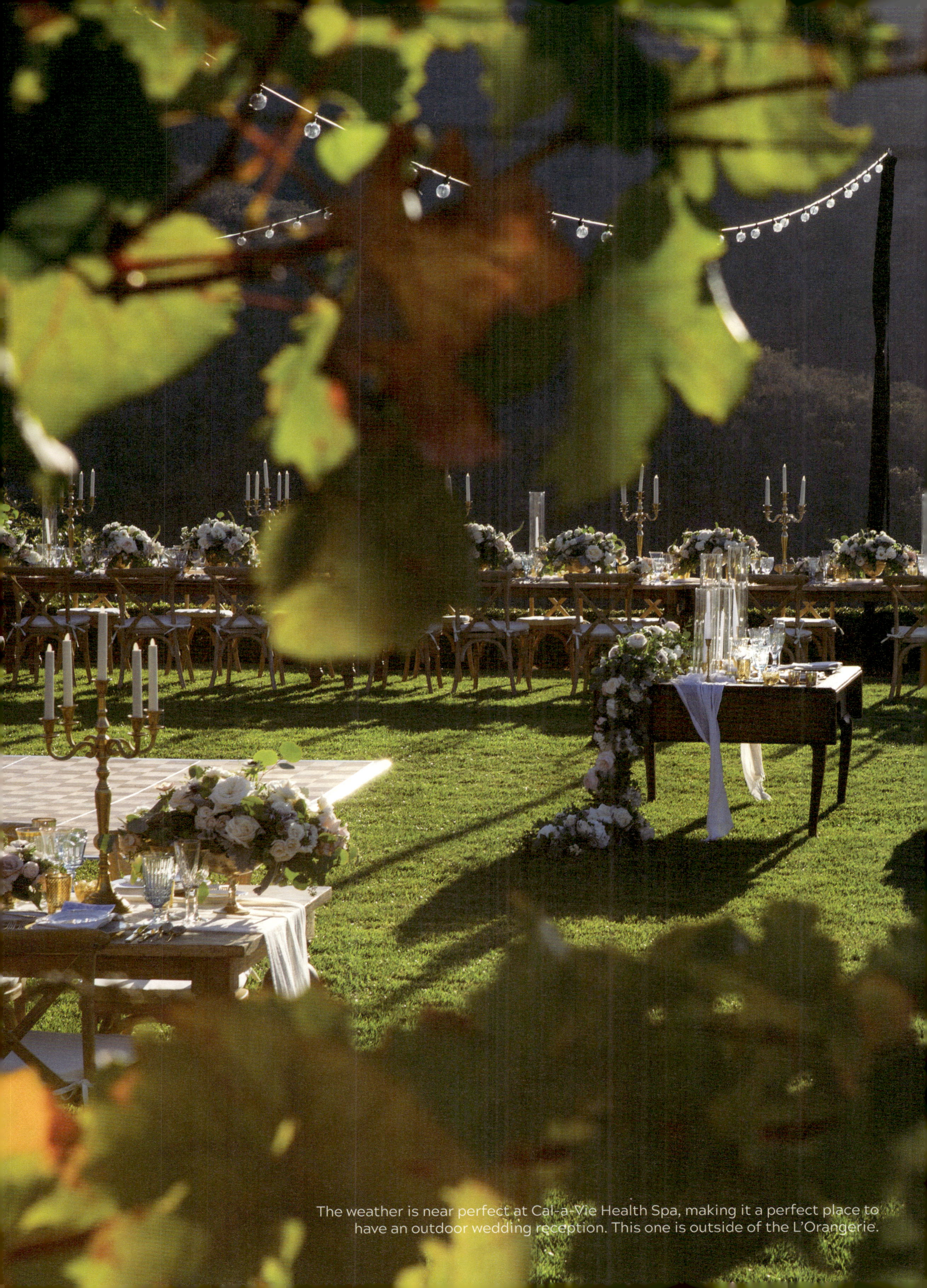

The weather is near perfect at Cal-a-Vie Health Spa, making it a perfect place to have an outdoor wedding reception. This one is outside of the L'Orangerie.

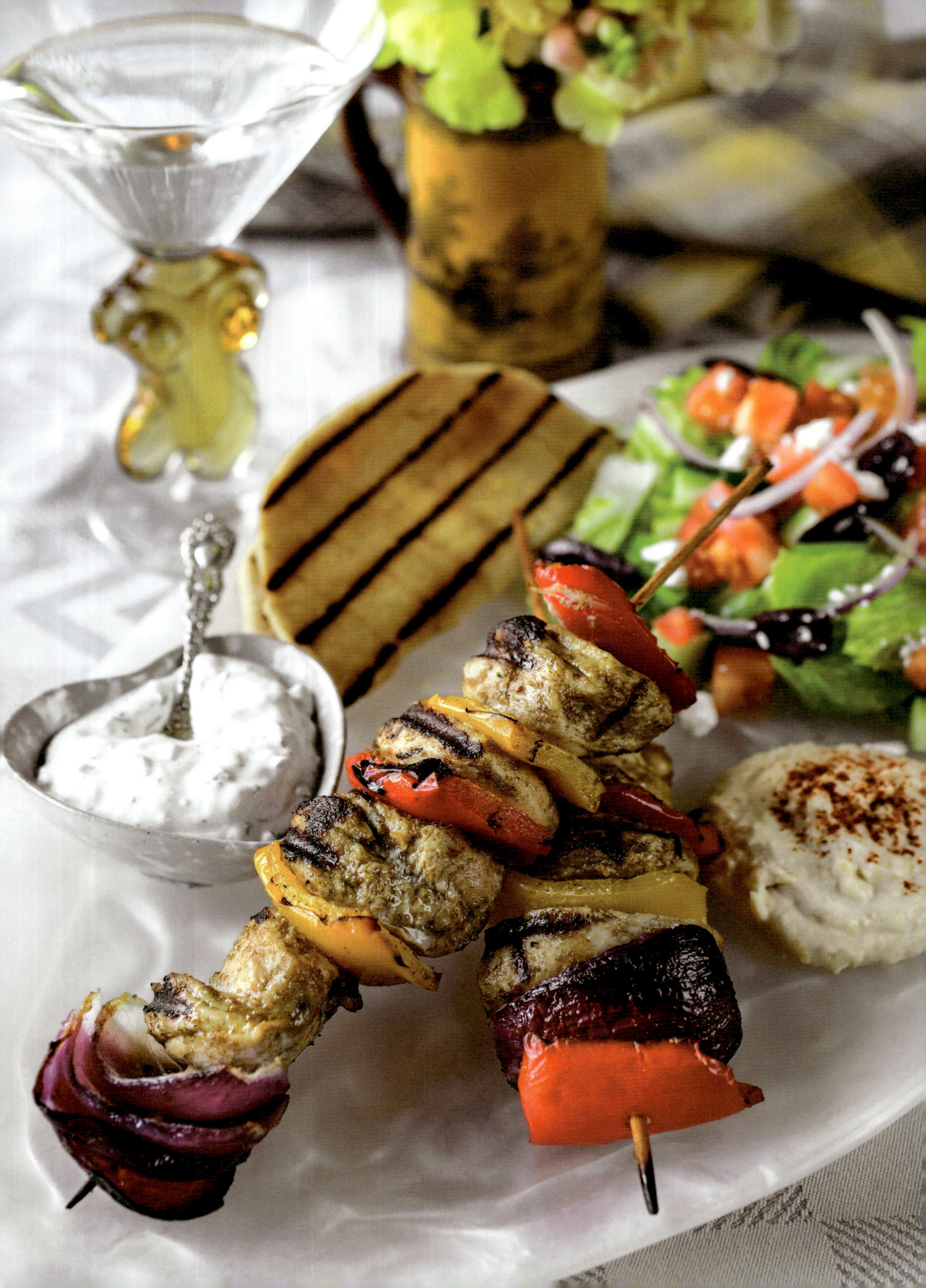

GRILLED CHICKEN KEBABS WITH
GARLIC FLATBREAD, TZATZIKI SAUCE, AND GREEK SALAD

SERVES 6

This Greek-inspired dish is fresh, colorful, and full of flavor. The chicken is marinated with rosemary, onion, garlic, cumin, and a little oil, then built onto skewers and served with homemade Tzatziki Sauce, Greek Salad, and fresh Garlic Flatbread. It's the perfect meal for your next outdoor BBQ.

GARLIC FLATBREAD

1 tablespoon dry active yeast

1 tablespoon honey

2 cups water at 105°F
(check with a thermometer)

2 cups high-gluten flour

2 cups organic whole wheat pastry flour

1 cup unbleached white flour

1½ tablespoons kosher salt

2 tablespoons extra-virgin olive oil

cornmeal

Combine the yeast, honey, and warm water in a small bowl. Stir to combine and let stand for 15 minutes at room temperature. It should become foamy. In a large bowl, combine the flours and salt and mix well. Set aside.

In a large electric mixer using the dough-hook attachment, add the yeast mixture. Start turning the yeast mixture on low while adding the flour mixture 1 cup at a time and alternating with the olive oil. The mixture should form into a ball. If it looks too dry, add a couple drops of water and keep mixing until it forms into a tight ball. If the mixture is too sticky, add a couple pinches of high-gluten flour until the mixture forms into a ball. Let the dough mix at low speed for 8 minutes. Remove the dough and knead for 1 minute on a floured flat surface to release any gases. Form into a ball and place in a large mixing bowl coated with non-stick cooking spray. Coat the dough lightly with the spray and cover the bowl with plastic wrap. Let rise at room temperature near a warm heat source (about 80-84°F) for 1½-2 hours. It should double in size.

Remove the dough and cut into 36 portions, about 4 ounces each. Using your hands, roll them into small dough balls about the size of golf balls and place on a baking sheet pan coated with non-stick spray. Lightly spray the tops and cover with a slightly damp towel and then plastic wrap. Chill overnight in the refrigerator.

CHICKEN KEBABS

2 cups fresh rosemary leaves

2 cups sliced yellow onions

6 garlic cloves, smashed

1 cup grapeseed oil

¼ cup cumin

12 chicken breasts (6 ounces each), skinless, boneless, each cut into 3 pieces

3 red bell peppers, cut into 2-inch squares

3 yellow bell peppers, cut into 2-inch squares

3 red onions, cut into 2-inch squares

12 9-inch long bamboo skewers

kosher salt

In a small bowl, combine the rosemary leaves, onion, garlic, oil, and cumin to make the marinade. Toss the chicken with the marinade and marinate for 6 hours in the refrigerator.

RED WINE VINAIGRETTE

1 cup red wine vinegar
⅓ cup honey
2 tablespoons Dijon mustard
1 teaspoon sea salt
½ cup water
1½ cups grapeseed oil

In a blender, combine all the ingredients except the grapeseed oil. While the blender is on high, slowly add the grapeseed oil until incorporated and emulsified. Set aside in the refrigerator.

GREEK SALAD

2 cups garbanzo beans (if using canned beans, rinse first)
2 cups chopped cucumber
2 cups chopped tomato
1 cup sliced red onion
1 cup Kalamata olives, halved
½ cup capers, rinsed
½ cup crumbled feta cheese
½ cup fresh oregano leaves
12 cups chopped romaine lettuce

In a large bowl, add all the ingredients and toss to combine. Set aside in the refrigerator.

TZATZIKI SAUCE

2 cups plain yogurt, strained
½ cup peeled, diced cucumber
1 tablespoon minced garlic
2 tablespoons chopped fresh dill
¼ cup extra-virgin olive oil
1 tablespoon fresh lemon juice
⅛ teaspoon cayenne pepper
1 teaspoon sea salt

In a small bowl, combine all the ingredients and mix until thoroughly incorporated. Set aside in the refrigerator.

GARLIC OIL

1 cup olive oil
6 garlic cloves, peeled

Preheat the oven to 350°F. In a small oven-safe saucepan or small baking dish, add the olive oil and garlic cloves. The garlic should be submerged in the olive oil. Cover with foil and place in the oven. Bake for 30 minutes, or until the garlic is soft. Refrigerate.

GRILLED GARLIC FLATBREAD

flour

Garlic Oil

grapeseed oil, optional

Preheat the grill to high heat. Remove the flatbread dough balls from the refrigerator. On a lightly floured surface, roll them out one at a time so they resemble thin round tortillas. Brush the tops with the Garlic Oil and place on the grill for one minute on each side so they have nice grill marks. If you don't have a grill, these can be done in a skillet with a small amount of grapeseed oil in the pan. Set aside, keeping the flatbreads warm.

GRILLED CHICKEN KEBABS

12 marinated chicken breast pieces

3 red bell peppers, cut into 2-inch squares

3 red onions, cut into 2-inch squares

3 yellow bell peppers, cut into 2-inch squares

12 9-inch long bamboo skewers

kosher salt

Remove the chicken from the refrigerator and discard the used marinade. Cut the breasts into large chunks. Build the skewers by placing a piece of chicken on first. Add a piece of red bell pepper, then a piece of chicken, followed by a piece of red onion, a piece of chicken, yellow bell pepper, and red onion. Continue building the skewers. Lightly season the skewers with salt and place on the grill for 10-15 minutes until chicken is ready. Check with a meat thermometer to see that it reaches 165°F. Remove when cooked and keep warm.

ASSEMBLY

8 cups Greek Salad

1 cup Red Wine Vinaigrette (add more if necessary)

12 pepperoncinis

1 cup Tzatziki Sauce

12 pieces Garlic Flatbread

When ready to serve, remove the Greek Salad from the refrigerator and toss with the Red Wine Vinaigrette. On a large platter, place the Grilled Chicken Kebabs, Greek Salad, pepperoncinis and the Garlic Flatbread. Serve with the Tzatziki Sauce on the side.

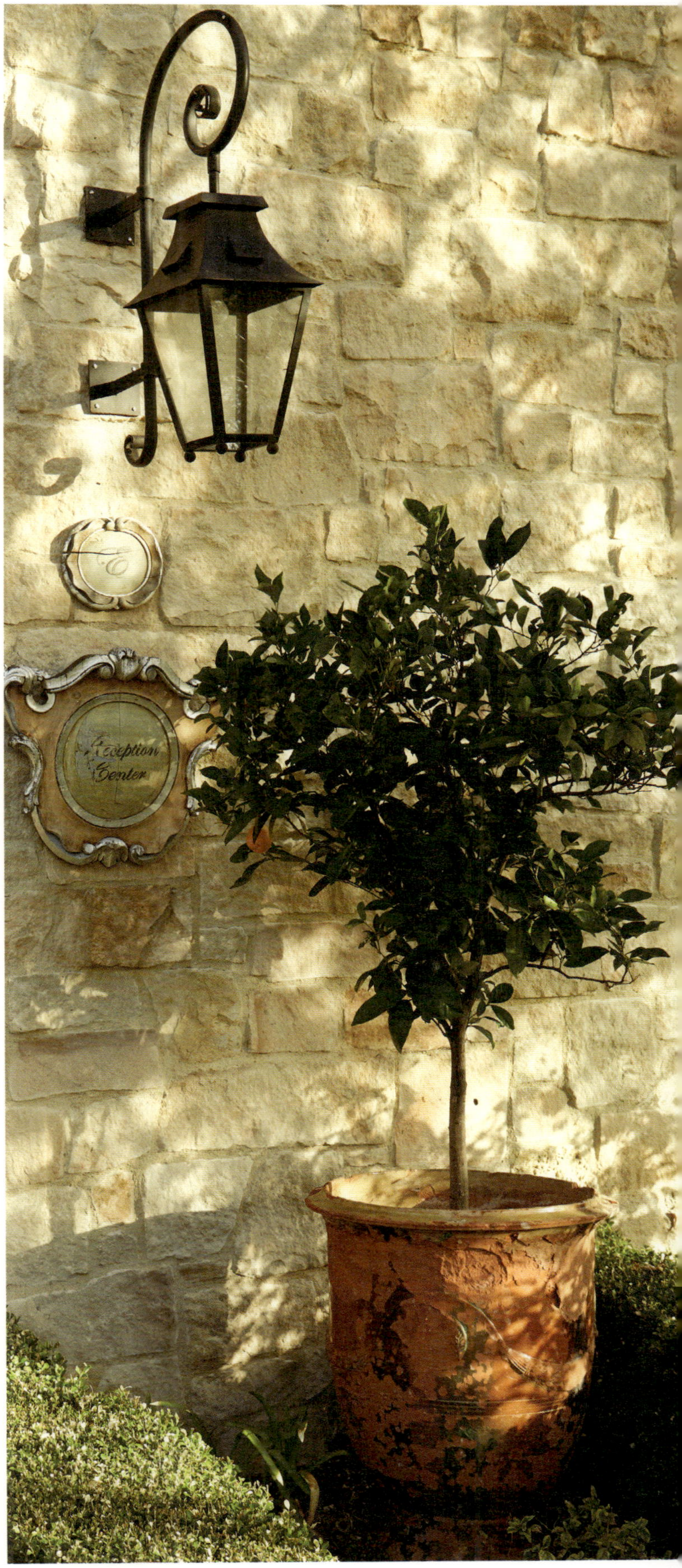

NUTRITION PER SERVING	Cal 417	Fat 19g	Protein 28g	Carbs 35g	Sugar 7g	Fiber 4g	Sod 414mg

CAL-A-VIE PIZZA THREE WAYS

For those who desire the comforting nostalgia of pizza while staying waistline friendly, our pizza recipe is an absolute must. Our homemade crust is well worth a little extra effort to take your pizza from ordinary to extraordinary. The fresh flavors and textures, which can only be achieved from a little labor of love, makes our pizza one of the most sought-after recipes from our guests. Pizza can be part of a healthy eating plan by having two petite slices as the side that accompanies a salad as your main entrée.

PIZZA DOUGH

YIELDS 32 8-INCH PIZZAS

DOUGH PREPARATION

- 1 tablespoon active dry yeast
- 1 tablespoon honey
- 2 cups water at 105°F (check with a thermometer)
- 2 cups high-gluten flour
- 2 cups whole wheat pastry flour
- 1 cup unbleached white flour
- 1½ tablespoons kosher salt
- 2 tablespoons extra-virgin olive oil
- cornmeal

Combine the yeast, honey, and warm water in a small bowl. Stir to combine and let stand for 15 minutes at room temperature. It should become foamy.

In a large bowl, combine the flours and salt and mix well. Set aside.

In a large electric mixer using the dough-hook attachment, add the yeast mixture. Start turning the yeast mixture on low while adding the flour mixture one cup at a time and alternating with the olive oil. The mixture should form into a ball. If it looks too dry, add a couple drops of water and keep mixing until it forms into a tight ball. If the mixture is too sticky, add a couple pinches of high-gluten flour until the mixture forms into a ball. Let the dough mix at low speed for 8 minutes. Remove the dough and knead for 1 minute on a floured flat surface to release any gases. Form into a ball and place in a large mixing bowl coated with non-stick cooking spray. Coat the dough lightly with the spray and cover the bowl with plastic wrap. Let rise at room temperature near a warm heat source (about 80-84°F) for 1½-2 hours. It should double in size.

Remove the dough and cut into 3-ounce portions. On a flat surface dusted with flour, use the palm of your hand to roll the dough into balls that are slightly bigger than a golf ball but smaller than a baseball. Place the dough balls on a baking sheet pan that has been sprayed with non-stick spray. Spray the tops of the balls, cover with a slightly damp dish towel, and then cover with plastic wrap. Chill overnight in the refrigerator.

Remove from the refrigerator and let sit at room temperature for about 15 minutes. Lightly spray a baking sheet with non-stick spray and dust with cornmeal. On a flat surface dusted with flour, roll out the dough balls using a rolling pin. Turn the dough 90 degrees after each roll so you will get perfect 8-inch circles. Place on the baking sheet.

Top the pizza dough with one of the recipes below and bake according to directions.

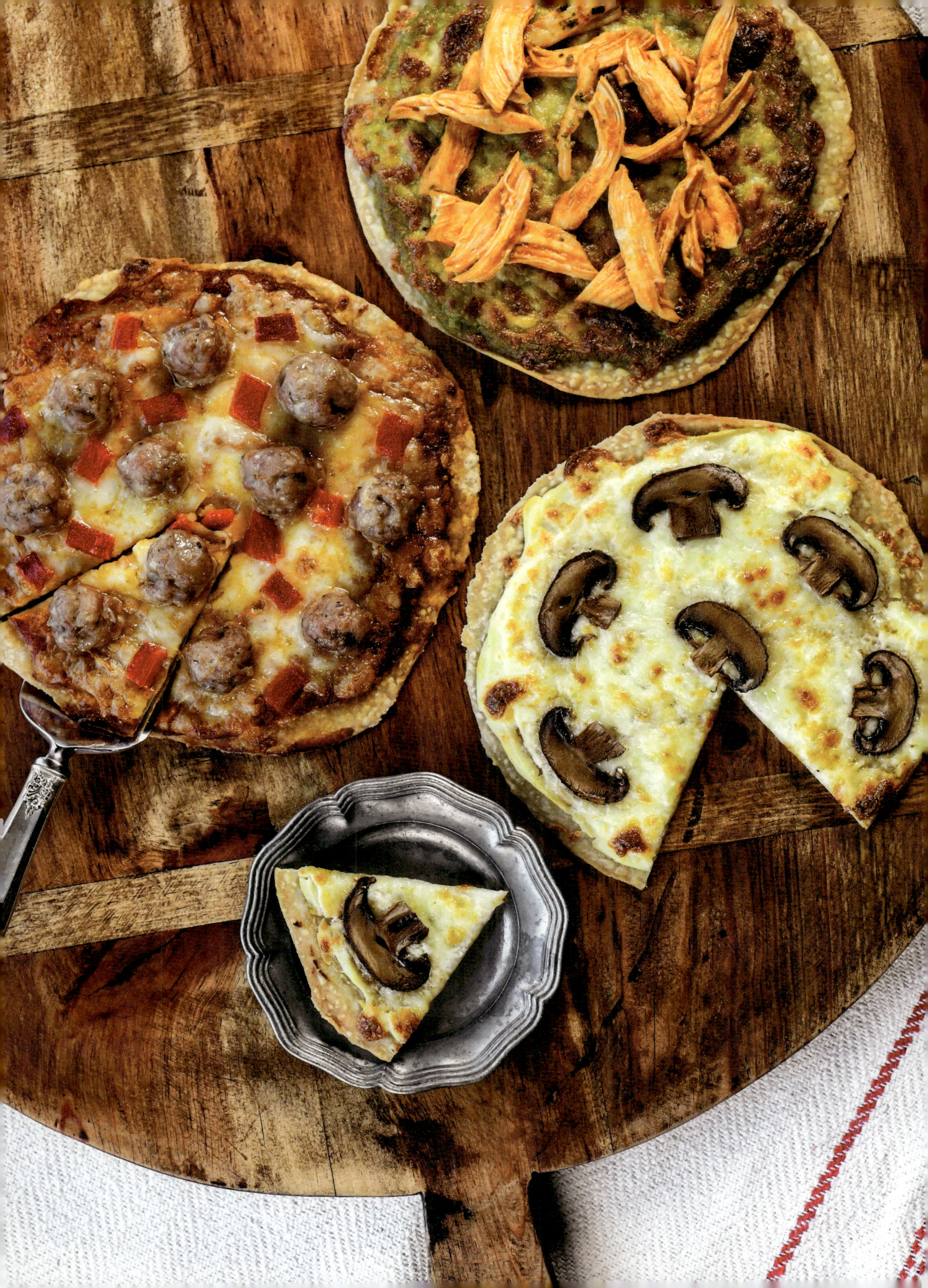

BBQ CHICKEN AND PESTO PIZZA

SERVES 3 (1/3 PIZZA)

JALAPEÑO PESTO

10 jalapeños, seeds and veins removed (more jalapeños can be added for personal taste)

6 garlic cloves

½ cup onion, cut into large pieces

½ cup whole almonds, toasted

¼ cup shredded Parmesan cheese

1 cup extra-virgin olive oil

1 teaspoon kosher or sea salt

In a blender, combine all of the ingredients and puree until smooth. Set aside.

BBQ SAUCE

1 teaspoon grapeseed oil

½ cup sliced onions

1½ garlic cloves, sliced

2 cups ketchup

1½ tablespoons apple cider vinegar

1½ tablespoons honey

¼ cup Worcestershire sauce

1½ tablespoons molasses

½ teaspoon freshly ground black pepper

½ teaspoon kosher or sea salt

In a medium saucepan over medium heat, add the grapeseed oil. Add the onions and garlic and sauté until caramelized, turning an amber color. Add the ketchup, vinegar, honey, Worcestershire sauce, and molasses. Simmer for 10 minutes. Stir in freshly ground black pepper and salt. Remove from the heat and cool.

In a blender, add the mixture and puree. Set aside.

BBQ CHICKEN

4 chicken breasts (6 ounces each)

kosher or sea salt

freshly ground black pepper

2 tablespoons grapeseed oil

1 cup BBQ Sauce

¼ cup shredded mozzarella cheese

Preheat the oven to 350°F. Season the chicken with salt and pepper. In a large sauté pan over medium heat, add the grapeseed oil. Add the chicken, and sauté on each side for about 2-3 minutes to develop a nice golden brown color. Transfer the chicken breasts to a baking sheet, and place in the oven for 4-6 minutes until the chicken reaches 165°F on a meat thermometer. Once the chicken is cool enough to handle, shred and mix with the BBQ sauce. Set aside.

Spread ¼ cup of the Jalapeño Pesto evenly over each pizza dough circle, leaving a ½-inch border. Sprinkle with a ¼ cup of mozzarella. Bake in the oven for 6 minutes. Remove and add ½ cup of shredded BBQ Chicken evenly over each pizza, and place back in the oven for an additional 4 minutes. Remove and let rest 1 minute before cutting into pieces.

NUTRITION PER SERVING	Cal 199	Fat 14g	Protein 7g	Carbs 12g	Sugar 5g	Fiber 1g	Sod 275mg

MARINARA AND TURKEY SAUSAGE PIZZA

SERVES 3 (1/3 PIZZA EACH)

MARINARA SAUCE

2 tablespoons extra-virgin olive oil

3 cups diced yellow onions

4 garlic cloves, minced

3 tablespoons tomato paste

½ cup dry red wine

3 pounds tomatoes (about 6 large tomatoes or 48 ounces canned)

1 tablespoon fennel seed

1 teaspoon chili flakes

1 teaspoon sea salt

1 teaspoon freshly ground black pepper

2 cups fresh basil, leaves torn

In a large sauce pot, over medium heat, add the olive oil. Add the onions and sauté for about 7 minutes. When the onions start to turn brown and caramelize, add the garlic and sauté for 1 minute. Add the tomato paste and stir until it turns brick red in color. Deglaze with the red wine and reduce by half. Add the tomatoes, fennel seed, chili flakes, salt, black pepper, and basil. Simmer for about 30 minutes. Transfer the tomato mixture to a blender and puree in batches until completely smooth. Set aside and let cool.

TIP: This recipe can be halved if you don't want any extra. However, if you keep it in a tightly covered container, it will store in your refrigerator for a week.

TOPPINGS

2 cups shredded mozzarella cheese

½ pound turkey sausage, rolled into small balls

3 red bell peppers, roasted, peeled, seeded, and diced

Preheat the oven to 350°F. Spread ¼ cup of the Marinara Sauce evenly over the pizza dough circle leaving a ½-inch border. Spread ¼ cup of mozzarella on top of the marinara. Place the small balls of turkey sausage over the mozzarella and sprinkle the red bell peppers evenly over the pizzas. Bake in the oven for 6 minutes. Rotate the pan and bake for an additional 4 minutes. Remove and let rest 1 minute before slicing into pieces.

NUTRITION PER SERVING	Cal 123	Fat 6g	Protein 8g	Carbs 8g	Sugar 2g	Fiber 1g	Sod 307mg

GARLIC AND MUSHROOM PIZZA

SERVES 3 (1/3 PIZZA EACH)

GARLIC OIL/ROASTED GARLIC

½ cup garlic cloves

1 cup extra-virgin olive oil

Preheat the oven to 350°F. Place garlic and olive oil in a small pan, cover with aluminum foil and place in the oven. Roast for 30 minutes or until the garlic is softened and roasted. Set aside and cool. Store in the refrigerator.

WHITE SAUCE AND ASSEMBLY

2 cups ricotta cheese

6 Roasted Garlic cloves

1 teaspoon sea salt

¼ teaspoon freshly ground black pepper

2 cups shredded mozzarella cheese

12 cremini or white button mushrooms, sliced

In a food processor, combine the ricotta cheese, Roasted Garlic, salt, and pepper and blend until completely smooth. Set aside.

Preheat the oven to 350°F. Brush the pizza dough with a tablespoon of Garlic Oil. Spread ¼ cup of the White Sauce evenly on top, leaving a ½-inch border. Sprinkle ¼ cup of mozzarella and place the sliced mushrooms over the mozzarella. Bake in the oven for 6 minutes. Rotate the pan and bake for an additional 4 minutes. Remove and let rest 1 minute before cutting into pieces.

NUTRITION PER SERVING	Cal 91	Fat 5g	Protein 4g	Carbs 7g	Sugar 1g	Fiber 1g	Sod 117mg

TURKEY BURGERS
ON HOMEMADE WHEAT BUNS WITH SWEET POTATO FRIES AND ALMOND COLESLAW

SERVES 8

A healthy (yet delicious) take on a classic American meal, this turkey burger is made even tastier with a light homemade Herb Mayonnaise and Sautéed Red Onions. Served with crisp Sweet Potato Fries and an Almond Coleslaw with our Citrus Vinaigrette, it is savory and filling and satisfies your burger cravings. Don't let the length of this recipe intimidate you. It's actually easy and well worth the effort.

Sweet potatoes come in many colors. The skin can be white, yellow, red, purple, or brown, and the flesh can be white, yellow, orange, or purple. However, in the United States, there are two main varieties: One has a golden skin with creamy white flesh and a crumbly texture, while the other is bright orange and sweet tasting.

HOMEMADE BURGER BUNS

YIELDS 8-10 BUNS

DOUGH PREPARATION

- 1 tablespoon dry active yeast
- 1 tablespoon honey
- 2 cups water at 105°F (check with a thermometer)
- 2 cups high-gluten flour
- 2 cups whole wheat pastry flour
- 1 cup unbleached white flour
- 1½ tablespoons kosher salt
- 2 tablespoons extra-virgin olive oil
- cornmeal

Combine the yeast, honey, and warm water in a small bowl. Stir and let stand for 15 minutes at room temperature. It should become foamy.

In a large bowl, combine the flours and salt and mix well. Set aside.

In a large electric mixer using the dough-hook attachment, add the yeast mixture. Start turning the yeast mixture on low while adding the flour mixture one cup at a time and alternating with the olive oil. The mixture should form into a ball. If it looks too dry, add a couple drops of water and keep mixing until it forms into a tight ball. If the mixture is too sticky, add a couple pinches of high-gluten flour until the mixture forms into a ball. Let the dough mix at low speed for 8 minutes. Remove the dough and knead for 1 minute on a floured flat surface to release any gases. Form into a ball and place in a large mixing bowl coated with non-stick cooking spray. Coat the dough lightly with the spray and cover the bowl with plastic wrap. Let rise at room temperature near a warm heat source (about 80-84°F) for 1½-2 hours. It should double in size.

Remove the dough from the bowl and cut into 8 to 10 evenly portioned dough balls about the size of a baseball. Place on a baking sheet lined with parchment paper and sprinkle with cornmeal. Press firmly on each dough ball with the palm of your hand, flattening them out to burger bun size. Spray the tops with non-stick spray, cover with plastic wrap and allow to rise for 1-2 hours until doubled in size.

Preheat the oven to 400°F. When the buns are ready, bake them on the middle rack for 15 minutes then lower the temperature to 325°F until the bottoms are golden brown, about 5-10 minutes more. Remove and cool on a rack for about an hour.

TIP: If you don't want to bake the buns immediately after you have formed them, they can be covered with a damp towel and then plastic wrap and chilled in the refrigerator overnight.

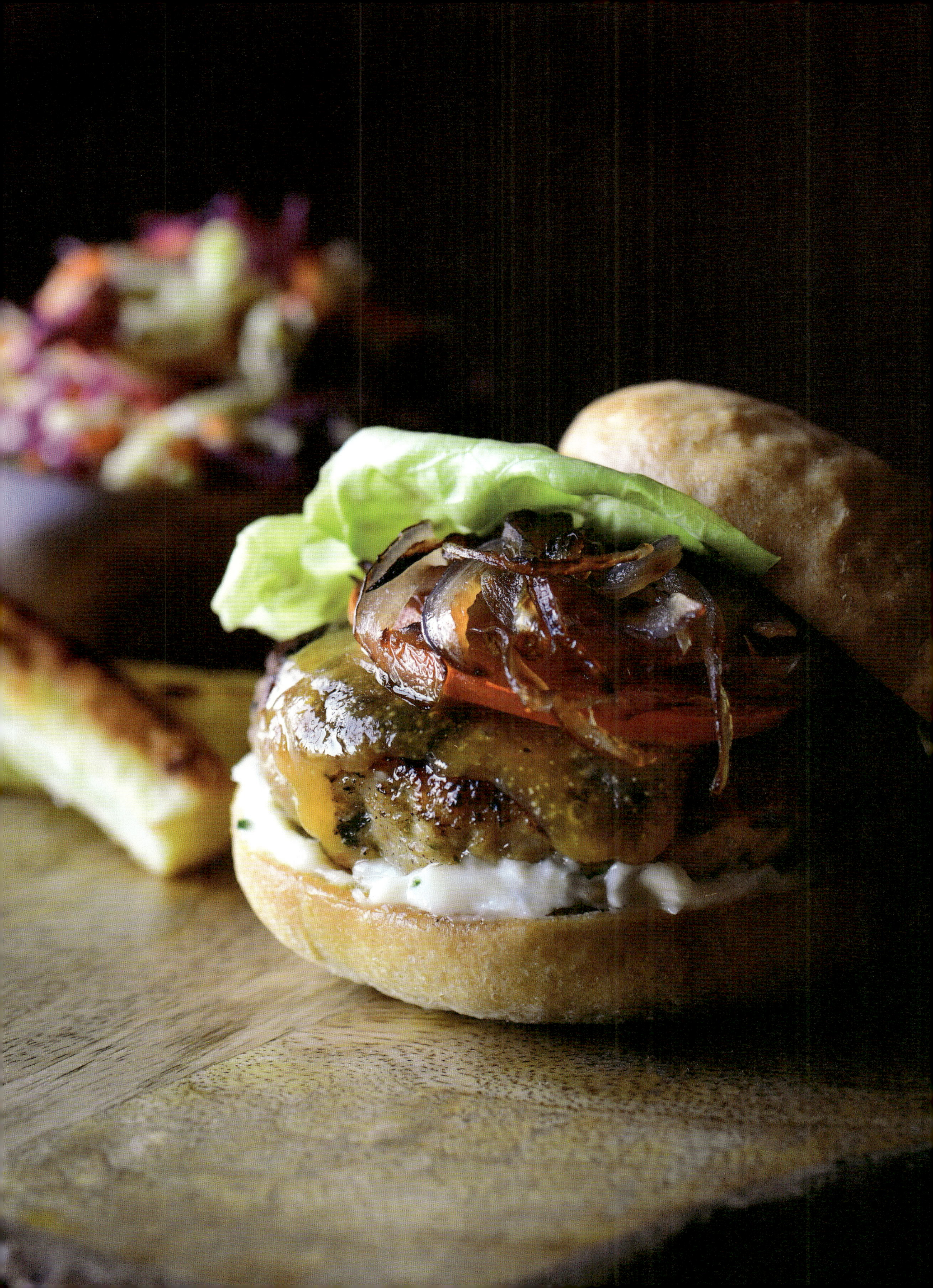

HERB MAYONNAISE

2 cups chopped fresh Italian parsley

1 cup fresh basil leaves

½ cup fresh tarragon leaves

2 tablespoons fresh thyme leaves

2 jars Spectrum® mayonnaise (we recommend the vegan, light-canola version)

2 tablespoons fresh lemon juice

2 teaspoons sea salt

½ teaspoon freshly ground black pepper

Puree all the herbs in a food processor until smooth. Scrape down and add the mayonnaise, lemon juice, salt, and pepper. Puree for another minute. Cover and chill in the refrigerator for at least 1 hour.

TIP: Our Herb Mayonnaise can be paired with just about any protein and also makes a nice dip to use with fresh vegetables. This recipe can also be halved if you don't want any extra. However, if you keep it in a tightly covered container, it will store in your refrigerator for a week.

ALMOND COLESLAW

2 cups thinly sliced red cabbage

4 cups thinly sliced green cabbage

2 cups peeled, grated carrots

2 cups chopped almonds, toasted

1 cup Citrus Vinaigrette (see recipe page 116)

In a large bowl, add all the ingredients and mix to combine. Cover and set aside in the refrigerator.

SAUTÉED RED ONIONS

2 teaspoons grapeseed oil

2 cups sliced red onions

In a medium sauté pan over medium-high heat, warm the oil. Add the red onions and slowly sauté for about 10 minutes, or until they turn a deep brown color. Remove from the stove, cover, and keep warm.

SWEET POTATO FRIES

2 large sweet potatoes, peeled, cut into 1x4-inch wedges (about 24 pieces)

2 tablespoons grapeseed oil

kosher salt and pepper

Preheat the oven to 400°F. In a large bowl, toss the sweet potato wedges with the oil. Lay on a baking sheet and roast for about 20-25 minutes, turning every 5 minutes until lightly browned. Remove from the oven and toss with salt and pepper to taste. Keep warm.

TURKEY BURGERS

2 pounds ground turkey

⅓ cup chopped fresh parsley

⅓ cup chopped green onions

1 egg

2½ tablespoons bread crumbs

1 teaspoon freshly ground black pepper

2 teaspoons kosher salt

2½ tablespoons Worcestershire sauce

2½ tablespoons balsamic vinegar

Mix all ingredients in a large bowl. Divide the meat mixture into 8 patties that are smooth and flat. Place on a parchment-lined baking sheet. In a large skillet coated with cooking spray over medium heat, add 4 of the patties about 1-inch thick, smooth, and flat. Cook for 5 minutes until crispy and browned, then flip to the other side for about 5 minutes more. Check to make sure the temperature in the middle is 165°F and the center is no longer pink. Set aside and keep warm. Repeat with the remaining 4 patties.

SERVE: Assemble the burgers and serve with Almond Coleslaw and a handful of Sweet Potato Fries.

NUTRITION PER SERVING	Cal 537	Fat 26g	Protein 31g	Carbs 47g	Sugar 9g	Fiber 7g	Sod 553mg

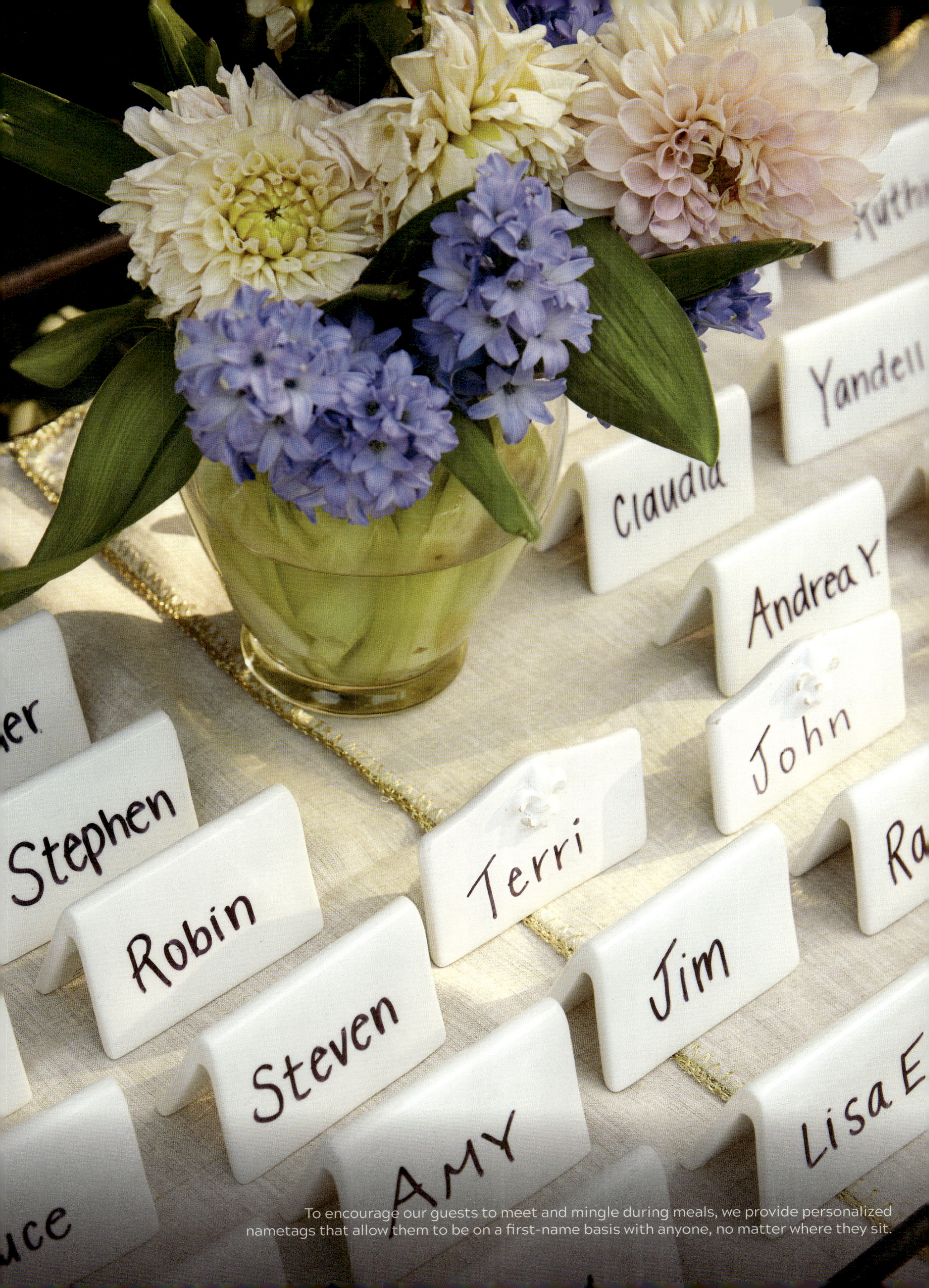

To encourage our guests to meet and mingle during meals, we provide personalized nametags that allow them to be on a first-name basis with anyone, no matter where they sit.

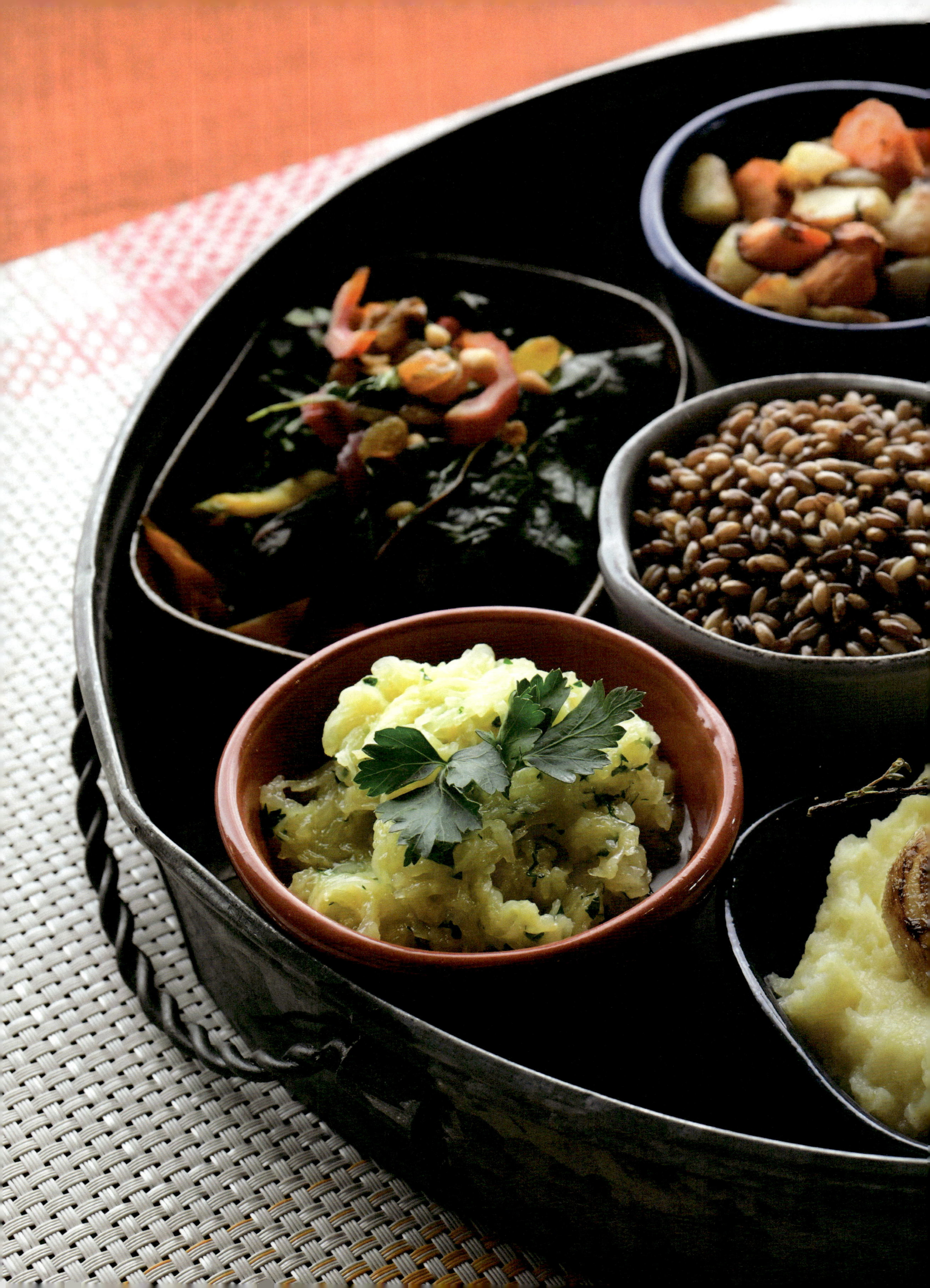

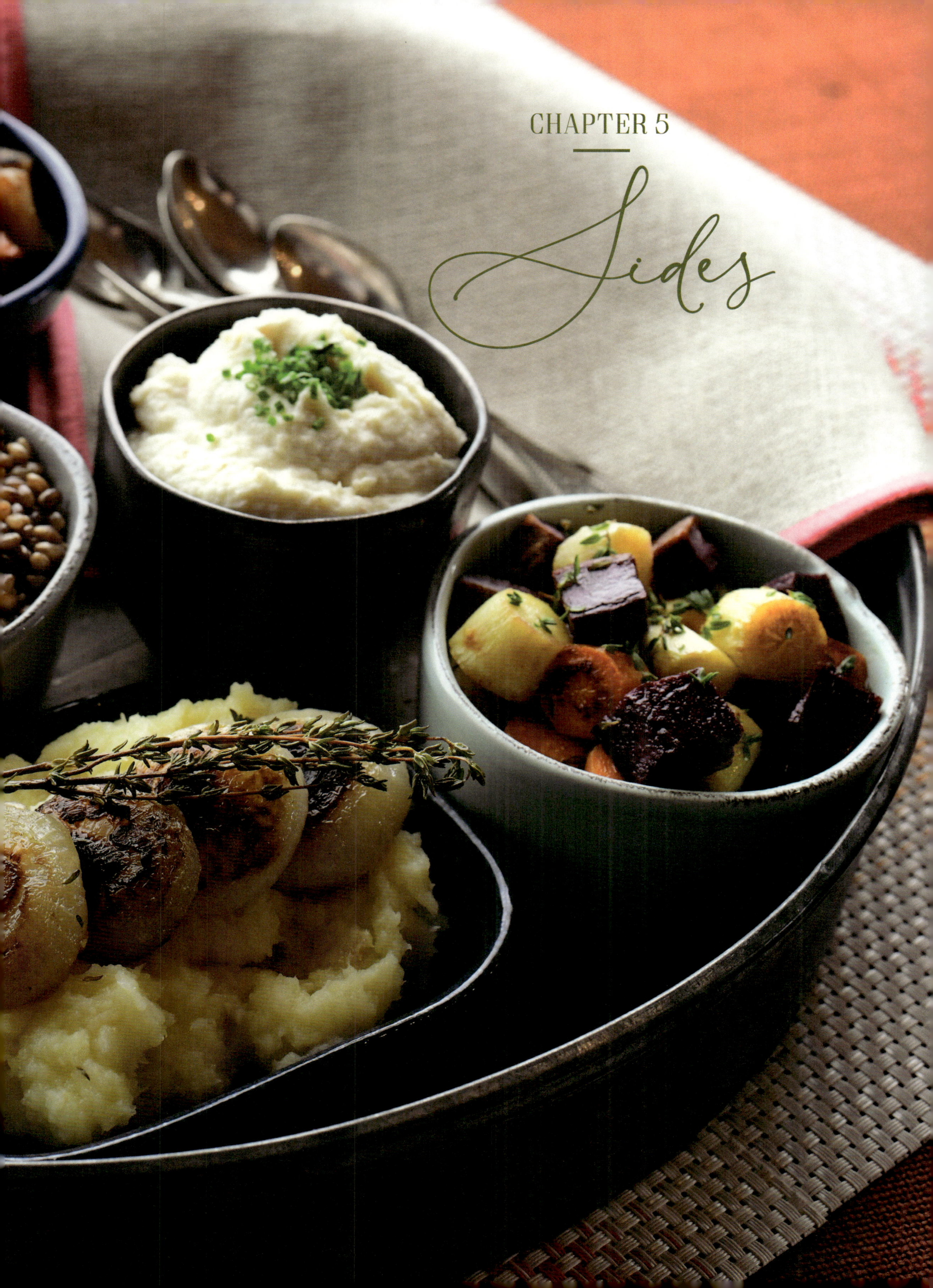

CHAPTER 5

Sides

CELERY ROOT MASH

SERVES 4 (YIELDS ABOUT 2 CUPS, ½ CUP PER SERVING)

Celery root, an ugly, knotted-up root vegetable also known as celeriac, can look a little intimidating at the grocery store. Don't underestimate how delicious it can be when served like mashed potatoes. This substitution helps to increase the fiber and decrease the total carbs of any meal.

- 1 pound celery root, peeled, ends trimmed, and cut into large, even-sized pieces
- 3 garlic cloves
- 1¼ teaspoon kosher or sea salt, plus more to taste
- diced fresh chives for garnish

In a medium pot, add the celery root pieces, garlic, and 1 teaspoon salt and cover with water. Bring to a boil and allow to cook for about 7-8 minutes until tender, so a knife can easily be inserted into the celery root. Drain, reserving about 1 cup of the cooking liquid. Return the cooked celery root to the hot pot and heat over medium-low heat until the excess water has evaporated.

Add the celery root to the bowl of a food processor. (You'll want to use this instead of a blender to avoid overprocessing.) Add ¼ teaspoon salt. Process, slowly adding the starchy cooking water, 1 tablespoon at a time, until a fluffy, smooth consistency is achieved (around ¾-1 cup total water). Taste and season with more salt as desired. Garnish with fresh chives.

NUTRITION PER SERVING	Cal 51	Fat 14g	Protein 3g	Carbs 39g	Sugar 6g	Fiber 8g	Sod 56mg

ROASTED ROOTS

SERVES 8

This is a colorful, flavorful side to pair with many entrées. Consider roasting a big batch of this to have on hand for a snack or to throw on a salad. The purple yams add so much sweetness, you'll think you are eating dessert instead of vegetables!

- 2 cups carrots, peeled, trimmed, and sliced 1-inch thick
- 2 cups parsnips, peeled, trimmed, and sliced 1-inch thick
- 2 cups purple yams, peeled, trimmed, and sliced 1-inch thick
- 8 sprigs fresh thyme
- 6 sprigs fresh rosemary
- ¼ cup extra-virgin olive oil
- kosher or sea salt to taste

Preheat the oven to 400°F. In a large bowl, toss the root vegetables, thyme, and rosemary sprigs with the olive oil and season with salt, to taste. Spread evenly on a baking sheet and roast in the oven for about 20 minutes, or until the roots are caramelized and soft. Remove and garnish with the roasted thyme leaves. Serve immediately.

TIP: For even cooking, it's important to try to cut the vegetables so they are similar in size.

NUTRITION PER SERVING	Cal 141	Fat 7g	Protein 1g	Carbs 19g	Sugar 3g	Fiber 4g	Sod 28mg

CARROT SUNCHOKE HASH

SERVES 4

Sunchokes, also known as Jerusalem artichokes, aren't actually related to artichokes at all. They are tubers of a species of sunflowers. But more important, they're a great source of inulin, a type of prebiotic fiber. Prebiotics help to feed the healthy bacteria in your gut, contributing to a healthy digestive system.

½ pound carrots, trimmed and peeled

½ pound sunchokes, trimmed and peeled

½ pound pearl onions (red or white), peeled and halved

2 tablespoons grapeseed oil

1 cup water

2 tablespoons finely chopped fresh parsley

Chop the carrots and sunchokes using the "oblique cut" technique. Holding the carrot or sunchoke across the cutting board and starting at one end, make a diagonal cut (also called a bias cut) about ½-inch in size and then roll the vegetable a quarter turn. Make another diagonal ½-inch cut and repeat, rotating the vegetable a quarter turn after every cut until you reach the end. This should result in similarly shaped and sized pieces.

Heat a large skillet over medium heat and add grapeseed oil. Once the oil is heated, add carrots, sunchokes, and pearl onions. Lower heat to medium-low and allow to slowly caramelize while regularly moving the vegetables around in the pan to cook evenly, about 20 minutes. If the vegetables are browning too quickly, lower the heat a bit more. Once everything has turned a deep golden brown, carefully add ¼ cup water. Allow the vegetables to cook in the water until it boils away and continue to add more water, ¼ cup at a time, until the vegetables have softened, about 5 minutes more.

Remove the pan from the heat and fold in the chopped parsley before serving warm.

NUTRITION PER SERVING	Cal 149	Fat 7g	Protein 2g	Carbs 20g	Sugar 11g	Fiber 4g	Sod 47mg

BLACK BARLEY

SERVES 4

Black barley is an heirloom variety of the healthy, high-fiber, high-protein cereal grain. Its dark exterior and chewy texture make it a visually appealing and palate-pleasing side. However, its most important benefit is that it can go from "farm to table" without processing or loss of nutrients since it doesn't need to be hulled.

½ cup black barley

2 cups water, plus more as needed

¼ teaspoon kosher or sea salt

Combine the barley, water, and salt in a small sauce pot. Bring to a boil. Cover and lower the heat to a simmer. Allow the barley to cook for 50 minutes over low heat. Check the softness of the grain and add more water and continue cooking if necessary. The barley should be tender and all water should be absorbed. Drain excess water if necessary. Serve warm.

NUTRITION PER SERVING	Cal 82	Fat 1g	Protein 3g	Carbs 17g	Sugar 0g	Fiber 4g	Sod 125mg

PARSNIP MASH AND CIPOLLINI ONIONS

SERVES 8

We often serve this recipe as the starch for our main entrée for dinner. Guests love how rich and creamy it is as a complement to any protein. You might have the urge to lick your plate before your server comes by at the end of your meal. We certainly won't stop you!

PARSNIP MASH

1 pound parsnips (about 4 medium), peeled, ends trimmed, and cut into large, even-sized pieces

1 herb sachet (5 sprigs fresh thyme plus 1 bay leaf, wrapped in cheesecloth and tied with butcher's twine)

¼ teaspoon kosher or sea salt plus more to taste

1½ tablespoons extra-virgin olive oil

In a medium saucepan, add the parsnips and herb sachet and cover with at least 2 inches of water. Bring to a boil and allow to cook for 5-7 minutes until tender and a knife can easily be inserted into the parsnips. Drain the parsnips, reserving about 1 cup of the cooking liquid. Discard the herb sachet. Return the cooked parsnips to the hot pot and heat over medium-low heat until the excess water has evaporated from the parsnips.

Add the parsnips to the bowl of a food processor (you'll want to use this instead of a blender to avoid overprocessing). Add the salt and olive oil. Process, adding the starchy cooking water 1 tablespoon at a time, until fluffy and smooth, about 5 tablespoons. Taste and season with more salt as needed. Set aside and keep warm.

CIPOLLINI ONIONS

1 tablespoon grapeseed oil

½ pound Cipollini onions (about 4 onions), root ends removed

1 small bunch fresh thyme sprigs

½ cup sherry wine

Preheat the oven to 350°F. Heat a medium oven-safe sauté pan over medium heat. Add the grapeseed oil. Once the oil is heated, add the onions and thyme and lower the heat to medium-low. Allow the onions to sizzle and slowly caramelize. Once the onion bottoms have achieved a nice, dark golden color, flip and cook slowly on the other side until golden brown (about 5-7 minutes on each side).

Turn off the stove and carefully add the sherry wine to deglaze the pan. Place the pan in the oven for 7 minutes or until the onions have cooked through.

Remove from the oven and allow the onions to cool until they can be handled. Cut the onions into quarters. Set aside and keep warm.

When ready to assemble, place a spoonful of Parsnip Mash on the plate and top with the braised Cipollini Onions.

TIP: Cipollini onions are not always readily available. Feel free to substitute any other small, pearl-like onions.

NUTRITION PER SERVING	Cal 117	Fat 4g	Protein 1g	Carbs 16g	Sugar 5g	Fiber 4g	Sod 68mg

SPAGHETTI SQUASH

SERVES 6

Cal-a-Vie cuisine highlights a moderate carbohydrate, high-fiber, plant-based diet. As an easy replacement for traditional pasta, spaghetti squash comes into play in early summer when our garden is exploding with hard squashes. We've even pickled our spaghetti squash and turned it into kimchi! This recipe makes a versatile "noodle" to pair with any of our sauces and proteins.

- 2 tablespoons plus 2 teaspoons extra-virgin olive oil, divided use
- 1 spaghetti squash (about 3 pounds), halved
- 4 garlic cloves
- 12 sprigs fresh thyme
- 1 lemon, zested
- 2 tablespoons minced fresh parsley
- 1 teaspoon kosher or sea salt

TIP: A 3-pound spaghetti squash yields about 5 cups cooked squash "noodles."

Preheat the oven to 350°F. Coat a baking sheet with 1 tablespoon olive oil. Using a spoon, remove the seeds from inside of the spaghetti squash and discard. Coat each cut side of the squash with 1 teaspoon olive oil. Evenly divide the garlic and thyme between each cavity of the squash. Carefully place the squash halves cut-side down on the oiled sheet tray, keeping the thyme and garlic inside the cavity. Place in the oven and roast for about 40 minutes until the skin has darkened and a knife can easily be inserted into the flesh of the squash. Remove from the oven.

Using a fork, scrape the thin strands of squash from the outer skin and place in a large bowl. Sprinkle with lemon zest, parsley, salt, and remaining 1 tablespoon of olive oil and toss well to evenly coat. Serve immediately.

NUTRITION PER SERVING	Cal 92	Fat 5g	Protein 1g	Carbs 13g	Sugar 1g	Fiber 2g	Sod 180mg

SWISS CHARD

SERVES 4

Swiss chard is related to the spinach and beet family and is well-known as a dark, leafy, green vegetable that's chock full of vitamins A and C as well as minerals including potassium. Cooking the whole plant, both stems and leaves, adds nutrition to your plate. The colorful stems contain anti-inflammatory betalains, which are responsible for the red, yellow, and purple hues of the chard.

- ¼ cup golden raisins, soaked in water overnight (or a minimum 4 hours), drained
- ¼ cup raw pine nuts
- 1 large or 2 small bunches Swiss chard
- 1 tablespoon extra-virgin olive oil
- ⅛ teaspoon kosher or sea salt

Preheat the oven to 350°F. On a baking sheet, lay the pine nuts in a single layer and bake for about 7 minutes, until golden and fragrant. Remove and set aside.

Using a knife, carefully remove the stems from the chard leaves. Slice the stems crosswise about ¼-inch thick and set aside. Chop the leaves into bite-sized, 1-inch pieces.

In a medium skillet over medium heat, warm the olive oil. Once hot, add the chard stems and sauté about 1 minute until slightly softened. Add the chard leaves and allow to wilt slightly. Add the roasted pine nuts and golden raisins. Continuously move the chard mixture so it doesn't burn. When wilted, remove from the heat and serve warm.

NUTRITION PER SERVING	Cal 130	Fat 9g	Protein 3g	Carbs 11g	Sugar 7g	Fiber 2g	Sod 246mg

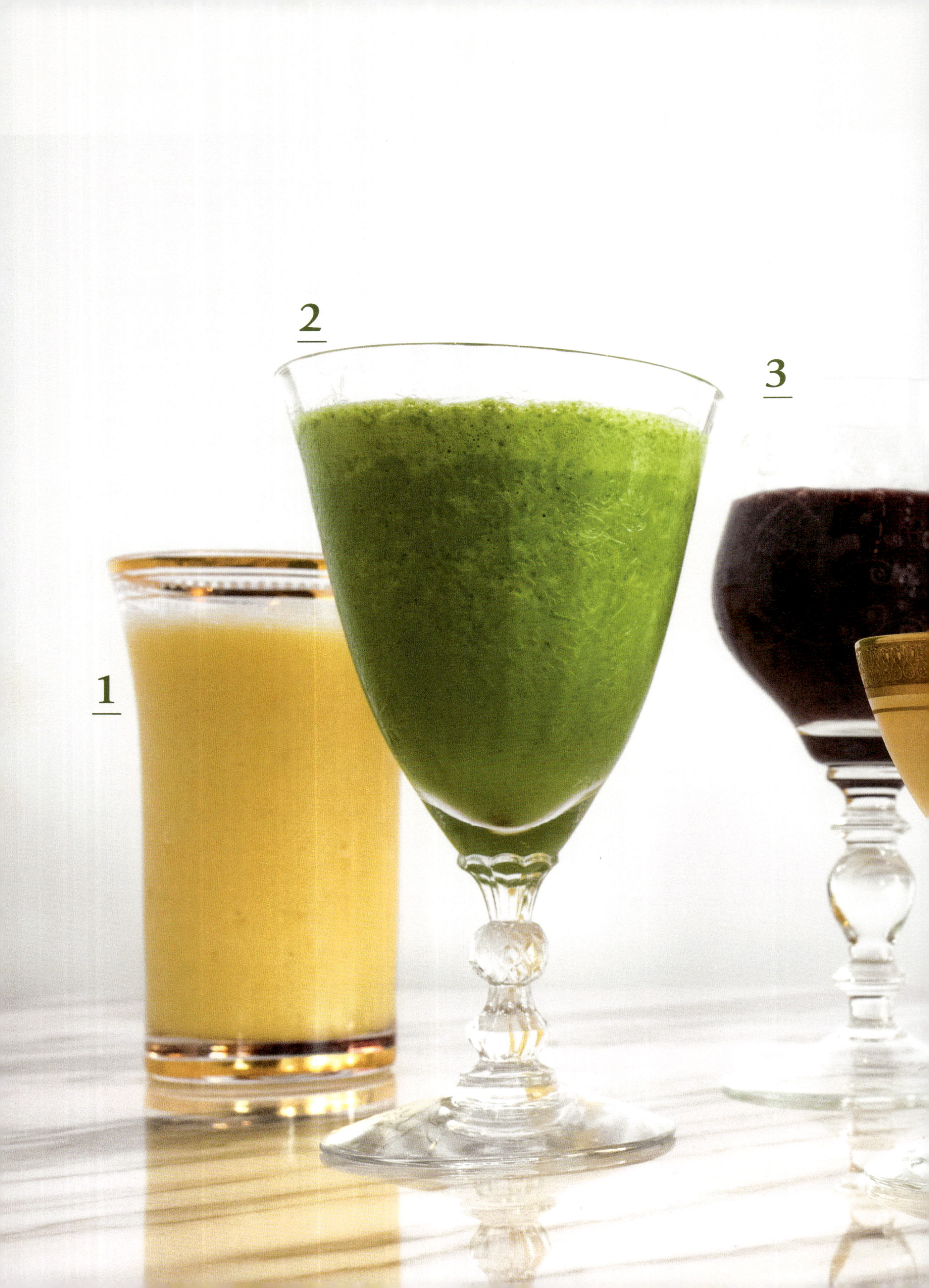
2
3
1

CHAPTER 6

Snacks and Smoothies

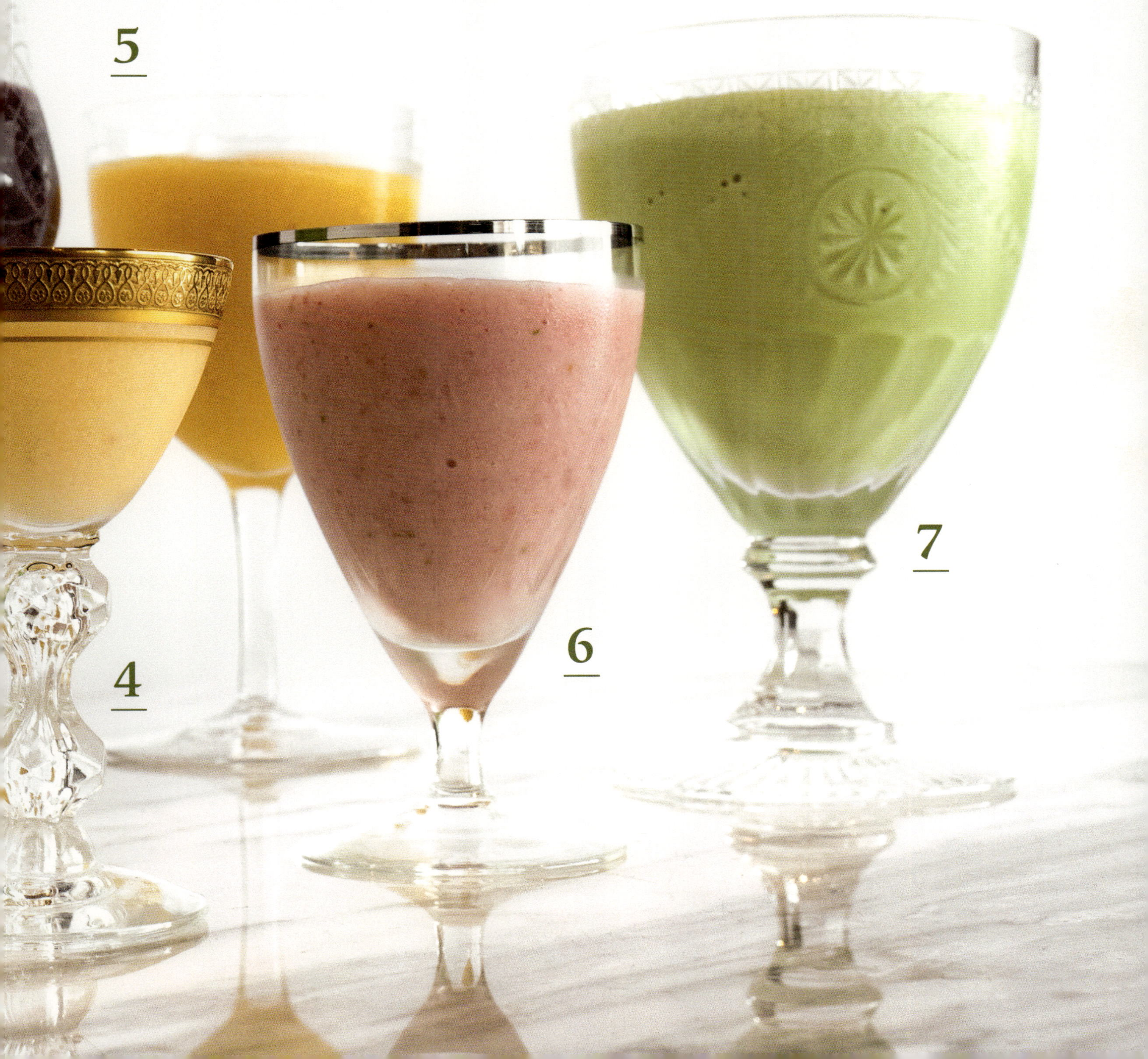

CAL-A-VIE HEALTH SPA SMOOTHIES

6 OUNCES = 1 SERVING

Smoothies can be notoriously high in sugar and calories, so we take out the guesswork and give you the tried-and-true Cal-a-Vie smoothie recipes that will keep you at your best. The key to a healthy smoothie is using real fruit and always having a protein to prevent a blood sugar crash. A smoothie can be used strategically to get a boost of phytonutrients when you're busy or on the go. Phytonutrients are the components of plants that are powerful defenders of health. The array of colors in fruits and vegetables are the phytonutrients that are known for fighting cancer and inflammation, strengthening immune health, protecting DNA and cells, and benefiting vascular health. These recipes are our guests' favorites and can be swapped for alternatives to create a new taste while suiting any dietary preference.

1 PINEAPPLE COCONUT SMOOTHIE

YIELDS 4 CUPS (5 SERVINGS)

1½ cups frozen sliced banana
2 cups frozen pineapple chunks
1½ cups organic coconut milk
1 tablespoon protein powder

In a blender, add all the ingredients and puree on high until completely smooth.

NUTRITION PER SERVING	Cal 155	Fat 3g	Protein 6g	Carbs 29g	Sugar 16g	Fiber 4g	Sod 33mg

2 GREEN SMOOTHIE

YIELDS 3 CUPS (4 SERVINGS)

1 cup frozen sliced banana
¼ avocado
2 cups curly leaf kale
1 teaspoon fresh chopped ginger
½ lemon, squeezed
2 cups coconut milk
¼ teaspoon kosher or sea salt
1 tablespoon protein powder

In a blender, add all the ingredients and puree on high until completely smooth.

NUTRITION PER SERVING	Cal 183	Fat 15g	Protein 8g	Carbs 17g	Sugar 4g	Fiber 4g	Sod 152mg

3 BLACKBERRY LEMON SMOOTHIE

YIELDS 4 CUPS (5 SERVINGS)

3 cups frozen blackberries
juice of one lemon
3½ cups almond milk
1 cup fresh spinach leaves
2 tablespoons honey
1 tablespoon protein powder

In a blender, add all the ingredients and puree on high until completely smooth. Strain through a fine mesh sieve to remove the blackberry seeds.

NUTRITION PER SERVING	Cal 117	Fat 3g	Protein 6g	Carbs 20g	Sugar 12g	Fiber 7g	Sod 125mg

4 BANANA ALMOND SMOOTHIE

YIELDS 4 CUPS (5 SERVINGS)

2 cups frozen sliced banana

⅓ cup almond butter

½ teaspoon ground cinnamon

2 cups almond milk

In a blender, add all the ingredients and puree on high until completely smooth.

NUTRITION PER SERVING	Cal 209	Fat 10g	Protein 7g	Carbs 27g	Sugar 12g	Fiber 6g	Sod 138mg

5 PEACH MAPLE SMOOTHIE

YIELDS 4 CUPS (5 SERVINGS)

3 cups frozen peaches

½ cup sliced banana

2 tablespoons maple syrup

2 cups almond milk

1 tablespoon protein powder

In a blender, add all the ingredients and puree on high until completely smooth.

NUTRITION PER SERVING	Cal 135	Fat 3g	Protein 6g	Carbs 25g	Sugar 18g	Fiber 4g	Sod 87mg

6 STRAWBERRY BANANA SMOOTHIE

YIELDS 4 CUPS (5 SERVINGS)

1½ cups sliced banana

2 cups frozen strawberries

1½ cups soy milk (almond or coconut milk can be substituted)

1 tablespoon protein powder

In a blender, add all the ingredients and puree on high until completely smooth.

NUTRITION PER SERVING	Cal 141	Fat 2g	Protein 6g	Carbs 26g	Sugar 14g	Fiber 4g	Sod 49mg

7 GREEN TEA MANGO SMOOTHIE

YIELDS 6 CUPS (8 SERVINGS)

3 cups Green Tea Ice Cream (see recipe page 271)

1 cup frozen mango chunks

2 cups soy milk (almond or coconut milk can be substituted)

1 tablespoon protein powder

In a blender, add all the ingredients and puree on high until completely smooth.

NUTRITION PER SERVING	Cal 134	Fat 4g	Protein 5g	Carbs 21g	Sugar 17g	Fiber 2g	Sod 52mg

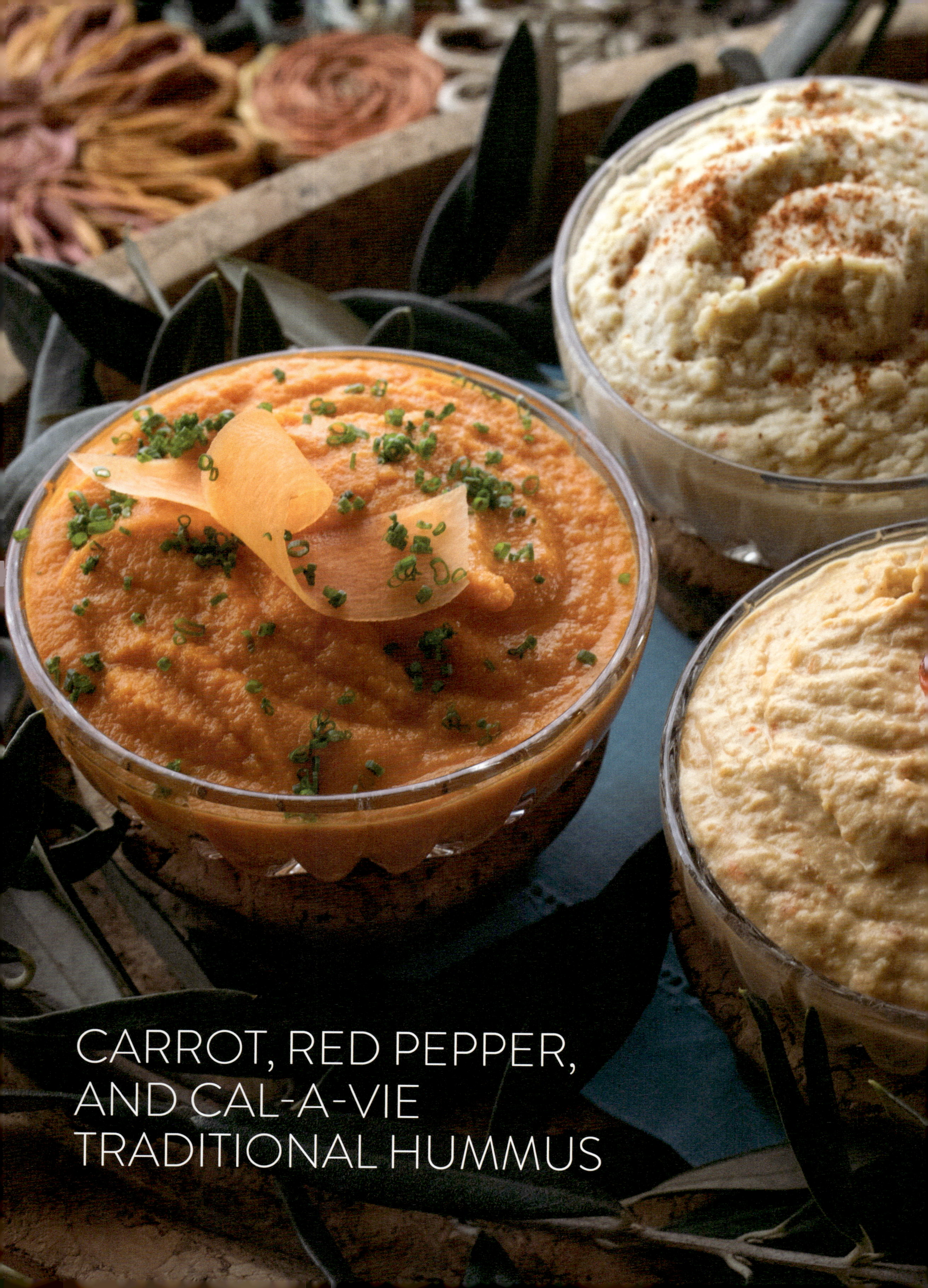

CARROT, RED PEPPER, AND CAL-A-VIE TRADITIONAL HUMMUS

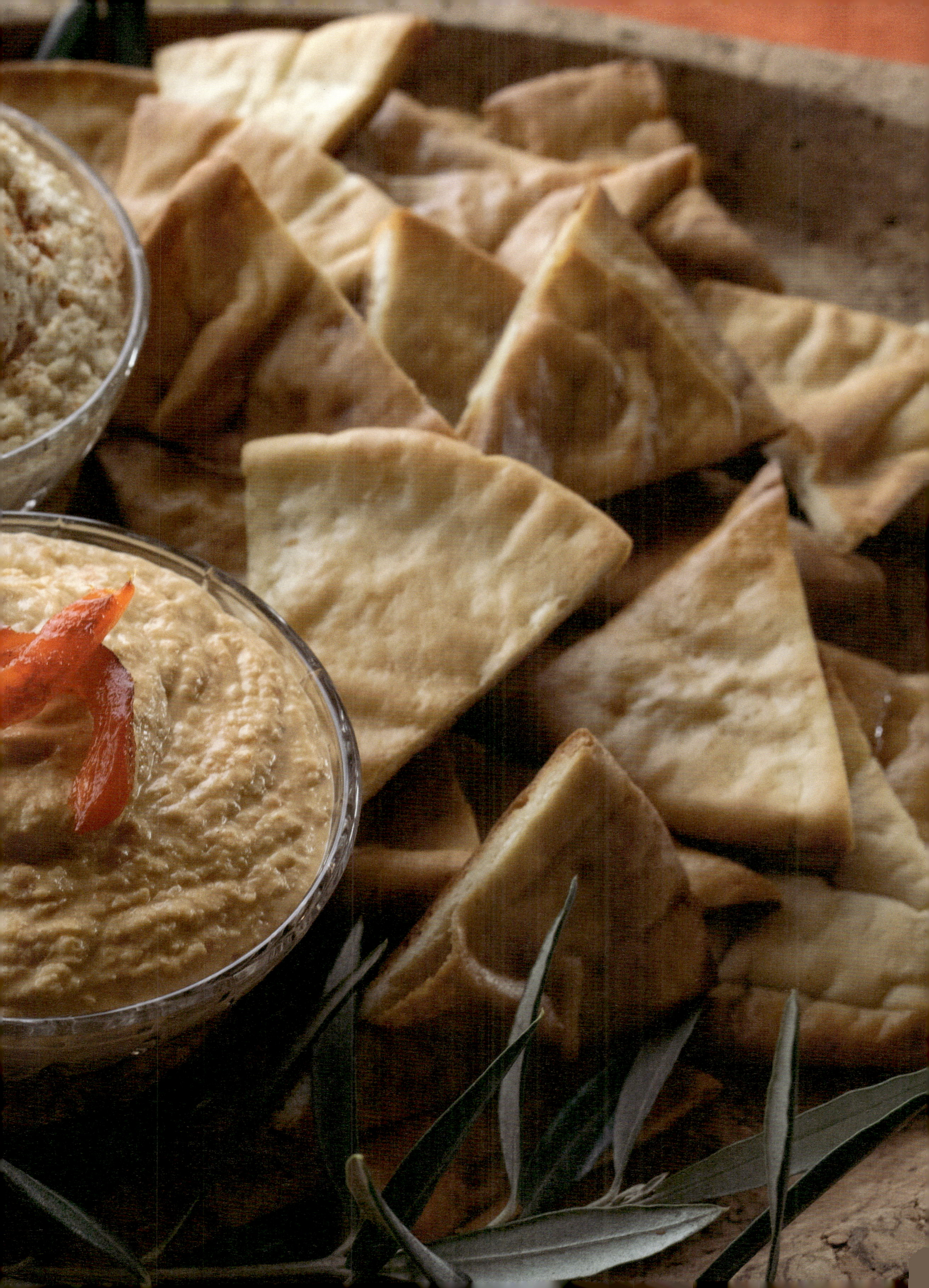

CARROT HUMMUS

SERVES 6

This brightly colored hummus is a great complement to any vegetable crudité. If you are looking to be creative, you can also make this a filling for deviled eggs instead of using mayo and yolk.

- 6 carrots, peeled and chopped into evenly sized, large pieces
- 2 garlic cloves
- 2 teaspoons fresh ginger, peeled and chopped
- ½ teaspoon paprika
- 2 tablespoons tahini
- 1 tablespoon fresh lemon juice
- kosher or sea salt

In a medium saucepan, add the carrots, garlic, and ginger. Cover with water and cook until tender. Drain and cool. Add the cooked carrot mixture, paprika, tahini, and lemon juice to a food processor and puree until smooth. Adjust the seasoning with salt to taste. Store in the refrigerator for 3-5 days.

NUTRITION PER SERVING	Cal 58	Fat 3g	Protein 2g	Carbs 8g	Sugar 3g	Fiber 2g	Sod 163mg

CAL-A-VIE TRADITIONAL HUMMUS

SERVES 8

You will be amazed at how good this traditional hummus tastes despite how simple the ingredients are. Our philosophy is pretty basic: If you start with fresh, high-quality ingredients, all you have to do is get out of the way and let them shine.

- 2 cups garbanzo beans, cooked (if using canned, drained)
- 3 tablespoons fresh lemon juice
- 2 garlic cloves
- ¼ cup tahini
- 3 tablespoons water
- ¼ cup extra-virgin olive oil
- 1 teaspoon kosher or sea salt
- ¼ teaspoon cayenne

In a food processor, combine all the ingredients. Puree until the hummus is smooth. If the hummus is too thick, add water, a tablespoon at a time, until reaching the desired consistency. Adjust the seasoning with additional salt to taste. Store in the refrigerator in an airtight container for 3-5 days.

NUTRITION PER SERVING	Cal 174	Fat 12g	Protein 5g	Carbs 13g	Sugar 2g	Fiber 4g	Sod 155mg

RED PEPPER HUMMUS

SERVES 6

Bell peppers are a great source of vitamins A, B6, and C, as well as folate. Use this hummus as a tasty dip or as a delicious spread in a wrap for some extra flavor and protein.

- 2 red bell peppers, roasted; stems, skins, and seeds removed
- 1 cup canned garbanzo beans, rinsed and drained
- 2 tablespoons fresh lemon juice
- 1 garlic clove
- 2 tablespoons tahini
- 2 tablespoons water
- 3 tablespoons extra-virgin olive oil
- ½ teaspoon kosher or sea salt

Using a food processor, add all the ingredients and puree until completely smooth. Adjust the seasoning with additional salt to taste. Store in the refrigerator in an airtight container for 3–5 days.

NUTRITION PER SERVING	Cal 139	Fat 10g	Protein 3g	Carbs 10g	Sugar 3g	Fiber 3g	Sod 202mg

BAKED PITA CHIPS

YIELDS 40 CHIPS (5 SERVINGS)

This recipe is a quick, easy way to transform a basic party snack into a homemade accompaniment that is full of flavor and much healthier than fried pita chips. These Baked Pita Chips pair wonderfully with our homemade hummus and salsas.

- 1 teaspoon sea salt
- 1 teaspoon smoked paprika
- 5 (5-inch-round) pitas, each cut into 8 wedges
- olive oil spray

Preheat the oven to 350°F. Combine the salt and smoked paprika in a small bowl and set aside. Place the pita wedges in a single layer on a baking sheet. Spray liberally with the olive-oil spray. Sprinkle the salt and paprika mixture over each pita wedge. Bake in the oven for 10–12 minutes, or until golden brown. Store in an airtight container.

NUTRITION PER SERVING	Cal 131	Fat 2g	Protein 5g	Carbs 26g	Sugar 0g	Fiber 4g	Sod 205mg

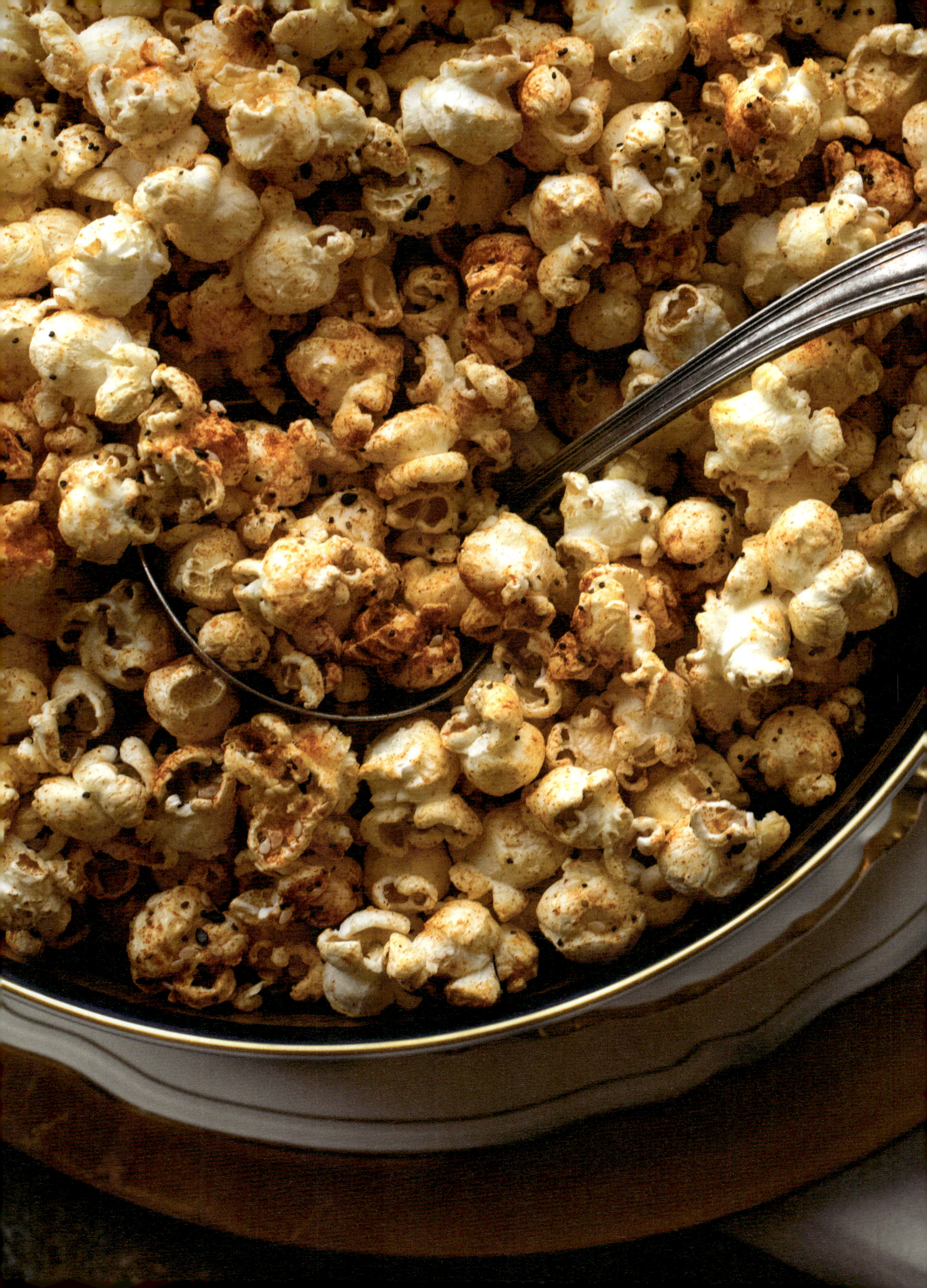

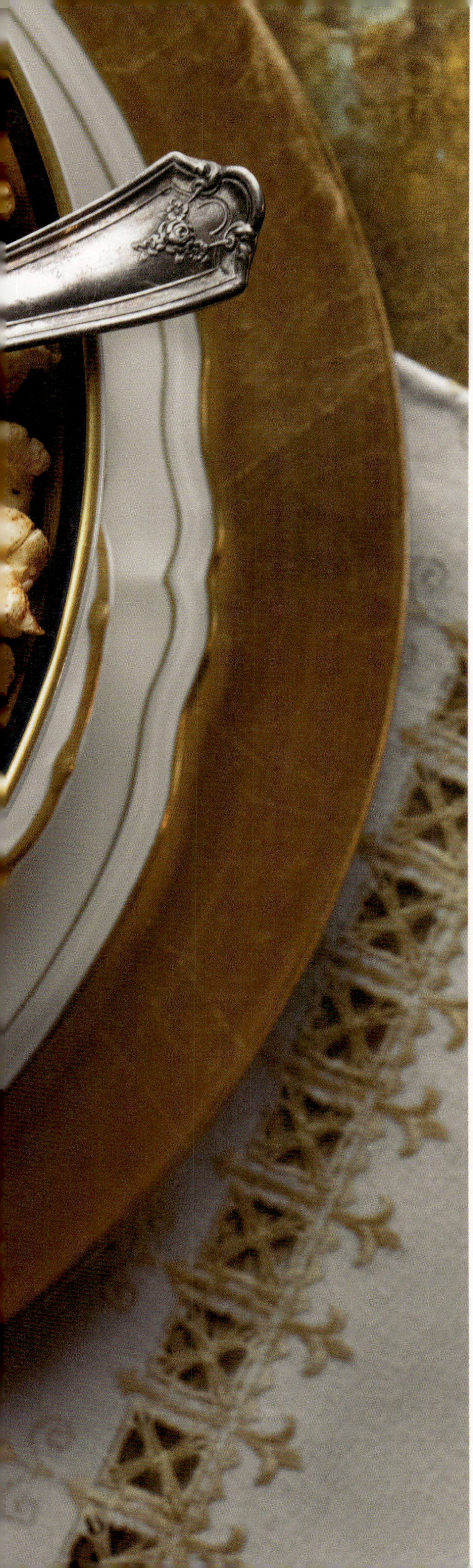

CAL-A-VIE POPCORN

SERVES 1

What makes our popcorn unique is the actual corn. We grow a variety that is strictly used for popping. We then put it through a special drying process to create the lightest, fluffiest, tastiest popcorn you could ever imagine.

SEASONING MIX

1 teaspoon white sesame seeds
½ teaspoon black sesame seeds
1 teaspoon smoked paprika
½ teaspoon sea salt
½ teaspoon celery seeds
½ teaspoon poppy seeds
¼ teaspoon garlic powder
¼ teaspoon freshly ground black pepper
⅛ teaspoon aji amarillo powder

In a small bowl, combine all the ingredients. Set aside.

POPCORN

1 cup popcorn, air popped
extra-virgin olive oil spray (1-3-second spray)
1 teaspoon Seasoning Mix

Once the corn is popped, spray it with olive oil and gently toss. Add the Seasoning Mix and adjust to taste.

NUTRITION PER SERVING	Cal	Fat	Protein	Carbs	Sugar	Fiber	Sod
	50	2g	1g	7g	0g	2g	5mg

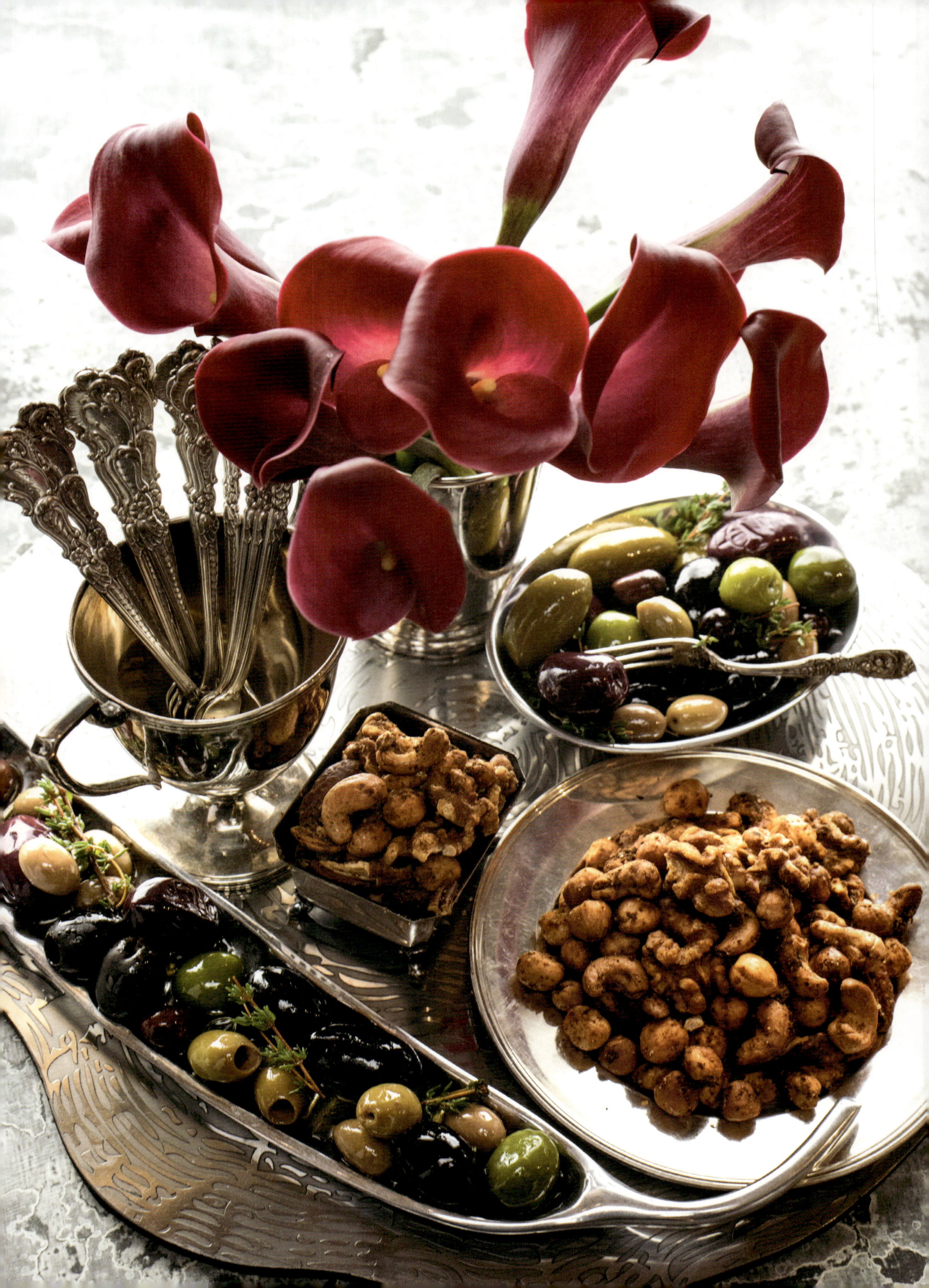

BARBECUE SPICED SNACK NUTS AND MARINATED OLIVES

YIELDS 2 CUPS (8 SERVINGS)

This snack mix features a combination of sweet and savory—with a little spicy kick—that creates a fusion of flavors for any occasion. Our health-conscious party planners love this recipe, as nuts are nutrient-dense foods that provide unique bioactive compounds. Nuts are cholesterol-free and include a natural compound called plant sterols, or phytosterols, which interfere with cholesterol absorption and thus help lower blood cholesterol when present in sufficient amounts. Other bioactive constituents of nuts—such as tocopherols, folic acid, selenium, and magnesium—are believed to have antioxidant, anti-inflammatory, or anti-carcinogenic properties, making nuts an exceptional food to support health and longevity.

Contrary to what you might expect, oil-roasted nuts are only slightly higher in fat and calories than dry-roasted nuts. This is because nuts are naturally high in fat (most of it good) and cannot absorb much more. When roasting nuts, use coconut oil rather than olive oil, which easily burns. It tolerates heat better to create a slowly roasted, golden nut.

BARBECUE SPICED SNACK NUTS

BARBECUE SEASONING MIX

- ½ cup coconut sugar
- ½ cup smoked paprika
- ¼ cup garlic powder
- ¼ cup onion powder
- ¼ cup celery seeds
- 3 tablespoons freshly ground black pepper
- 2 teaspoons dried mustard
- 3 tablespoons dried thyme
- 2 tablespoons dried basil
- 3 tablespoons sea salt

Mix all ingredients together. Set aside. Store in an airtight container.

SPICED NUTS

- 8 teaspoons coconut oil, divided use
- ½ cup walnut halves
- ½ cup pecan halves
- ½ cup whole cashews
- ½ cup whole hazelnuts
- 8 teaspoons of Barbecue Seasoning Mix, divided use

Preheat the oven to 350°F. In a skillet over medium heat, add 2 teaspoons coconut oil. When hot, add only the walnut halves and 2 teaspoons of the Barbecue Seasoning Mix. Stir 1-2 minutes until lightly browned. Remove and then add 2 teaspoons coconut oil, pecan halves, and 2 teaspoons seasoning mix, then stir 1-2 minutes and remove. Repeat the process for the cashews and hazelnuts. Then mix all the nuts together. Place on a baking sheet and toast in the oven for 5 minutes. Remove and cool. Store in an airtight container.

NUTRITION PER SERVING	Cal 206	Fat 19g	Protein 4g	Carbs 8g	Sugar 2g	Fiber 2g	Sod 9mg

MARINATED OLIVES

SERVES 20

Olives are grown in trees all over the world including Cal-a-Vie. We have dozens of olive trees on our grounds. For this recipe we use three varieties from the Mediterranean region: Kalamata—which are large black or brown olives that come from southern Greece, Picholine—which are small, bright green olives from Morocco or southern France, and Castelvetrano—which are sweet, meaty, green olives that come from Sicily.

Olives are considered a fruit since they are formed from the ovary of the olive flower and produce seeds or pits.

- 1 cup whole Kalamata olives, pitted
- 1 cup whole Picoline olives, pitted
- 1 cup whole Castelvetrano olives, pitted
- 2 cups extra-virgin olive oil (or enough to cover olives)
- 1 tablespoon red chili flakes
- 2 garlic cloves, sliced
- 9 sprigs fresh thyme
- 1 bay leaf

In a large bowl, combine all of the ingredients and mix thoroughly. Store in an airtight container in the refrigerator. When serving, drain the olives to remove the excess olive oil.

TIP: Homemade marinated olives should be stored in the refrigerator and will keep in the refrigerator for two weeks in an airtight container.

NUTRITION PER SERVING	Cal 38	Fat 4g	Protein 0g	Carbs 1g	Sugar 0g	Fiber 1g	Sod 132mg

REVITALIZER

YIELDS 23 4-OUNCE SERVINGS

Mornings at Cal-a-Vie usually start with an invigorating 2-mile hike and then some fun exercise classes. To keep your energy level up, we always serve a morning snack of grilled vegetables which includes our Revitalizer. A small cup of our special drink provides just the right amount of added nutrition to keep you going until lunch is served. We get requests for this recipe every week, and we are happy to provide it so you can keep your mornings going at home. It's also a great way to get your daily serving of vegetables in!

---

2 quarts organic tomato juice
3 cups water
1 cup chopped carrots
1 cup chopped celery
1 cup chopped fennel
½ cup chopped onions
½ cup fresh basil leaves
½ cup fresh parsley leaves
1 bay leaf
½ cup fresh thyme
kosher salt to taste

In a large saucepan over high heat, combine the ingredients and bring to a boil. Reduce the heat to low and simmer for 1 hour, stirring occasionally.

Remove from the heat and press the mixture through a strainer over a bowl to catch the liquid. Discard the solids. Add salt to taste.

Serve hot or cold.

TIP: You can add chili flakes, ground flax seeds, and freshly ground black pepper. Freeze any extra in 1-cup amounts for later use.

NUTRITION PER SERVING	Cal 22	Fat 4g	Protein 4g	Carbs 16g	Sugar 3g	Fiber 1g	Sod 20mg

BAKED CORN TORTILLA CHIPS

YIELDS 40 PIECES (6 SERVINGS)

There's not a better way to pair our homemade salsas and hummus than with a homemade hot and crispy tortilla chip right out of the oven. Baking tortilla chips in a light spray of oil gives the same beautiful golden color and perfect crunch, while offering a much healthier alternative to traditionally fried tortilla chips.

- 5 organic thin yellow corn tortillas
- olive oil spray
- sea salt

Preheat the oven to 350°F. Cut the corn tortillas in quarters and then cut the quarters in half, creating 8 pieces per tortilla. Lay the cut tortillas on a baking sheet in a single layer, making sure not to overlap. Spray with olive oil and sprinkle with salt to taste. Bake for 9 minutes or until crisp.

NUTRITION PER SERVING	Cal 45	Fat 1g	Protein 1g	Carbs 9g	Sugar 0g	Fiber 1g	Sod 47mg

ROASTED TOMATILLOS SALSA

YIELDS 2 CUPS (8 SERVINGS)

No Southern California culinary dining experience would be complete without an occasional taste of Mexico. We love making this dish in-house from the fresh tomatillos and jalapeños growing in our garden during the summer. This refreshing salsa can be served as a snack or used to complement grilled chicken or seafood.

- 1 pound tomatillos, husked and thoroughly washed
- 1½ tablespoons plus 3 teaspoons grapeseed oil, divided use
- 1½ teaspoons kosher or sea salt, divided use and more to taste
- 1 teaspoon minced garlic
- ½ small onion, thinly sliced
- 1 jalapeño, stem and seeds removed, sliced in half lengthwise
- 1 bunch fresh cilantro, roughly chopped

Preheat the oven to 350°F. Toss the tomatillos with one tablespoon grapeseed oil and ½ teaspoon salt to coat evenly. Spread evenly on a baking sheet so the tomatillos have plenty of space. Roast in the oven for 20-30 minutes, until softened and lightly browned in spots. Roast longer if needed. Remove and set aside.

In a medium saucepan over medium heat, add ½ tablespoon of grapeseed oil. Once hot, add the garlic and sauté until lightly browned and softened. Set the garlic aside. Wipe the pan clean and return to medium heat. Add 1 teaspoon of grapeseed oil and add onions. Sauté the onions, stirring occasionally until caramelized to a deep golden color, about 10 minutes. Remove the onions and set aside. Wipe the pan clean and return to medium heat again with 1 teaspoon grapeseed oil. Add the jalapeños cut side down and allow to cook until lightly browned. Turn the jalapeños over and continue cooking until softened. Remove and set aside.

In a food processor, add the tomatillos, garlic, onion, and cilantro. Add 1 teaspoon of salt and 1 teaspoon of grapeseed oil. Process well. Add as much jalapeño as desired and process until no large chunks remain. Taste and season with salt and more jalapeños, processing after each addition, until the desired level of flavor and heat has been achieved. Place in an airtight container and refrigerate for up to 1 week.

NUTRITION PER SERVING	Cal 47	Fat 3g	Protein 1g	Carbs 4g	Sugar 3g	Fiber 1g	Sod 172mg

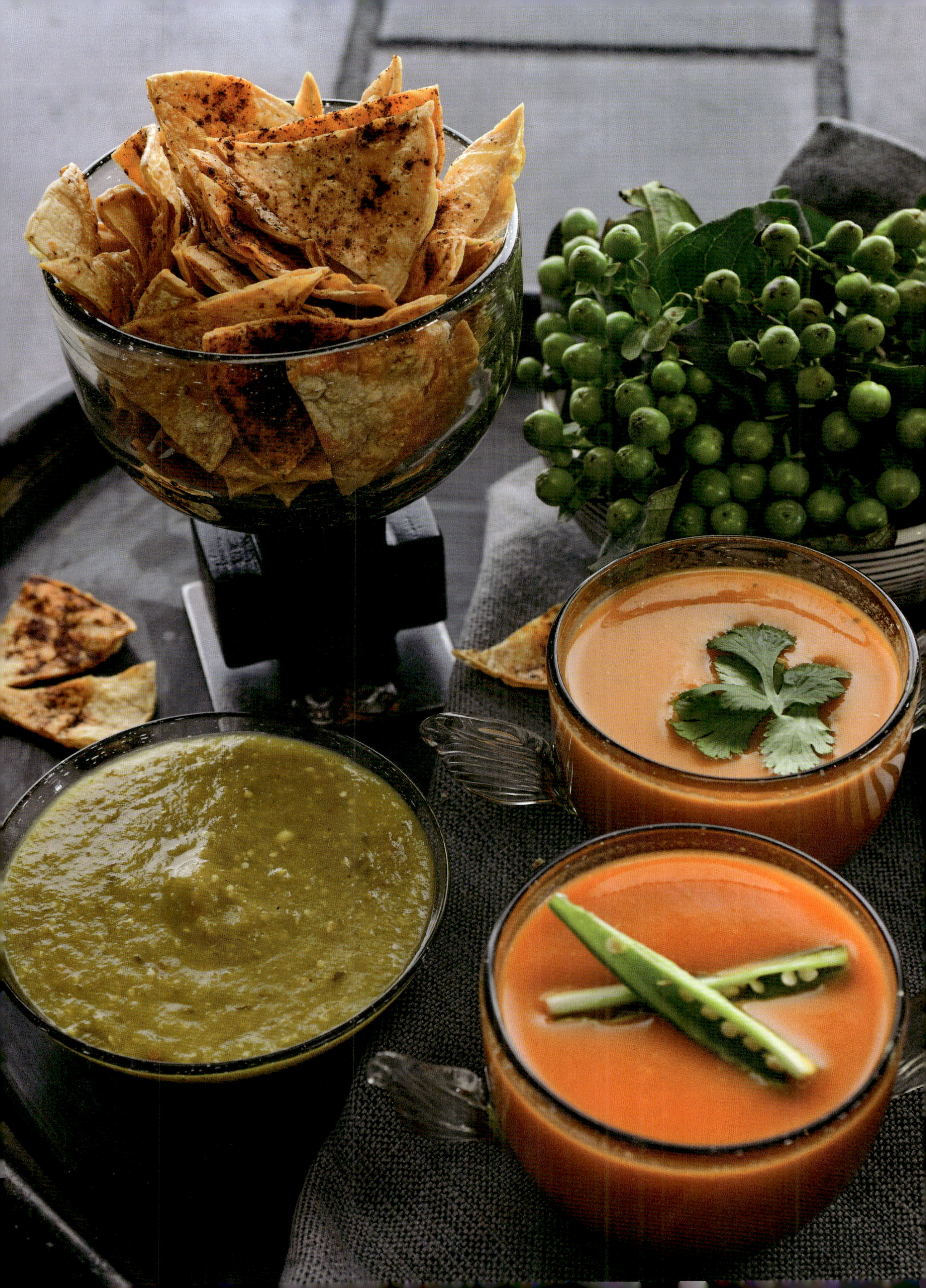

MEDIUM SALSA

YIELDS ABOUT 2 QUARTS (32 SERVINGS)

Our chef is sharing the secret recipe to Cal-a-Vie's simple yet absurdly flavorful salsa, which we promise will outshine any store-bought version. It's wonderful with eggs, tacos, or our homemade Baked Pita Chips (see recipe page 207). Our dieticians encourage using fresh garlic in recipes, as research shows it has numerous health benefits and is recognized as a medicinal food. When fresh garlic is chopped or crushed, the enzyme alliinase converts alliin into allicin, which is responsible for the aroma of fresh garlic. This allicin may also prevent oxidative damage to DNA in the body, thereby protecting against disease. For higher concentrations of allicin, use fresh garlic cloves and allow chopped garlic to sit for 5 minutes to allow the allicin to fully develop before adding into your recipe.

16 Roma tomatoes, tops removed

1 jalapeño pepper, stem and seeds removed

2 teaspoons grapeseed oil, divided use

3 garlic cloves, chopped

¼ cup thinly sliced yellow onions

kosher or sea salt

In a medium saucepan over high heat, cover the tomatoes and jalapeño with water. Bring to a boil and then lower the heat to a simmer for 10-15 minutes until the tomato skins are falling off. Remove from the heat and drain. When cool enough to handle, remove any loose skins from the tomatoes and discard.

While the tomatoes and peppers are cooking, add 1 teaspoon of grapeseed oil to a small sauté pan over medium heat. Once oil is hot, add the garlic and sauté until just softened and starting to brown, about 3 minutes. Add the remaining teaspoon of grapeseed oil and the sliced onions. Sauté until the onions begin to caramelize, about 5 minutes. Remove from the heat.

In a blender combine the tomatoes, jalapeño, garlic, and onions and process until smooth. Store in the refrigerator in an airtight container for up to a week.

NUTRITION PER SERVING	Cal 9	Fat 0g	Protein 0g	Carbs 1g	Sugar 1g	Fiber 0g	Sod 74mg

HOT SALSA

YIELDS ABOUT 2 QUARTS (32 SERVINGS)

This takes our traditional salsa recipe and adds some intense heat by using árbol chili peppers. These peppers are rated at 50,000-65,000 on the Scoville heat-unit scale, equivalent to a 7-8 on a 1-10 spiciness scale. Their spicy residue can linger on your hands, so be sure to wear gloves or wash your hands well after cooking with them.

16 Roma tomatoes, tops removed

3 árbol chili peppers, stems removed

2 teaspoons grapeseed oil, divided use

3 garlic cloves, chopped

¼ cup thinly sliced yellow onion

kosher or sea salt

In a medium saucepan over high heat, cover the tomatoes and chiles with water. Bring to a boil and then lower the heat to simmer for 10-15 minutes until the tomato skins are falling off. Remove from the heat and drain. When cool enough to handle, remove any loose skins from the tomatoes and discard.

While the tomatoes and chilies are cooking, add one teaspoon of grapeseed oil to a small sauté pan over medium heat. Once oil is hot, add the garlic and sauté until just softened and starting to brown, about 3 minutes. Add the remaining teaspoon of grapeseed oil and the sliced onions. Sauté until the onions begin to caramelize, about 5 minutes. Remove from the heat.

Roughly chop the tomatoes and add to a blender along with the garlic, onion, and two of the chilies. Puree until the salsa is smooth. Taste for heat and flavor, and add the last chili if desired. Add salt to taste. Keep in an airtight container in the refrigerator for up to one week.

NUTRITION PER SERVING	Cal 10	Fat 0g	Protein 0g	Carbs 2g	Sugar 1g	Fiber 0g	Sod 86mg

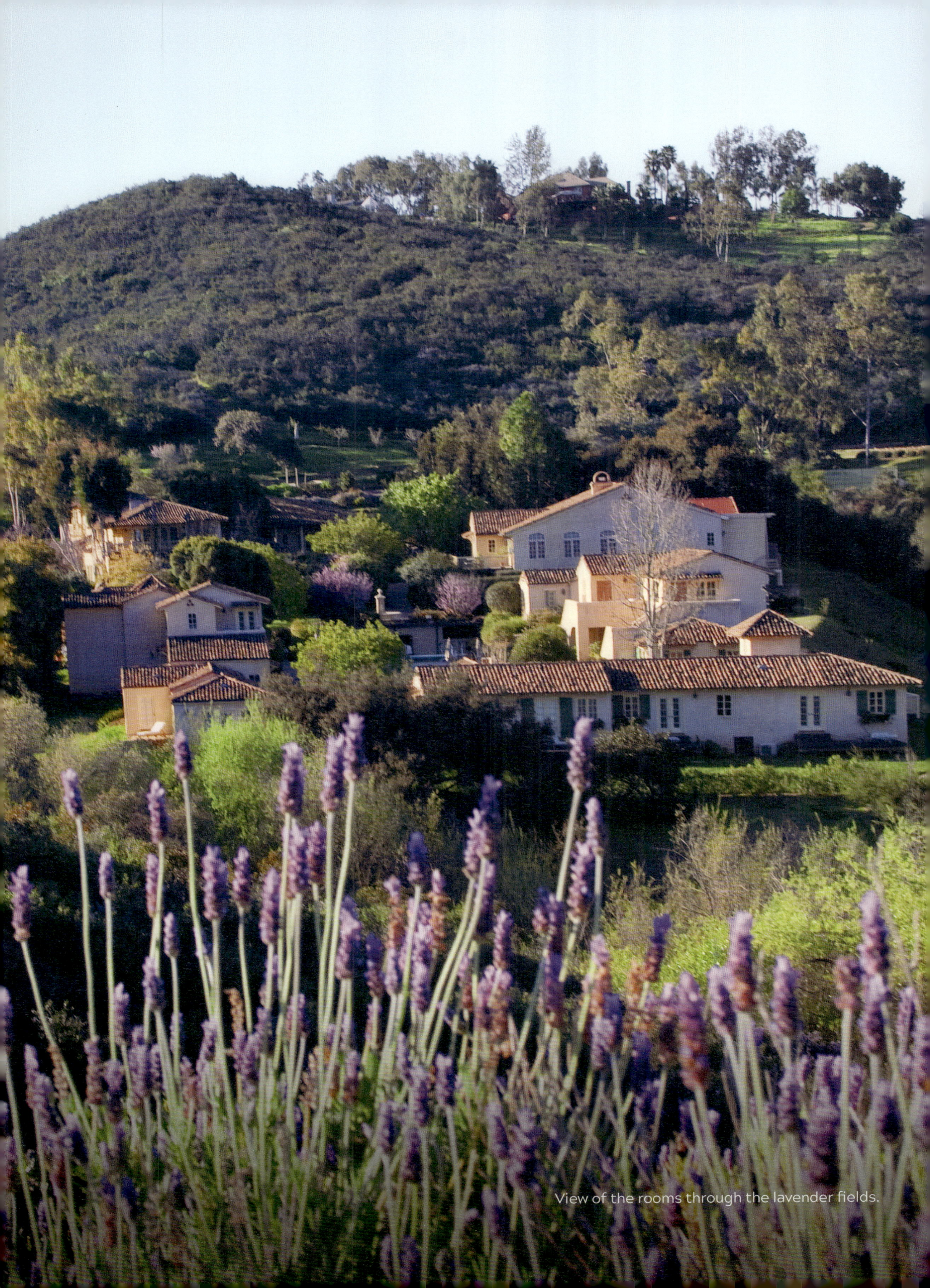

View of the rooms through the lavender fields.

COCONUT ALMOND PROTEIN BARS

MAKES ABOUT 16 BARS

These high-protein bars make a healthy, tasty mid-morning or afternoon snack. We use PurePaleo™ protein powder, which doesn't have any aftertaste and blends well with other ingredients. If you can't find it locally, it can be ordered on the Internet.

PROTEIN BAR

1 cup almond butter
½ cup almond flour
1 teaspoon vanilla extract
1 tablespoon honey or maple syrup (optional)
2 tablespoons (1 scoop) PurePaleo™ Natural Vanilla Flavor Protein powder
1 teaspoon ground cinnamon
⅓ cup dried unsweetened cranberries
⅓ cup chopped pistachio nuts
¼ cup chopped toasted walnuts
dash of Himalayan salt or sea salt
½ cup shredded unsweetened coconut

TOPPING

½ cup shredded unsweetened coconut

In a food processor with the metal blending blade, combine all Protein Bar ingredients and mix until sticky and blended. The mixture will start to pull together into a dough ball.

In an 8 x 8-inch baking pan covered with a sheet of parchment paper, spread the dough with a spatula. Sprinkle the top with shredded coconut and press down. Place in the refrigerator and let chill for at least an hour before cutting into bars.

DO NOT SUBSTITUTE a blender or a Vitamix for a food processor, since the dough will become gummy and hard to get out of the machine.

The moisture content in store-bought almond butter can vary greatly from brand to brand and can affect the texture of the bars.

TIP: If you're a chocolate lover, add ¼ cup of organic cacao nibs to the mix. These are nature's original chocolate chips. They are made from crushed cacao beans, which also add antioxidants, powerful nutrients, and fiber to the bars.

NUTRITION PER SERVING	Cal 160	Fat 14g	Protein 6g	Carbs 5g	Sugar 1g	Fiber 3g	Sod 20mg

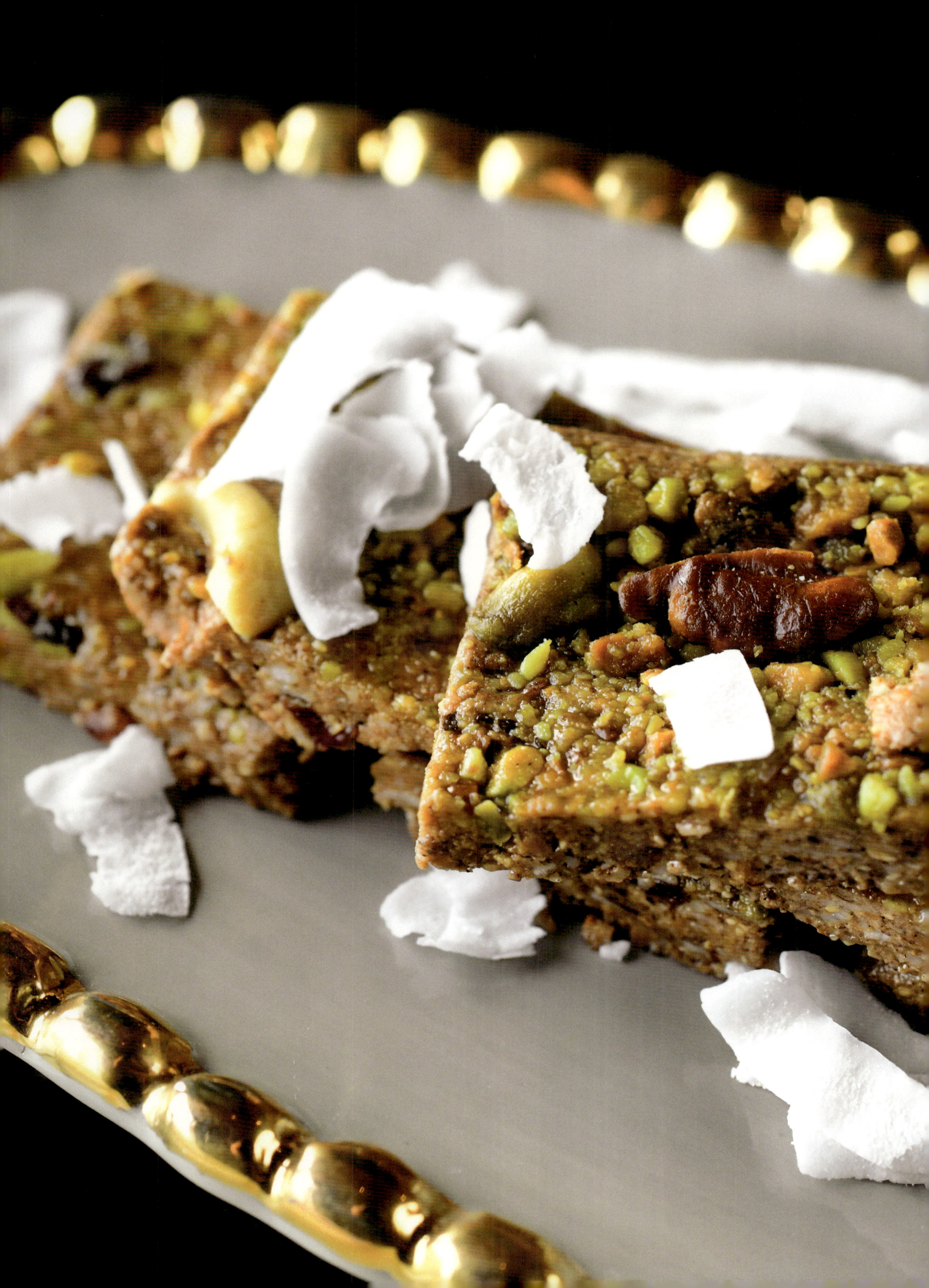

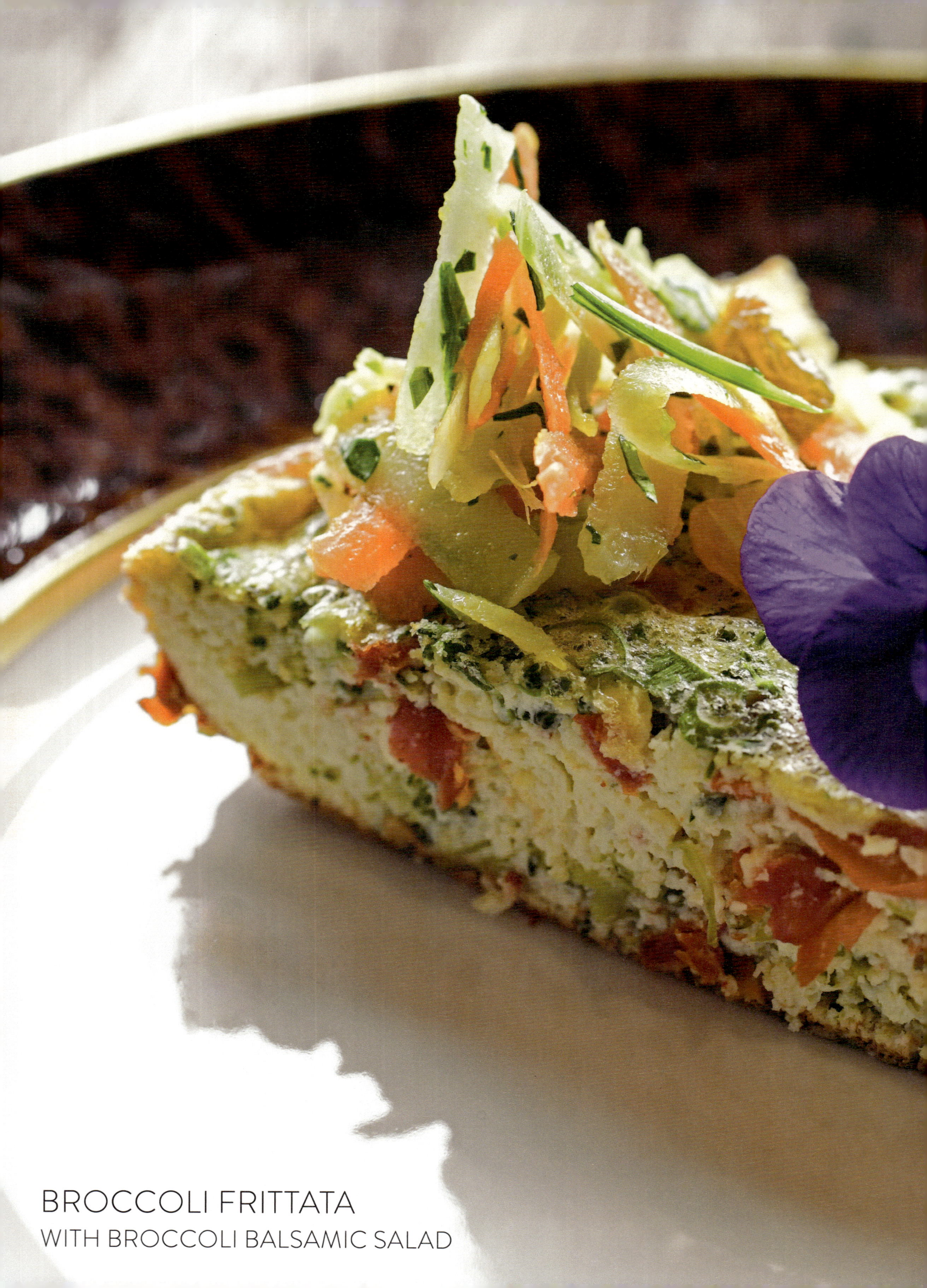

BROCCOLI FRITTATA
WITH BROCCOLI BALSAMIC SALAD

CHAPTER 7

Breakfast

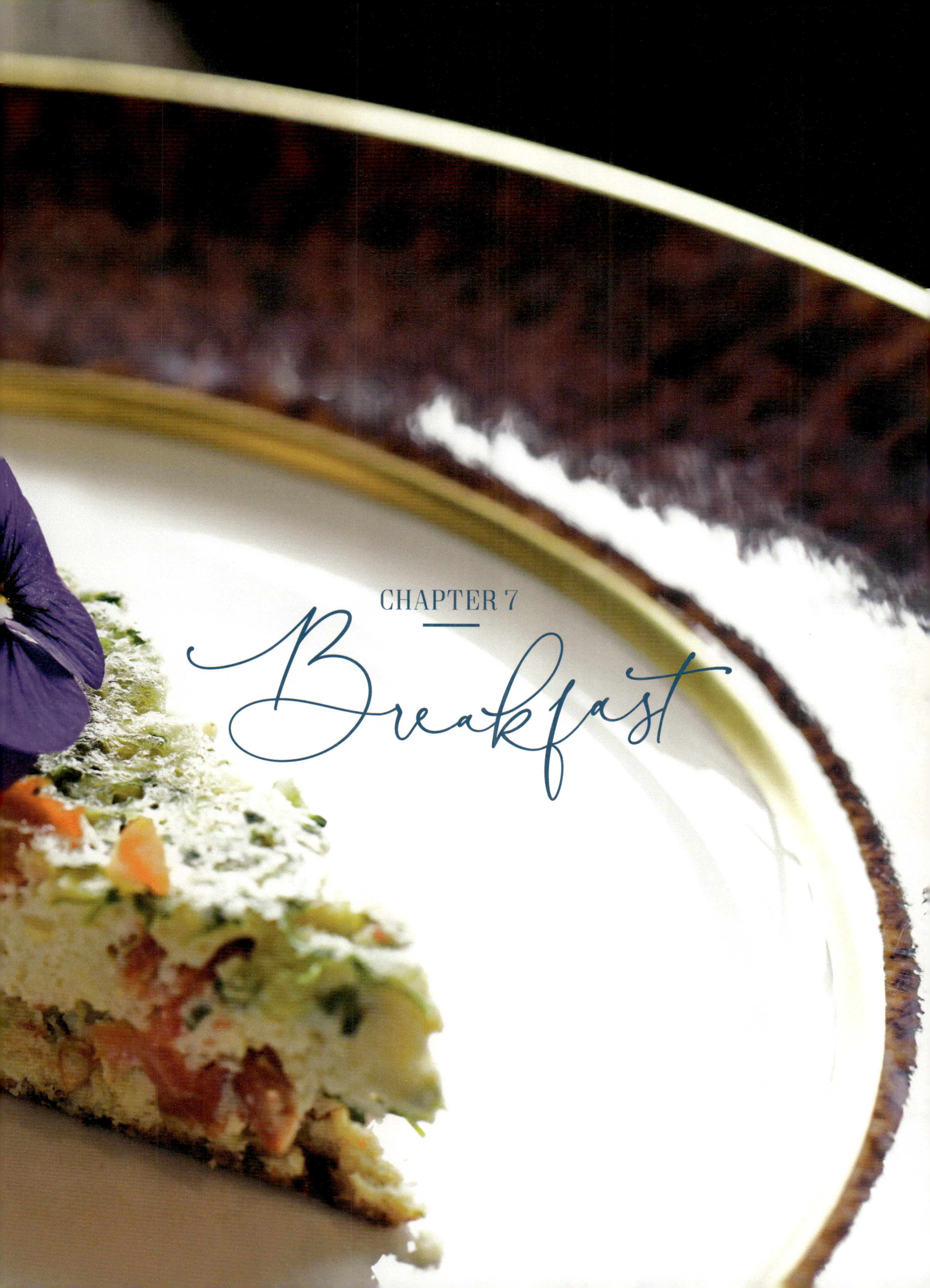

BROCCOLI FRITTATA
WITH BROCCOLI BALSAMIC SALAD

SERVES 6

This frittata and salad combo is a great way to use both the florets and the stalk of your broccoli. It's full of sulforaphane which is a cancer-fighting, detox-enhancing compound that is formed when raw broccoli is cut and then allowed to sit for a few minutes before being eaten. If you eat the broccoli shortly after it's cut, you'll get the maximum amount of sulforaphane in your body. Of course, don't forget to chew well for optimal digestion.

CASHEW CREAM (ALSO A DAIRY SUBSTITUTE)

⅓ cup raw cashews

1 cup warm water

In a small bowl, soak the cashews in the water for a minimum of 1 hour. In a blender, combine the cashews and water to reach a creamy consistency similar to half and half. Set aside in the refrigerator.

WHITE BALSAMIC VINAIGRETTE

¼ cup white balsamic vinegar

1 tablespoon honey

½ tablespoon Dijon mustard

2 tablespoons water

¼ teaspoon sea salt

¼ cup plus 2 tablespoons grapeseed oil

In a small bowl, whisk all the ingredients until smooth. Set aside.

BALSAMIC BROCCOLI SALAD

1 broccoli stalk, trimmed and julienned (florets are for the frittata)

2 large carrots, peeled, trimmed, and julienned

¼ cup chopped fresh parsley

¼ cup golden raisins

¼ cup White Balsamic Vinaigrette

In a large bowl, combine the broccoli, carrots, parsley, raisins, and vinaigrette. Set aside in the refrigerator.

TIP: To shorten the preparation time, purchase a bag of broccoli slaw from the produce section of the grocery store and then mix with parsley, raisins, and White Balsamic Vinaigrette.

BROCCOLI FRITTATA

6 large eggs

⅓ cup Cashew Cream
(you can substitute whole fat milk)

1½ teaspoons grapeseed oil

1 small head of broccoli, florets only, cut into small bite-sized pieces

¼ cup chopped sun-dried tomatoes

2 tablespoons sliced green onions or fresh chives

2 tablespoons chopped fresh parsley

1 teaspoon sea salt

½ teaspoon freshly ground black pepper

¼ cup plus 2 tablespoons grapeseed oil

Preheat the oven to 350°F. Place an 8-inch oven-proof skillet (preferably a black, cast-iron one) in the oven to warm. In a small bowl, whisk the eggs and Cashew Cream. Add the broccoli, sun-dried tomatoes, green onions, and parsley and stir to combine. Set aside.

Remove the heated skillet from the oven and add ½ teaspoon of grapeseed oil so the bottom and sides are evenly coated. Pour in the egg mixture, sprinkle with salt and pepper, and place a lid on the pan. Return to the oven, allow the pan to sit 1 minute, and turn the temperature down to 300°F. Check on the frittata after 5 minutes to make sure the edges are not burning. If burning, turn the oven down to 250°F. Cook another 5-10 minutes until the eggs are no longer runny and completely set. Remove from the oven, allow to set a few minutes, then slice into serving pieces. Top with a serving of Broccoli Balsamic Salad.

NUTRITION PER SERVING	Cal	Fat	Protein	Carbs	Sugar	Fiber	Sod
	158	11g	9g	9g	3g	3g	105mg

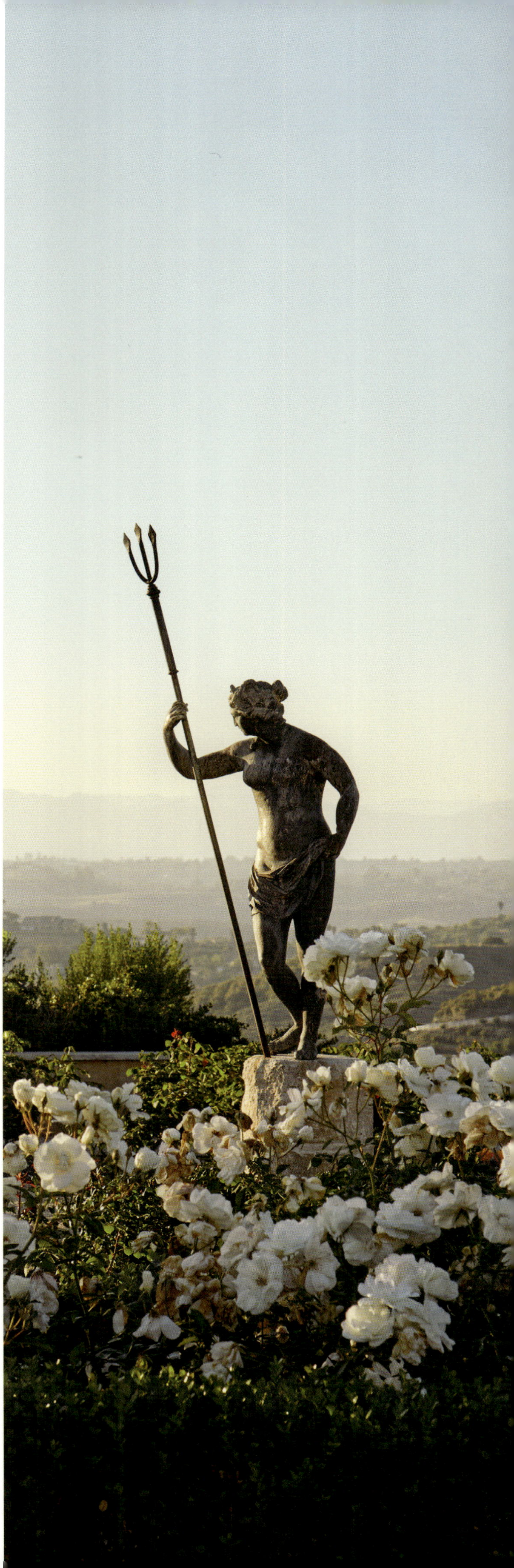

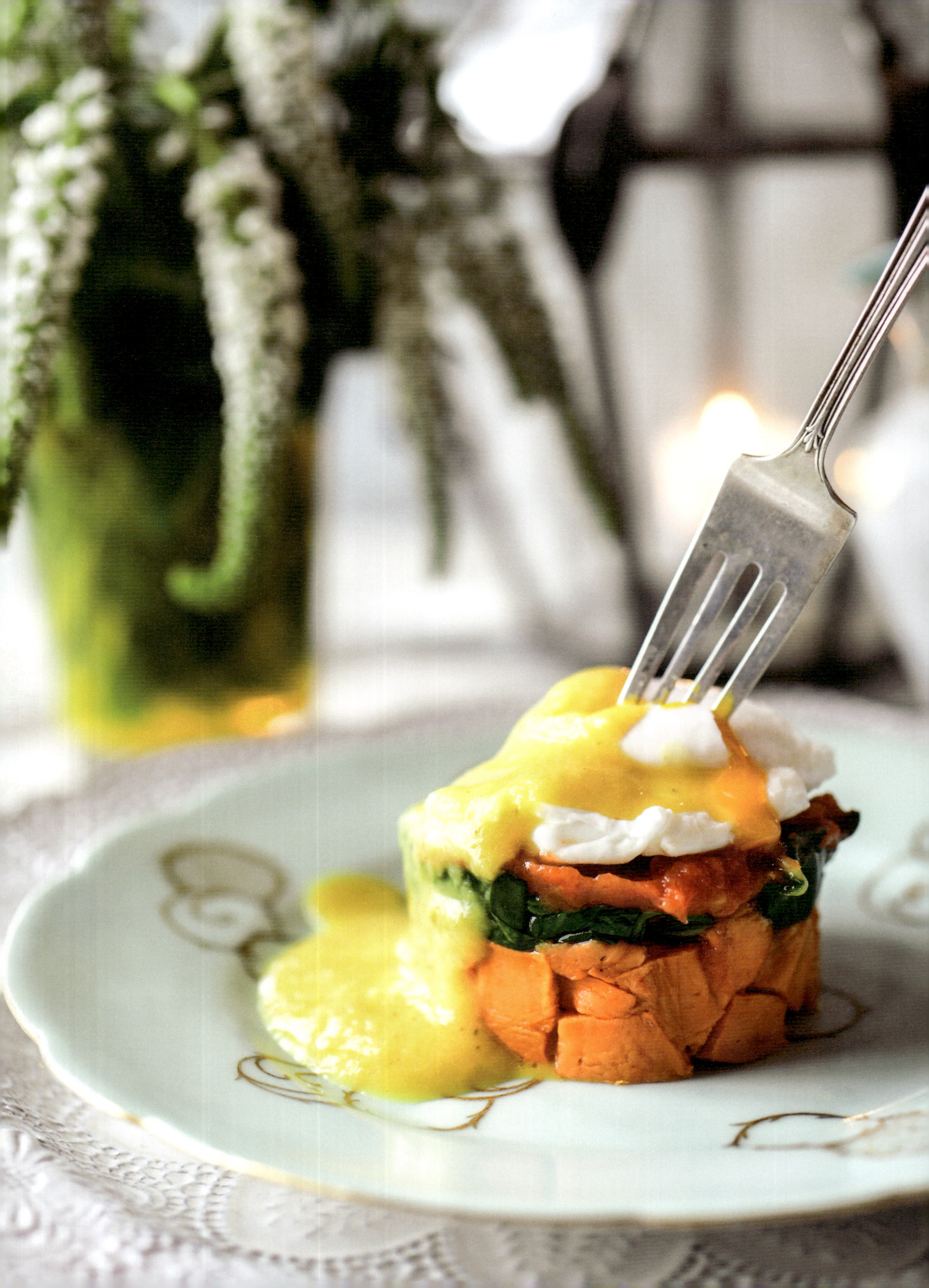

EGGS BENEDICT TOWERS

SERVES 6

Guests always comment on how delicious breakfasts at Cal-a-Vie taste, especially after an invigorating morning hike! Sweet potatoes are a great upgrade to traditional potatoes, and even though they taste sweeter, they actually have a lower glycemic index. Sweet potatoes also are a great source of beta-carotene and have more potassium than a banana. Our Yellow Pepper Hollandaise Sauce is a healthier, dairy-free substitute to traditional Hollandaise. You can make the Tomato Jam and the Yellow Pepper Hollandaise Sauce ahead of time, then reheat when ready to serve.

TOMATO JAM

YIELDS ABOUT 2 CUPS

8 tomatoes, tops removed and halved (any type of red, firm tomatoes will work–we recommend using Roma)

1 tablespoon grapeseed oil

2 sprigs fresh thyme

1½ teaspoons kosher salt

In a food processor, add the tomatoes and pulse until broken down, but still chunky (about 10-20 pulses).

In a large skillet over medium heat, warm the grapeseed oil. When hot, add the tomatoes, thyme, and salt and allow to reduce until most of the liquid in the pan disappears. Remove from the stove, discard the thyme sprigs, keep warm, and set aside.

YELLOW PEPPER HOLLANDAISE SAUCE

YIELDS ABOUT 1 CUP

¼ cup grapeseed oil

5 yellow bell peppers, cored, seeded, and roughly chopped to about 2-inch pieces

½ teaspoon kosher or sea salt

In a large skillet over medium heat, warm the oil. When the oil is hot, add the yellow peppers and salt. Allow the peppers to cook until they sweat, are softened, and are lightly browned.

In a blender, add the yellow pepper mixture and process until completely smooth. Cover to keep warm. Set aside.

ROASTED SWEET POTATO HASH

2 pounds red garnet yams or sweet potatoes, peeled and chopped in ½-inch cubes

2 teaspoons grapeseed oil

Preheat the oven to 350°F. In a large bowl, combine the yams and grapeseed oil. Spread evenly in a single layer on a baking sheet. Use more than one baking sheet if necessary so as not to overcrowd. Roast in the oven for 20-30 minutes until softened and browned. Keep warm and set aside.

SAUTÉED SPINACH

1 teaspoon grapeseed oil

16 ounces baby spinach

In a large sauté pan over medium heat, warm the oil. Add the spinach and stir, turning it regularly so it doesn't stick to the pan. When wilted, remove from the heat. Cover to keep warm, and set aside.

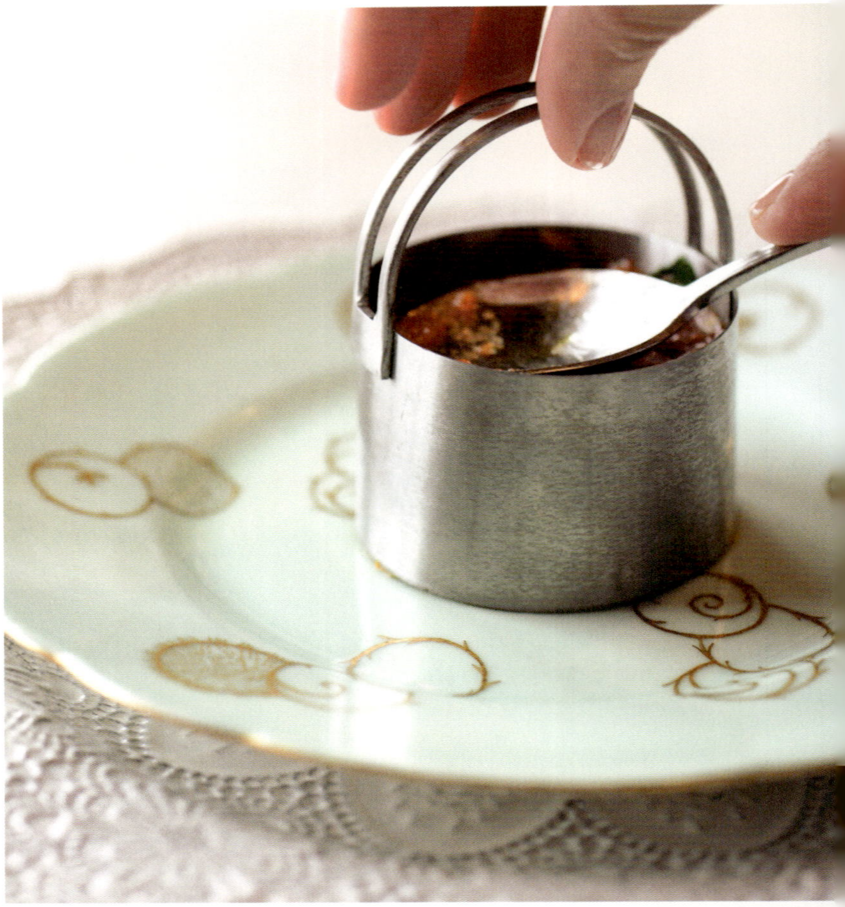

EGGS BENEDICT TOWERS ASSEMBLY

2 tablespoons white distilled vinegar

16 cups water

12 organic eggs

1½ cups Sweet Potato Hash

6 ounces Sautéed Spinach

½ cup Tomato Jam

1 cup Yellow Pepper Hollandaise Sauce

In a large stock pot over high heat, add the vinegar and water and bring to a rolling boil. Stir the water with a spoon to create a light circular current and gently crack 6 eggs into the water. Lower the heat to a very light boil. Set a timer for 4 minutes and gently remove the eggs from the water with a slotted spoon when time is up. While the eggs are cooking, build the Eggs Benedict Towers.

To create the Eggs Benedict Towers: Place a 3-inch ring mold on a serving plate. Spoon about ¼ cup of Sweet Potato Hash in the bottom and lightly tap down to make sure it's secure. Spoon on top about 2 tablespoons of Sautéed Spinach and lightly tap down again. Spoon about 2 teaspoons of Tomato Jam on top and spread to the edges. Then carefully remove the ring mold.

Repeat to build a second tower on the same plate. Place one poached egg on top of each tower. Pour about 2 tablespoons of Yellow Pepper Hollandaise over the eggs and serve.

Repeat the process on the remaining plates.

> TIP: If not using raw chopped yams right away, keep them in the refrigerator submerged in water. This recipe can also be used as a side dish with just about any protein.

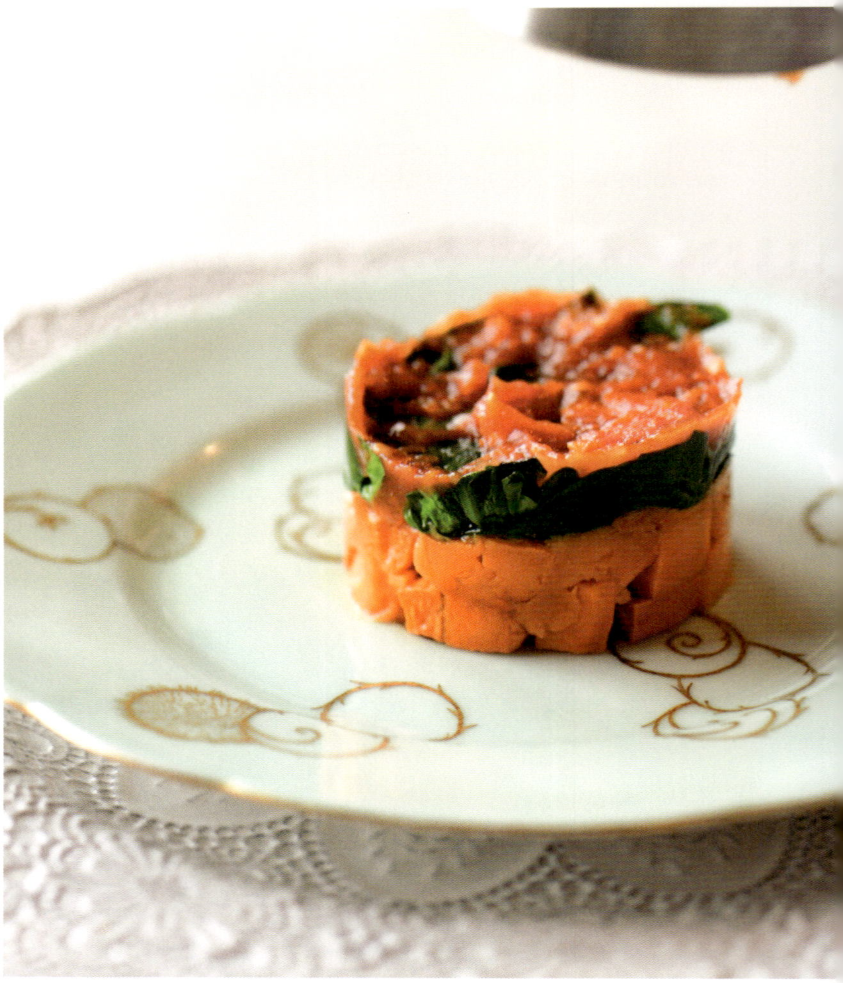

NUTRITION PER SERVING	Cal 316	Fat 20g	Protein 14g	Carbs 22g	Sugar 4g	Fiber 4g	Sod 523mg

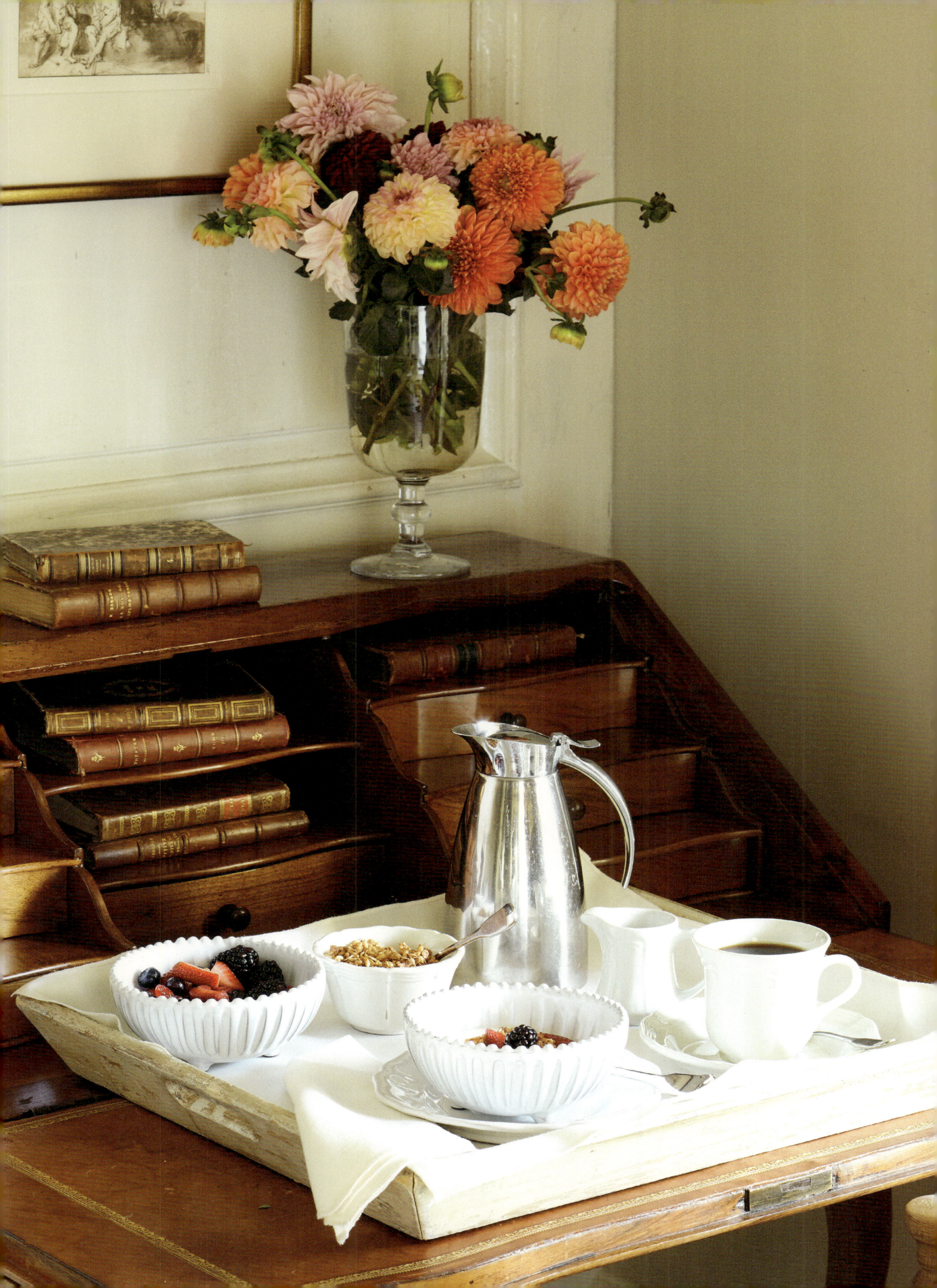

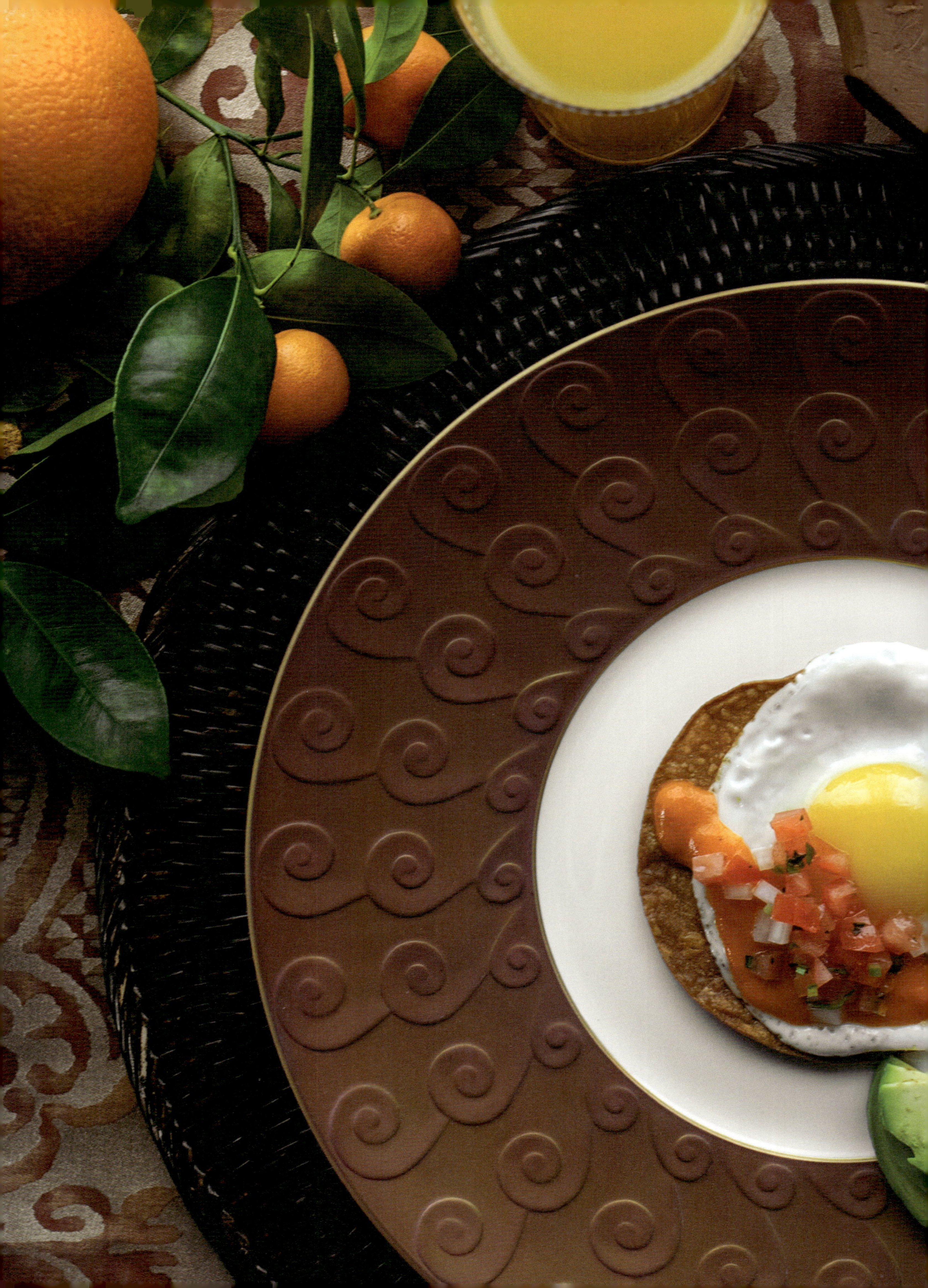

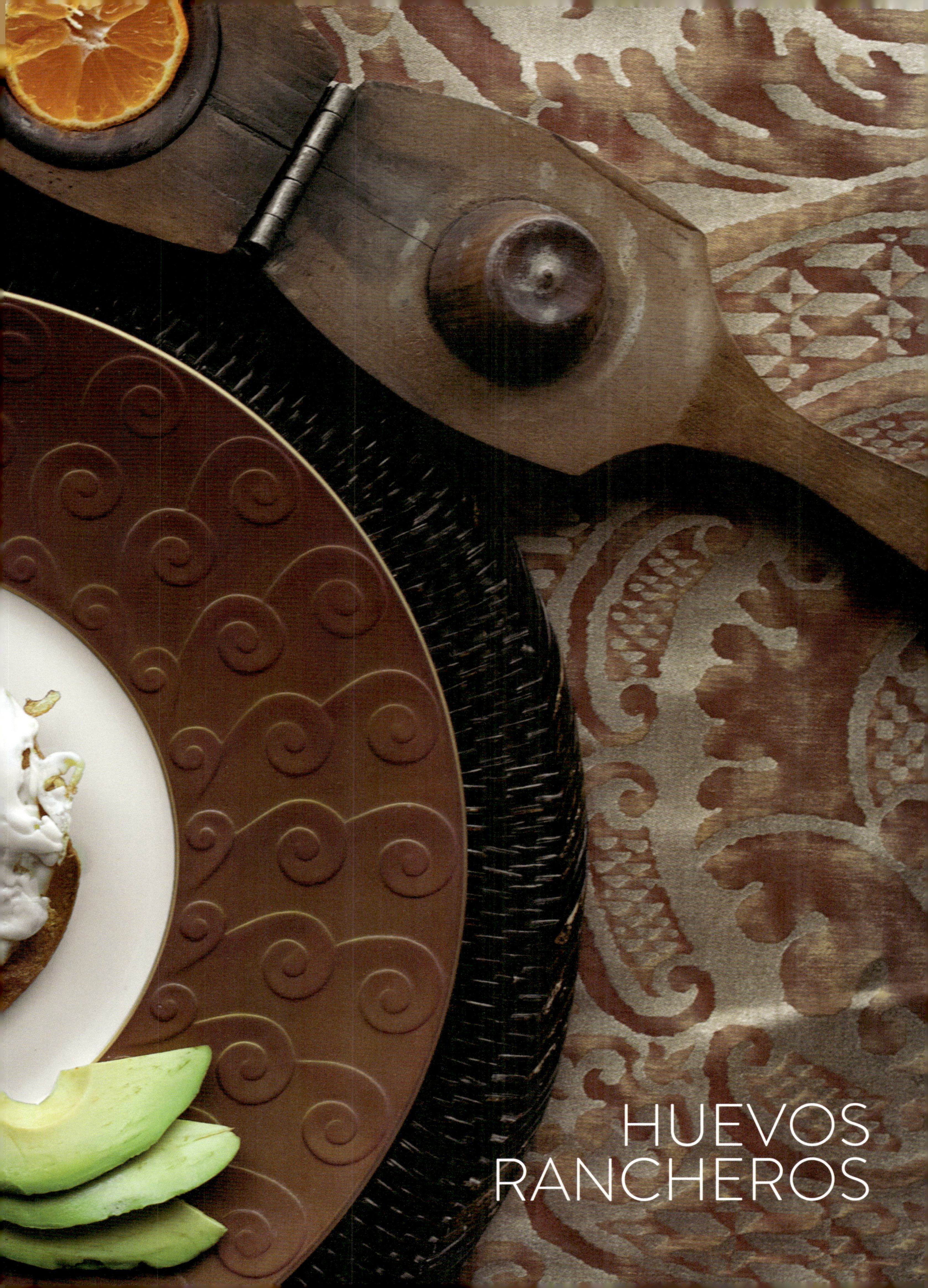

HUEVOS RANCHEROS

HUEVOS RANCHEROS

SERVES 8

This recipe is inspired by our cooks in the kitchen, many of whom learned how to make salsa from their grandmothers when they were children. This recipe is also a great way to enjoy an egg for breakfast with some extra healthy fat, flavor, and vegetables! For a cooking class, we demonstrated this recipe as an appetizer by cutting the tortillas into 3-inch circles with a mold and using quail eggs instead of chicken eggs.

PICO DE GALLO YIELDS ABOUT 1 CUP

1 cup Roma tomatoes, seeded and diced
¼ cup diced red onion
2 tablespoons minced jalapeño
3 tablespoons minced fresh cilantro
2 tablespoons fresh lime juice
kosher or sea salt to taste

In a small bowl, add all the ingredients and combine thoroughly. Season with salt to taste. Set aside in the refrigerator.

RANCHERO SALSA

2 tablespoons grapeseed oil
2 garlic cloves, peeled and quartered
¼ cup yellow onion, chopped into 1-inch pieces
1 yellow bell pepper, core removed, seeded, and cut into 1-inch pieces
1 red bell pepper, core removed, seeded, and cut into 1-inch pieces
4 Roma tomatoes, tops removed and chopped into 1-inch pieces
2 dried chilies de arbol, stems removed
1 teaspoon kosher or sea salt, plus more to taste

In a medium saucepan over medium-high heat, add the oil. When the oil is hot, add the garlic and onion and stir constantly for about 1-2 minutes. Add the bell peppers and cook another 1-2 minutes, until just starting to soften. Add tomatoes and dried chilies, stir, and cover. Lower the heat and allow to simmer for about 5 minutes until the tomatoes begin to break down and the peppers soften. Once tomatoes are mushy, remove the chilies de arbol and set aside. Transfer the rest of the mixture to a blender. Add 1 chile and 1 teaspoon salt. Blend until fully smooth. Taste and add more salt as needed and an additional chile if more heat is desired. Set aside in the refrigerator.

TOASTED TOSTADA SHELL

8 thin organic yellow corn tortillas

Preheat the oven to 350°F. Lay the tortillas on a baking sheet making sure they don't overlap. Bake for about 9 minutes, or until crisp. Cool and reserve.

HUEVOS RANCHEROS ASSEMBLY

8 Toasted Tostada Shells
1 cup shredded mozzarella cheese (or similar mild cheese)
8 teaspoons grapeseed oil, divided use
8 large organic eggs
2 cups Ranchero Salsa
1 cup Pico de Gallo
2 ripe avocados, pits removed, peeled, and sliced or chopped

Place 1 Toasted Tostada Shell on each serving plate and top each with 1 tablespoon of cheese. Set aside.

In a medium skillet over medium heat, add 2 teaspoons of grapeseed oil. Once the oil is hot, carefully crack 4 eggs into the pan and allow to lightly fry, covered, for about 90 seconds until the whites are cooked and the yolk is still soft. Remove from heat and place one egg on each tostada shell. Return pan to heat with 2 teaspoons grapeseed oil and repeat process, working in batches of 4 eggs at a time.

Top the eggs with ¼ cup Ranchero Salsa, 2 tablespoons Pico de Gallo, and avocado. Serve immediately.

NUTRITION PER SERVING	Cal 276	Fat 18g	Protein 10g	Carbs 21g	Sugar 4g	Fiber 5g	Sod 504mg

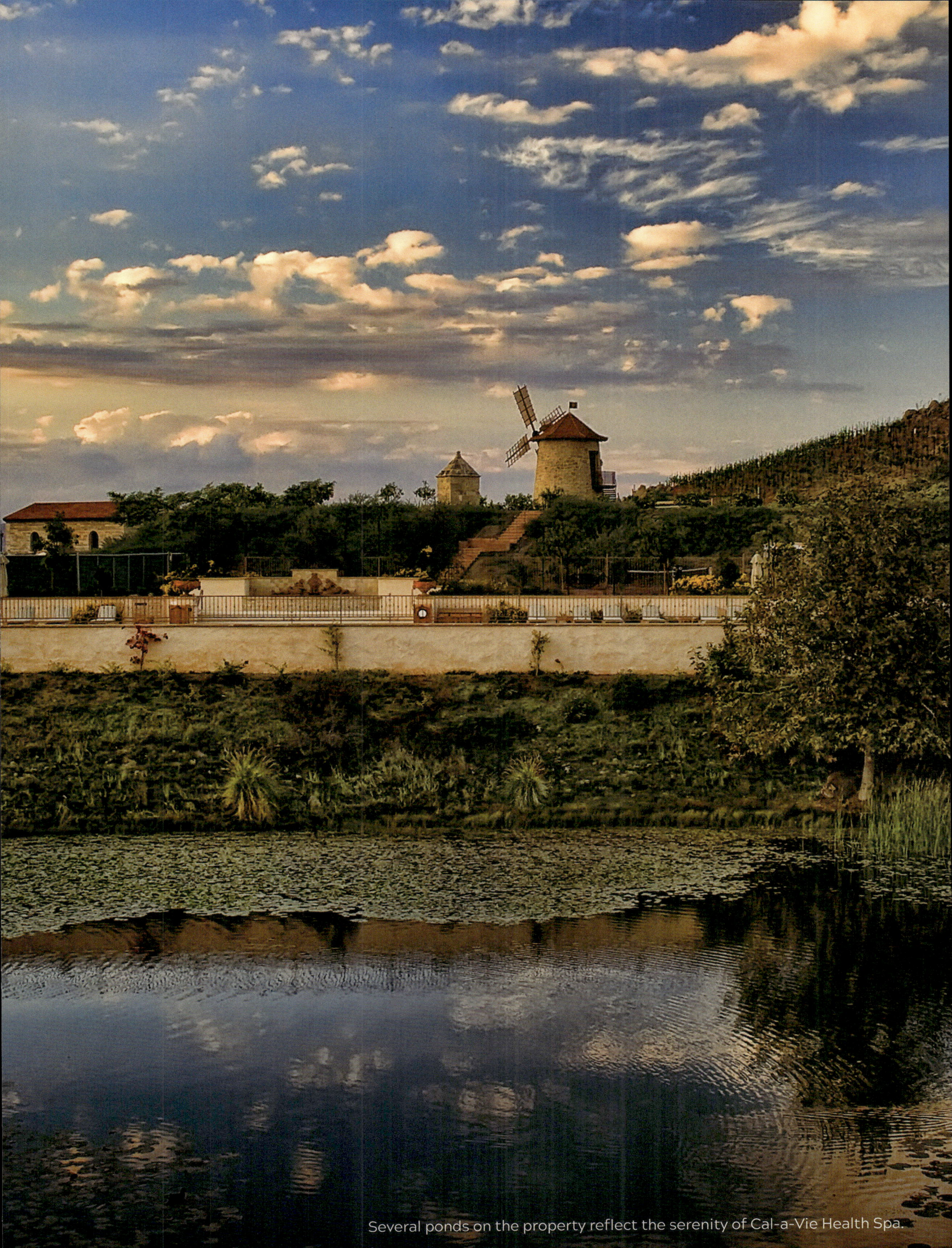

Several ponds on the property reflect the serenity of Cal-a-Vie Health Spa.

PANCAKES
WITH BLUEBERRY COMPOTE

MAKES 18 4-INCH PANCAKES

This is a great recipe to make on the weekends or when you have guests over. Be creative with this basic recipe. We serve it with Blueberry Compote, but you can add just about any berry or Fruit Compote. (See Steel Cut Oatmeal recipe page 236.) Spread a little nut butter on your pancakes for some extra protein to improve the glycemic index of this meal.

BLUEBERRY COMPOTE

YIELDS ABOUT 1 CUP

1 cup blueberries

¼ cup organic refined cane sugar

2 tablespoons water

1 teaspoon fresh lemon juice

In a medium skillet over medium heat, mix blueberries, sugar, and water. Allow to come to a boil and shake the pan occasionally until the blueberries begin to burst in 3-5 minutes. Remove from the heat, stir in the lemon juice, and set aside.

PANCAKES

2 eggs

¼ cup grapeseed oil

2 cups Glutino® All-Purpose Gluten Free Flour

1 teaspoon baking soda

1 teaspoon baking powder

½ teaspoon salt

2 cups soy milk (or any non-dairy milk)

¼ cup honey

In a large bowl, whisk eggs and grapeseed oil together until foamy and light. Add the flour, baking soda, baking powder, salt, milk, and honey, and whisk until batter is smooth.

Heat a large skillet or griddle over medium heat and lightly grease with oil or cooking spray. Use a ladle to pour about ¼ cup batter onto the griddle and cook until the edges become dry and small bubbles appear. Flip the pancake and cook the other side until lightly golden. Continue with remaining batter.

Drizzle 2-3 tablespoons of Blueberry Compote on top of the pancakes and serve immediately.

TIP: This recipe can be cut in half, or extra pancakes can be stored in the freezer for a morning treat on another day.

NUTRITION PER SERVING	Cal 126	Fat 4g	Protein 3g	Carbs 20g	Sugar 9g	Fiber 2g	Sod 158mg

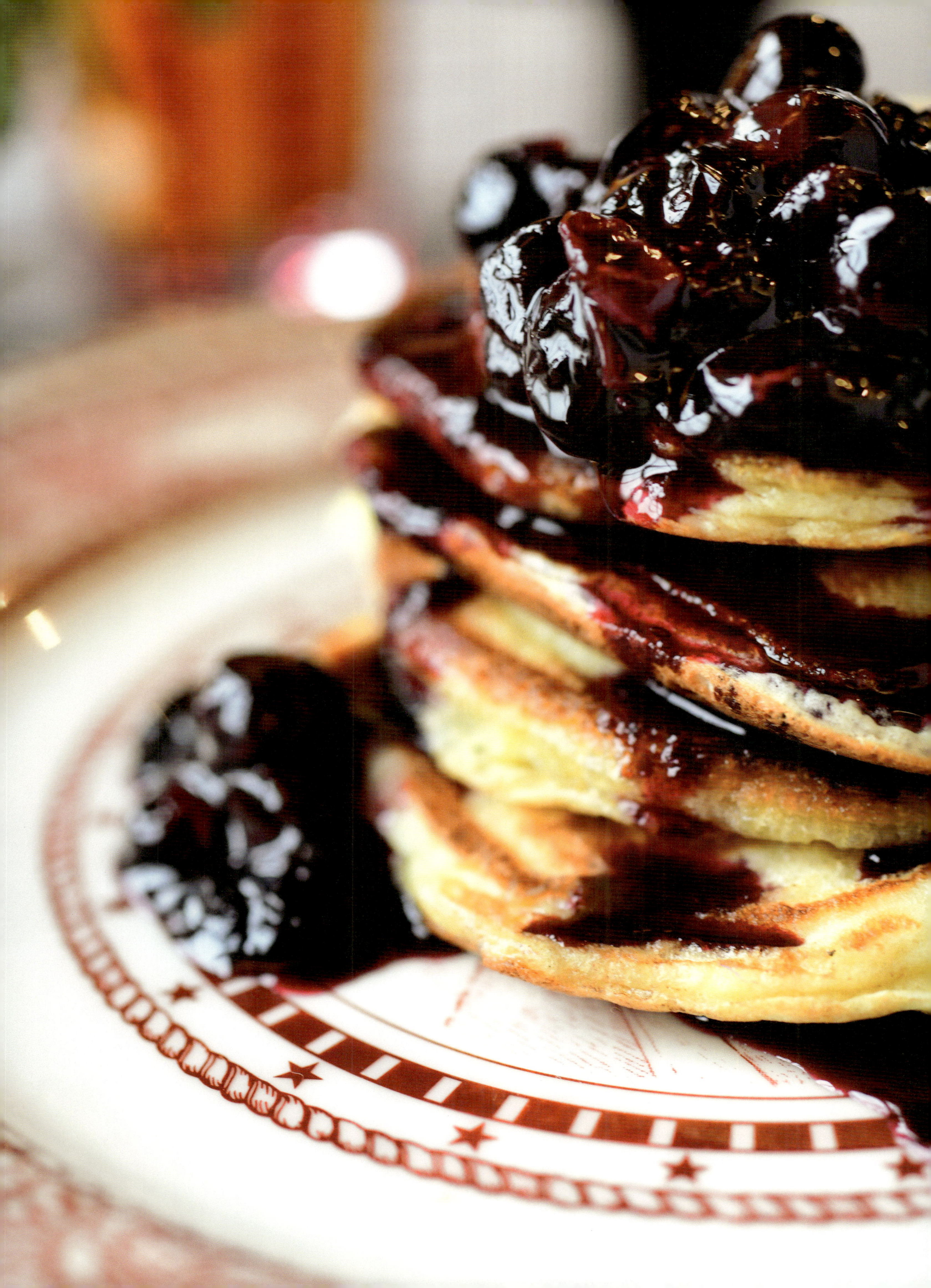

WAFFLES
WITH STRAWBERRY SAUCE AND MAPLE SYRUP

MAKES 10 WAFFLES

If you are trying to make these waffles healthy, skip the whipped cream and syrup and substitute fresh fruit and nut butter. If you choose to use milk and butter, make sure to pick the organic, grass-fed variety.

STRAWBERRY SAUCE

2 cups hulled and sliced strawberries

¼ cup organic refined cane sugar

2 tablespoons water

1 teaspoon fresh lemon juice

In a medium saucepan over medium heat, combine the strawberries, sugar, and water. Bring to a boil, then reduce the heat and simmer 20 minutes. Remove from the heat. Stir in the lemon juice. At this point, the sauce can be pureed in a blender or serve as is with chunks of strawberries. Set aside.

WAFFLES

1¾ cups unbleached, all-purpose flour

¼ cup light brown sugar

2 teaspoons baking powder

¼ teaspoon kosher salt

¼ cup unsalted butter
(substitute with ¼ cup grapeseed oil for dairy-free)

1½ cups milk (substitute with almond, soy, or coconut milk for dairy-free)

2 teaspoons apple cider vinegar

2 large eggs, separated

1 teaspoon vanilla extract

maple syrup

blueberries and raspberries for garnish

Heat a waffle iron and lightly grease with grapeseed oil or cooking spray. In a medium bowl, sift together the flour, light brown sugar, baking powder, and salt. Set aside. In a small pan over low heat, warm the butter (or oil), milk, and vinegar until just heated and the butter has melted, whisking to combine. Do not let milk come to a boil. Allow to cool slightly.

In a large bowl, whisk together the warmed milk and butter mixture, egg yolks, and vanilla. In a small, clean bowl, whisk egg whites until foamy, and soft peaks form. Set aside.

Slowly add dry ingredients into wet ingredients, working in batches and mixing well to combine before adding more. Gently fold in whipped egg whites until combined, but do not overmix to avoid deflating egg whites. Add about ¼ cup of batter to the waffle iron and cook until golden brown. Top with fresh berries. Drizzle with Strawberry Sauce and maple syrup.

NUTRITION PER SERVING	Cal	Fat	Protein	Carbs	Sugar	Fiber	Sod
	201	7g	5g	30g	12g	1g	150mg

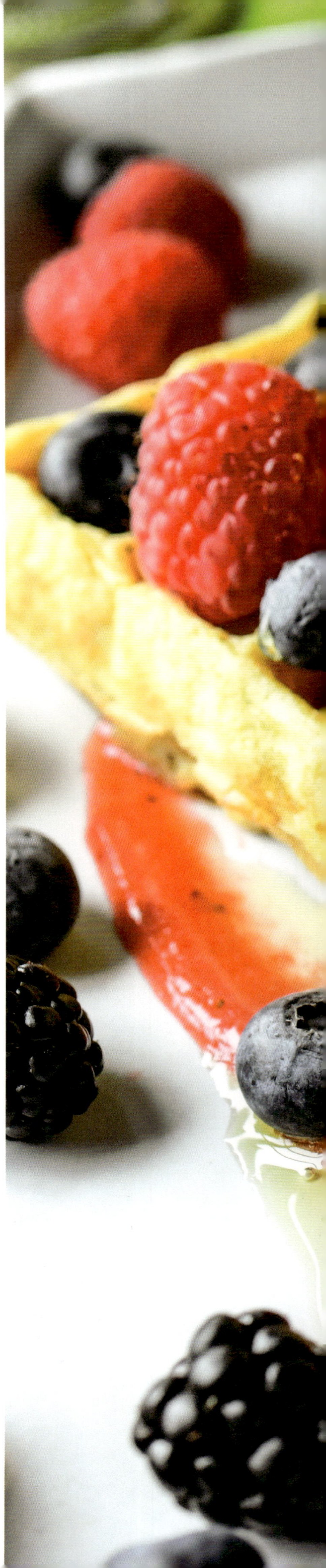

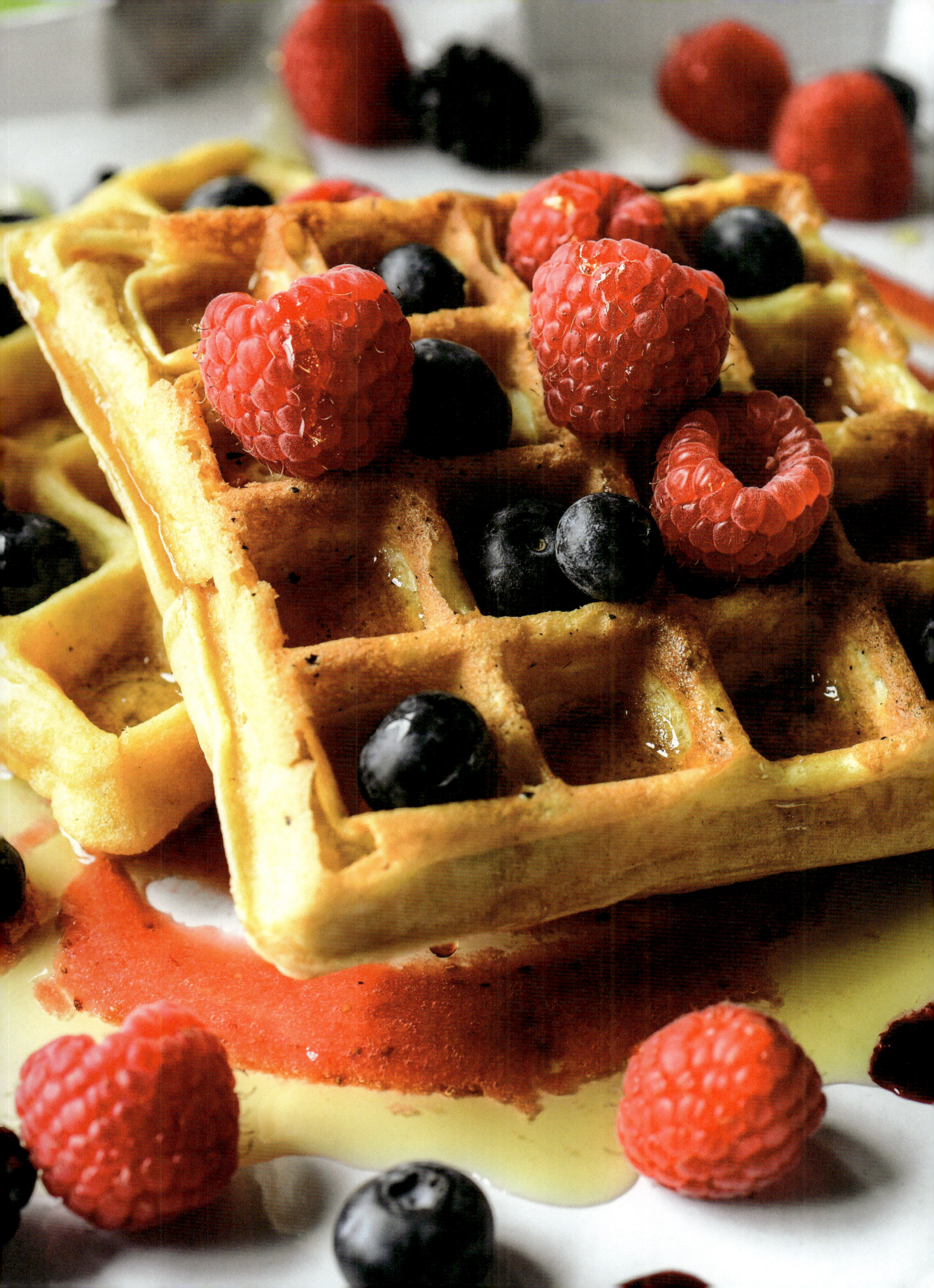

STEEL-CUT OATMEAL
WITH FRUIT COMPOTE

MAKES 4 SERVINGS

If you don't have time to wait 45 minutes for your steel-cut oats to cook, try soaking them overnight. Steel-cut oats have a chewier texture and a much lower glycemic index than regular rolled or instant oats. Cinnamon in the fruit compote and pecans on top of the oatmeal help to improve blood sugars.

STEEL-CUT OATMEAL

6 cups water

2 cups Bob's Red Mill® Gluten Free Steel Cut Oats

In a medium saucepan over high heat, add the water and oats. Bring to a boil. Lower the heat to a simmer and cook, covered, for about 45 minutes. Remove and keep warm.

FRUIT COMPOTE

¼ teaspoon grapeseed oil

1 pound apples or peaches (about 3 pieces of fruit), cored, pitted, and diced to about ¼-inch pieces (we recommend Pink Lady, Honeycrisp, or Gala apples)

1 teaspoon ground cinnamon

¼ cup maple syrup

½ cup pecans, toasted and chopped

In a medium saucepan over medium heat, add the oil. Once hot, add the fruit and allow to soften, stirring regularly, for about 5 minutes. Add cinnamon and maple syrup and stir, making sure to coat all the fruit. Continue cooking for an additional 1-2 minutes and remove from heat.

Serve about ¾ cup of oats topped with ¼ cup Fruit Compote and chopped pecans.

NUTRITION PER SERVING	Cal	Fat	Protein	Carbs	Sugar	Fiber	Sod
	348	12g	7g	58g	25g	8g	19mg

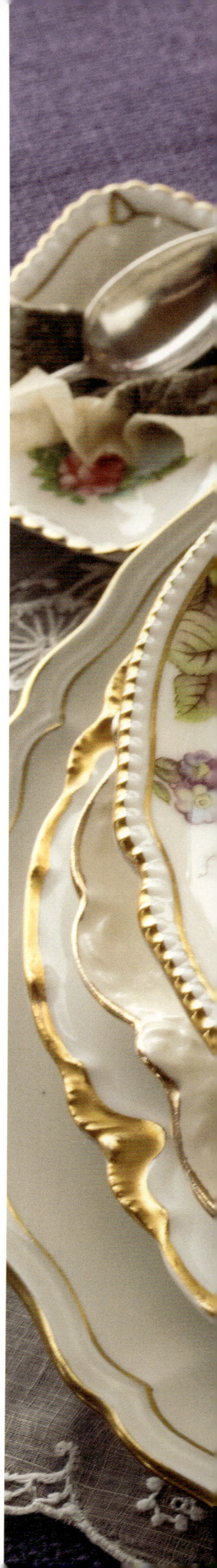

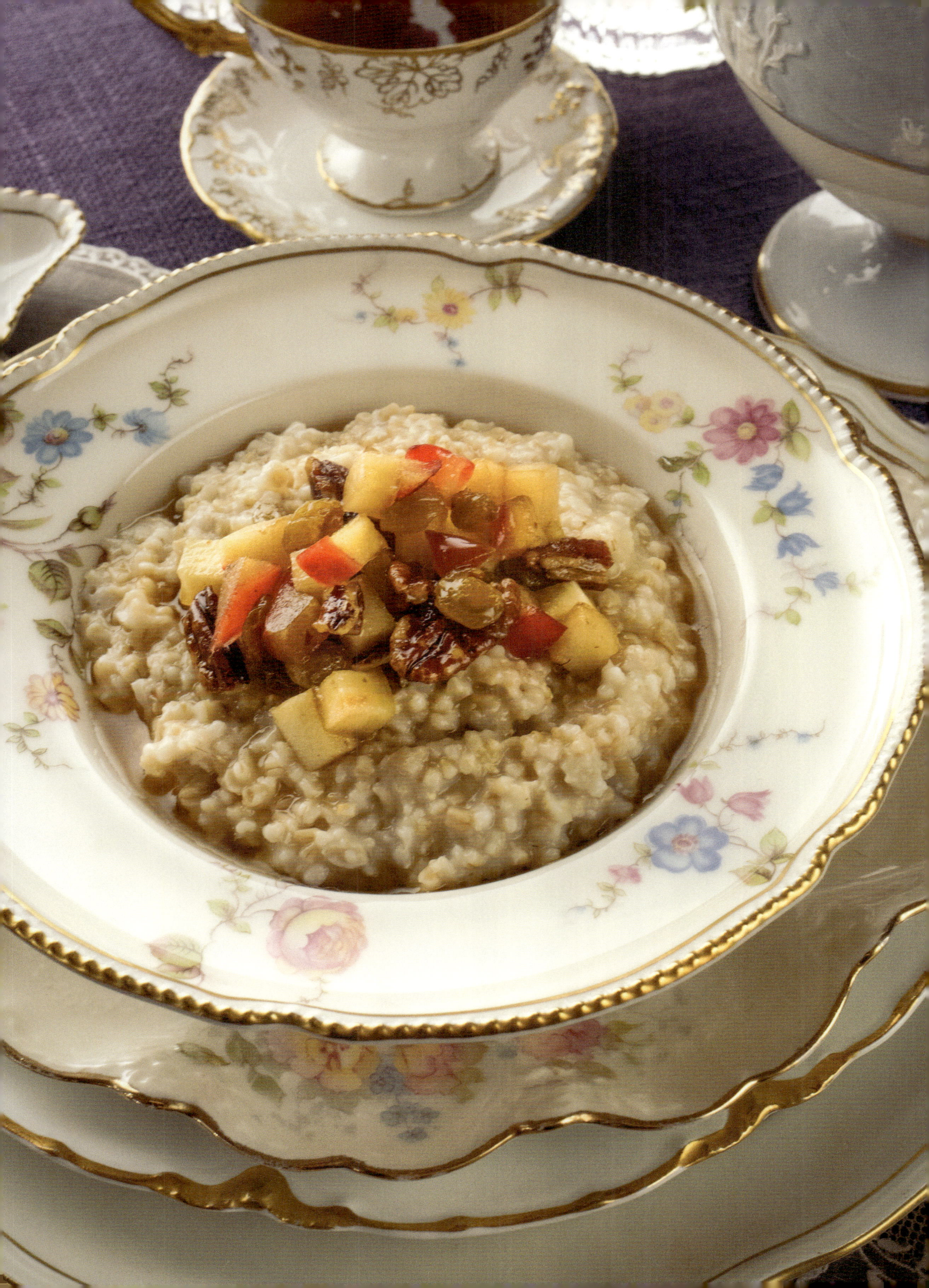

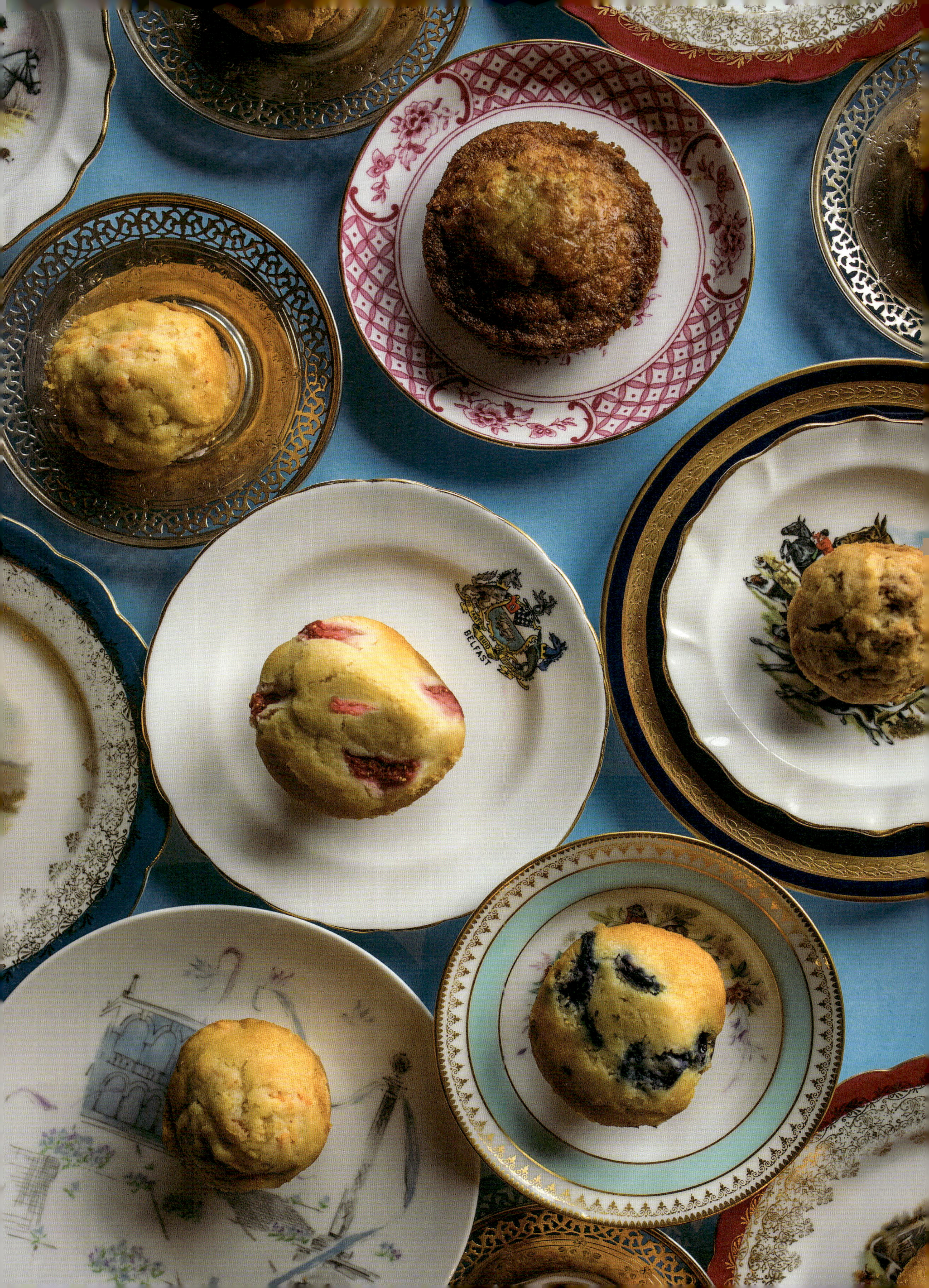
BELFAST

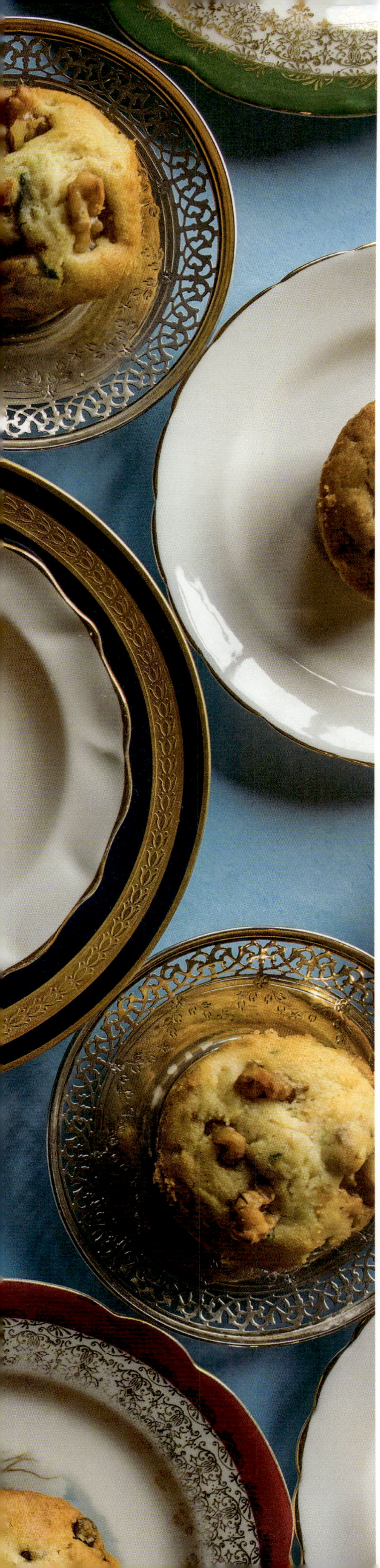

WELCOME BANANA MUFFINS

MAKES 18 2-INCH MUFFINS

This famous muffin is what welcomes each guest when they arrive and settle into their rooms every week. In the kitchen, we affectionately call it the "Welcome Muffin." Choose riper bananas for a sweeter muffin.

¾ cup Glutino® All-Purpose Gluten Free Flour
½ teaspoon baking soda
⅛ teaspoon kosher or sea salt
2 tablespoons grapeseed oil
½ cup sugar
1 egg, lightly beaten
2 ripe bananas, lightly mashed

Preheat the oven to 350°F. Lightly grease a muffin tin.

In a large bowl, whisk to combine flour, baking soda, and salt. Add in remaining ingredients and gently stir, being careful not to over-mash the bananas.

Evenly portion the batter into a prepared muffin tin. Bake for 12 minutes, then rotate the pan and continue to bake for an additional 2-4 minutes, until golden brown. A toothpick inserted into the center of a muffin should come out clean. Allow to cool in the tin a few minutes before removing.

TIP: For Banana Bread: Double the recipe to make a loaf of banana bread. Adjust the baking time to at least 40 minutes, but check with a toothpick inserted into the center for doneness.

NUTRITION PER SERVING	Cal	Fat	Protein	Carbs	Sugar	Fiber	Sod
	68	2g	1g	13g	7g	1g	52mg

ZUCCHINI MUFFINS

MAKES 18 2-INCH MUFFINS

This is our version of your favorite zucchini bread, served in just the right portions. Zucchini is a classic vegetable that is often found in both savory and sweet baked goods.

¼ cup grapeseed oil
½ cup sugar
¼ cup soy or other non-dairy milk
1 egg
¾ cup Glutino® All-Purpose Gluten Free Flour
½ teaspoon baking soda
¼ teaspoon kosher or sea salt
¾ cup shredded zucchini, skin on

Preheat the oven to 350°F. Lightly grease a muffin tin.

In a small bowl, whisk together the grapeseed oil, sugar, soy milk, and egg. Set aside. In a large bowl, combine the flour, baking soda, and salt and whisk well. Add the wet ingredients to the dry ingredients and mix just to combine, making sure not to leave any dry lumps in the batter. Gently fold in the shredded zucchini. Do not overmix.

Evenly portion the batter into the prepared muffin tin. Bake for 20 minutes, rotating pan halfway through baking, until golden brown. A toothpick inserted into the center of a muffin should come out clean. Allow to cool for 5 minutes in the tin and then remove and finish cooling on a wire rack.

NUTRITION PER SERVING	Cal 72	Fat 4g	Protein 1g	Carbs 10g	Sugar 6g	Fiber 1g	Sod 59mg

APPLE SPICE MUFFINS

MAKES 18 2-INCH MUFFINS

People love our muffins and are always surprised they are gluten-free. The secret is using a gluten-free flour blend, and in many of our muffins, adding ricotta cheese to help improve the overall texture and moistness. Apple Spice Muffins are perfect to serve in the fall as the weather starts to cool.

2 tablespoons grapeseed oil
½ cup sugar
½ cup ricotta cheese or coconut yogurt
1 egg
1 tablespoon soy milk (or other non-dairy milk)
½ teaspoon vanilla extract
1 cup Glutino® All-Purpose Gluten Free Flour
¼ teaspoon baking powder
¼ teaspoon baking soda
¼ teaspoon kosher or sea salt
½ teaspoon allspice
½ teaspoon ground cinnamon
½ cup shredded apple, peeled (we recommend Pink Lady, Honey Crisp, Gala, or Fuji varieties)

Preheat the oven to 350°F. Lightly grease a mini-muffin tin.

In a small bowl, whisk together the grapeseed oil, sugar, ricotta cheese, egg, soy milk, and vanilla extract. Set aside. In a large bowl, combine the flour, baking powder, baking soda, salt, allspice, and cinnamon and whisk well. Add the wet ingredients to the dry ingredients and mix just to combine, making sure not to leave any dry lumps in the batter. Once combined, gently fold in the shredded apple. Do not overmix.

Once the batter is mixed, evenly portion the batter into prepared muffin tin. Bake for 20 minutes, rotating the pan halfway through baking, until golden brown. A toothpick inserted into the center of a muffin should come out clean. Allow to cool for 5 minutes in the tin and then remove and finish cooling on a wire rack.

NUTRITION PER SERVING	Cal 77	Fat 3g	Protein 2g	Carbs 12g	Sugar 6g	Fiber 1g	Sod 58mg

CARROT APPLE MUFFINS

MAKES 18 2-INCH MUFFINS

We love upgrading the nutrition in our muffins by sneaking in fresh fruit and vegetables whenever possible. If you don't have time to shred apples and carrots by hand on a grater, consider using a kitchen gadget such as a Saladmaster© machine.

¼ cup grapeseed oil

½ cup sugar

¼ cup soy or other non-dairy milk

1 egg

¾ cup Glutino® All-Purpose Gluten Free Flour

½ teaspoon baking soda

¼ teaspoon kosher or sea salt

½ cup shredded apple, peeled (we recommend Pink Lady, Honey Crisp, Gala, or Fuji varieties)

½ cup shredded carrot

Preheat the oven to 350°F. Lightly grease a mini-muffin tin.

In a small bowl, whisk together the grapeseed oil, sugar, soy milk, and egg. In a large bowl, combine the flour, baking soda, and salt and whisk well. Set aside. Add the wet ingredients to the dry ingredients and mix just to combine, making sure not to leave any dry lumps in the batter. Gently fold in the shredded apple and carrot. Do not overmix.

Once batter is mixed, evenly portion batter into prepared muffin tin. Bake for 12-15 minutes, rotating pan halfway through baking, until golden brown. A toothpick inserted into the center of a muffin should come out clean. Allow to cool for 5 minutes in the tin and then remove and finish cooling on a wire rack.

NUTRITION PER SERVING	Cal 75	Fat 3g	Protein 1g	Carbs 11g	Sugar 6g	Fiber 1g	Sod 62mg

MACADAMIA CHOCOLATE MUFFINS

YIELDS 36 2-INCH MUFFINS

If you are trying to steer clear of soy, dairy, or gluten, this recipe will hit the spot. You can find Enjoy Life® chocolate chips at your local health food store. Regular semi-sweet chocolate chips often have soy lecithin in them and can contain trace amounts of gluten due to cross contamination. Always read your labels carefully.

2 cups Glutino® All-Purpose Gluten Free Flour

½ teaspoon baking powder

½ teaspoon baking soda

¼ teaspoon ground cinnamon

¼ teaspoon ground cloves

¼ teaspoon kosher or sea salt

1 cup organic unrefined cane sugar

½ cup coconut yogurt

1 egg

¼ cup coconut oil

½ cup Enjoy Life® gluten free chocolate chips

½ cup macadamia nuts, toasted and finely chopped

Preheat the oven to 350°F. In a small bowl, combine the flour, baking powder, baking soda, cinnamon, cloves, and salt and mix thoroughly. In a separate bowl, combine the sugar, coconut yogurt, egg, and coconut oil and mix well. Set aside. Gently fold the wet ingredients into the dry ingredients until completely combined. Add the chocolate chips and macadamia nuts. Evenly portion the batter into a greased muffin tin, and bake for about 12-15 minutes. A toothpick inserted into the center of a muffin should come out clean. Allow to cool for 5 minutes in the tin and then remove and finish cooling on a wire rack.

NUTRITION PER SERVING	Cal 92	Fat 5g	Protein 1g	Carbs 12g	Sugar 7g	Fiber 1g	Sod 42mg

LEMON BLUEBERRY MUFFINS

MAKES 36 2-INCH MUFFINS

Lemon zest not only has the wonderful aromatic compounds from the essential oils of the peel, it also is loaded with Vitamin C. Make sure to buy organic blueberries as they are always on the "Dirty Dozen" list (See page 276.) of fruits that are usually treated in the fields with pesticides or other chemicals.

- ½ cup grapeseed oil
- 1 cup sugar
- 2 lemons, zested and juiced
- 1 cup coconut yogurt or coconut milk or non-dairy sour cream
- 2 eggs
- 1 teaspoon vanilla extract
- 2 cups Glutino® All-Purpose Gluten Free Flour
- ½ teaspoon baking soda
- ½ teaspoon kosher or sea salt
- 1 pint blueberries

In a small bowl, whisk together the grapeseed oil, sugar, lemon juice, zest, yogurt, eggs, and vanilla extract. Set aside. In a large bowl, combine the flour, baking soda, and salt and whisk well. Add the wet ingredients to the dry ingredients and mix just to combine, making sure not to leave any dry lumps in the batter. Gently fold in the blueberries. Do not overmix.

Once batter is mixed, evenly portion the batter into the prepared muffin tins. Bake for 20 minutes, rotating the pans halfway through baking, until golden brown. A toothpick inserted into the center of a muffin should come out clean. Allow to cool for 5 minutes in the tin and then remove and finish cooling on a wire rack.

TIP: Try different brands of gluten free flour since the flavor and texture of your muffins can vary with the brand.

NUTRITION PER SERVING	Cal 91	Fat 4g	Protein 1g	Carbs 13g	Sugar 7g	Fiber 1g	Sod 48mg

LEMON POPPYSEED MUFFINS

MAKES 18 2-INCH MUFFINS

Poppy seeds come in black, blue, and white varieties. Visually, blue or black serves as a great color contrast for most baked goods. Don't worry, there are very few opiates in poppy seeds.

- ¼ cup grapeseed oil
- ½ cup sugar
- 1 lemon, zested and juiced
- ½ cup Greek yogurt
- 1 egg
- ½ teaspoon vanilla extract
- 1 cup Glutino® All-Purpose Gluten Free Flour
- 1 tablespoon poppy seeds
- ¼ teaspoon baking soda
- ⅛ teaspoon kosher or sea salt

Preheat the oven to 350°F. Lightly grease a muffin tin.

In a small bowl, whisk together the grapeseed oil, sugar, lemon juice, zest, Greek yogurt, egg, and vanilla extract. Set aside. In a large bowl, combine the flour, poppy seeds, baking soda, and salt and whisk well. Add the wet ingredients to the dry ingredients and mix just to combine, making sure not to leave any dry lumps in the batter. Do not overmix.

Once batter is mixed, evenly portion batter into prepared muffin tin. Bake for 20 minutes, rotating pan halfway through baking, until golden brown. A toothpick inserted into the center of a muffin should come out clean. Allow to cool for 5 minutes in the tin and then remove and finish cooling on a wire rack.

NUTRITION PER SERVING	Cal 87	Fat 4g	Protein 2g	Carbs 12g	Sugar 6g	Fiber 1g	Sod 38mg

COCONUT PISTACHIO MUFFINS

MAKES 18 2-INCH MUFFINS

The pistachios and shredded coconut give this muffin a fantastic texture. They also add fiber, protein, and fat to slow digestion and offset the sugar in this recipe.

- ¼ cup grapeseed oil
- ½ cup sugar
- ½ teaspoon lemon zest
- 1 egg
- ½ teaspoon vanilla extract
- 1 cup Glutino® All-Purpose Gluten Free Flour
- ¼ teaspoon baking powder
- ¼ teaspoon baking soda
- ¼ teaspoon kosher or sea salt
- ¼ teaspoon ground cinnamon
- ⅛ teaspoon ground nutmeg
- ¼ cup pistachios, toasted and chopped
- ¼ cup shredded unsweetened coconut flakes
- ¼ cup Greek yogurt

Preheat the oven to 350°F. Lightly grease a muffin tin.

In a small bowl, whisk together the grapeseed oil, sugar, lemon zest, egg, and vanilla extract. Set aside. In a large bowl, combine the flour, baking powder, baking soda, salt, cinnamon, and nutmeg and whisk well. Add the wet ingredients to the dry ingredients and mix just to combine, making sure not to leave any dry lumps in the batter. Gently fold in the pistachios and coconut flakes. Do not overmix.

Evenly portion the batter into the prepared muffin tin and top each muffin with about 1 teaspoon of coconut flakes. Bake for 20 minutes, rotating pan halfway through baking, until golden brown. A toothpick inserted into the center of a muffin should come out clean. Allow to cool for 5 minutes in the tin and then remove and finish cooling on a wire rack.

NUTRITION PER SERVING	Cal 79	Fat 5g	Protein 2g	Carbs 8g	Sugar 4g	Fiber 1g	Sod 35mg

STRAWBERRY LEMON MUFFINS

MAKES 18 2-INCH MUFFINS

Choose strawberries in season for the best flavor, and make sure they are organic. Folding them in gently is key to making sure you can still see the strawberries in your final product.

- 2 tablespoons grapeseed oil
- ½ cup sugar
- 1 lemon, zested and juiced
- ½ cup Greek yogurt or ricotta cheese
- 1 egg
- ½ teaspoon vanilla extract
- 1 cup Glutino® All-Purpose Gluten Free Flour
- ¼ teaspoon baking powder
- ¼ teaspoon baking soda
- ¼ teaspoon kosher or sea salt
- ½ cup strawberries, sliced

Preheat the oven to 350°F. Lightly grease a muffin tin.

In a small bowl, whisk together the grapeseed oil, sugar, lemon juice, zest, Greek yogurt or ricotta cheese, egg, and vanilla extract. Set aside. In a large bowl, combine the flour, baking powder, baking soda, and salt and whisk well. Set aside. Add the wet ingredients to the dry ingredients and mix just to combine, making sure not to leave any dry lumps in the batter. Gently fold in the strawberries. Do not overmix.

Once batter is mixed, evenly portion batter into prepared muffin tin. Bake for 20 minutes, rotating pan halfway through baking, until golden brown. A toothpick inserted into the center of a muffin should come out clean. Allow to cool for 5 minutes in the tin and then remove and finish cooling on a wire rack.

NUTRITION PER SERVING	Cal 72	Fat 2g	Protein 2g	Carbs 12g	Sugar 6g	Fiber 1g	Sod 56mg

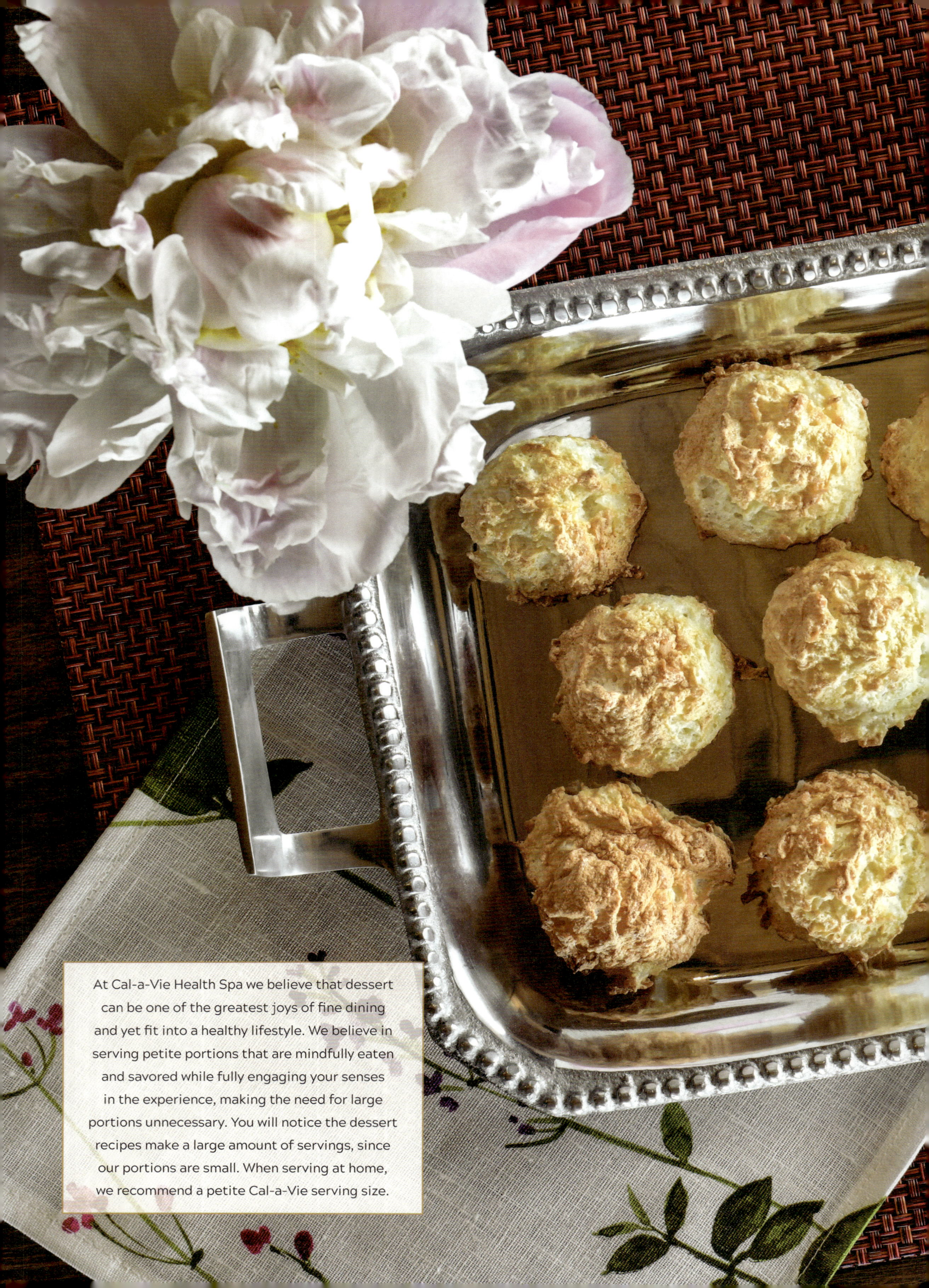

At Cal-a-Vie Health Spa we believe that dessert can be one of the greatest joys of fine dining and yet fit into a healthy lifestyle. We believe in serving petite portions that are mindfully eaten and savored while fully engaging your senses in the experience, making the need for large portions unnecessary. You will notice the dessert recipes make a large amount of servings, since our portions are small. When serving at home, we recommend a petite Cal-a-Vie serving size.

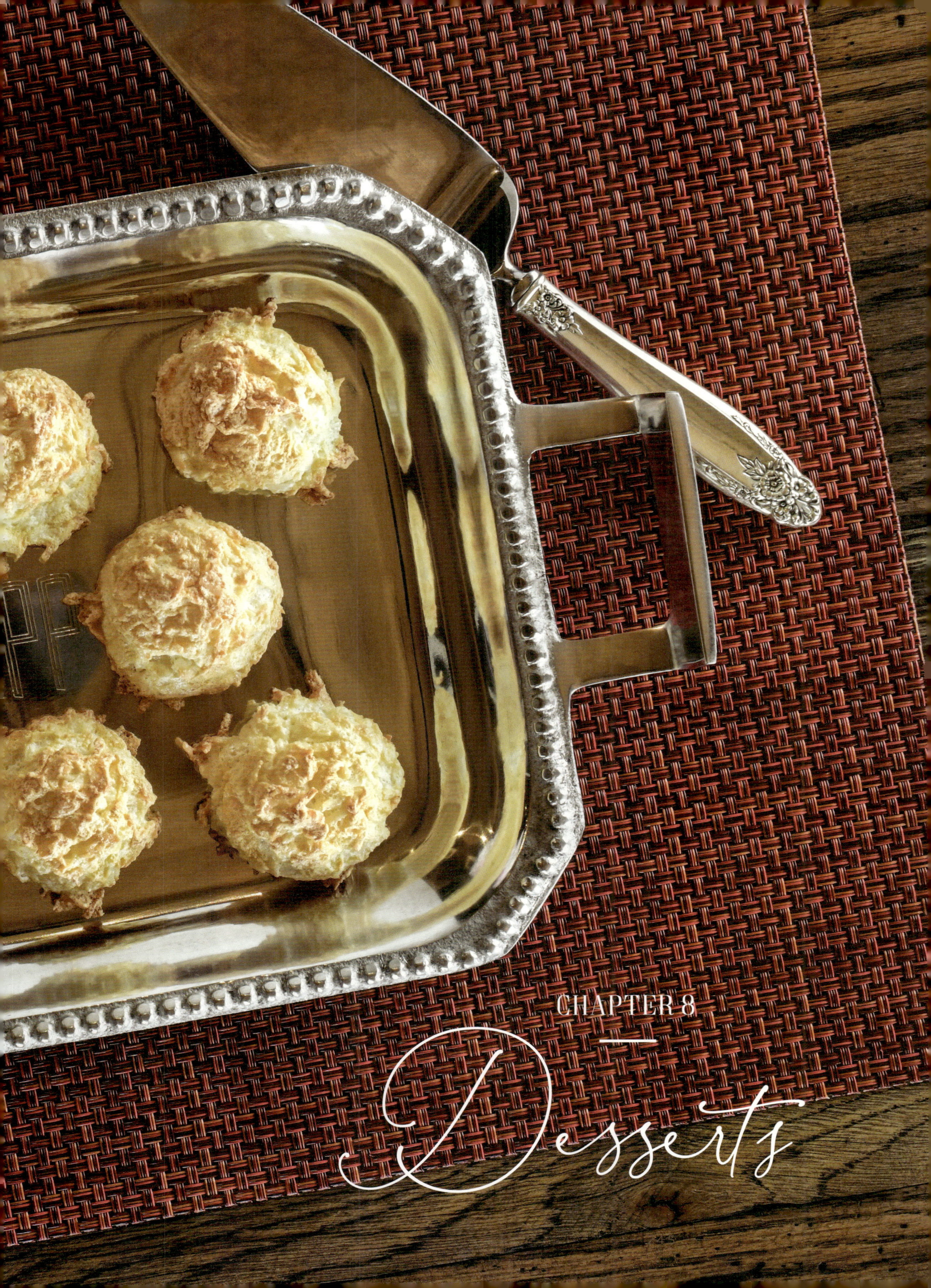

CHAPTER 8

Desserts

COCONUT MACAROON

YIELDS 2 DOZEN

Hmm...is it macaroon or macaron? Macarons are pronounced "mack-ah-ROHN" and are usually made into little colorful, round, layered cookies that have a variety of sweet fillings. Macaroons, on the other hand, are pronounced "mach-ah-ROON" and are fairly dense, ambiguously shaped dollops of coconut-filled cookies baked to a golden brown. Cal-a-Vie's are the second variety, and they're a sweet treat to end a meal and are remarkably low in calories.

2 cups unsweetened coconut flakes

3 egg whites

½ cup organic cane sugar, divided use

Preheat the oven to 350°F. In a mixer with the whip attachment, whip the egg whites to soft peaks. With the mixer still whipping, add ¼ cup of the sugar, making certain it is fully incorporated before adding the next ¼ cup. Whip the meringue until stiff peaks are formed, about 3-5 minutes. Gently fold the coconut flakes into the meringue. Using a small ice cream scoop, drop the dough in rounds onto a baking pan lined with a silicone sheet. Bake for 15-20 minutes until lightly browned. Cool on the pan for a few minutes to let the macaroons set, and then gently take them off. Keep stored in an airtight container.

NUTRITION PER SERVING	Cal	Fat	Protein	Carbs	Sugar	Fiber	Sod
	64	5g	1g	6g	5g	1g	8mg

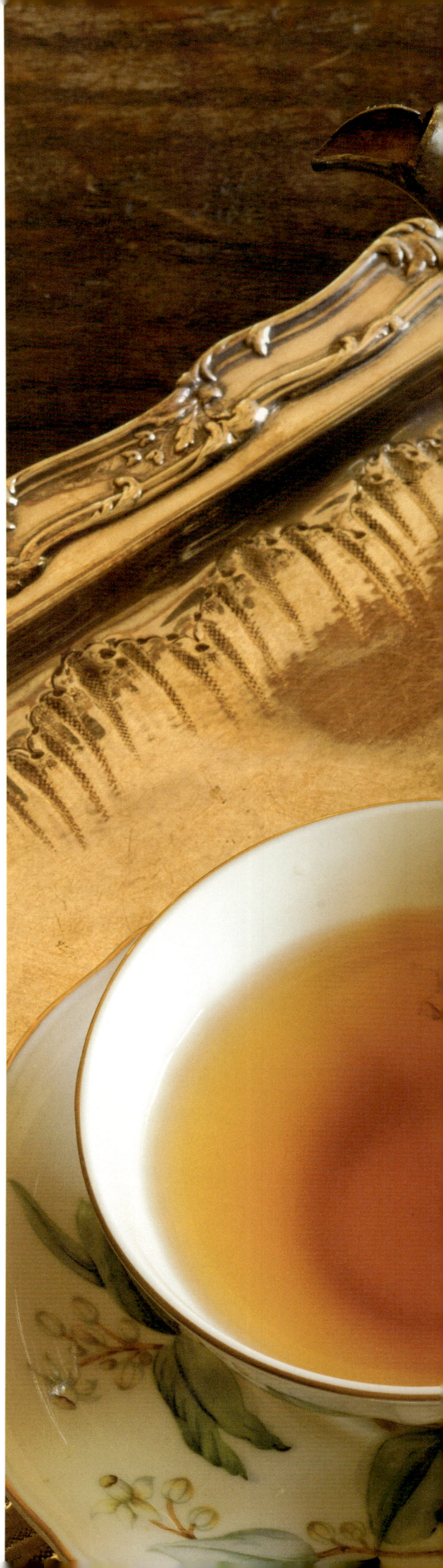

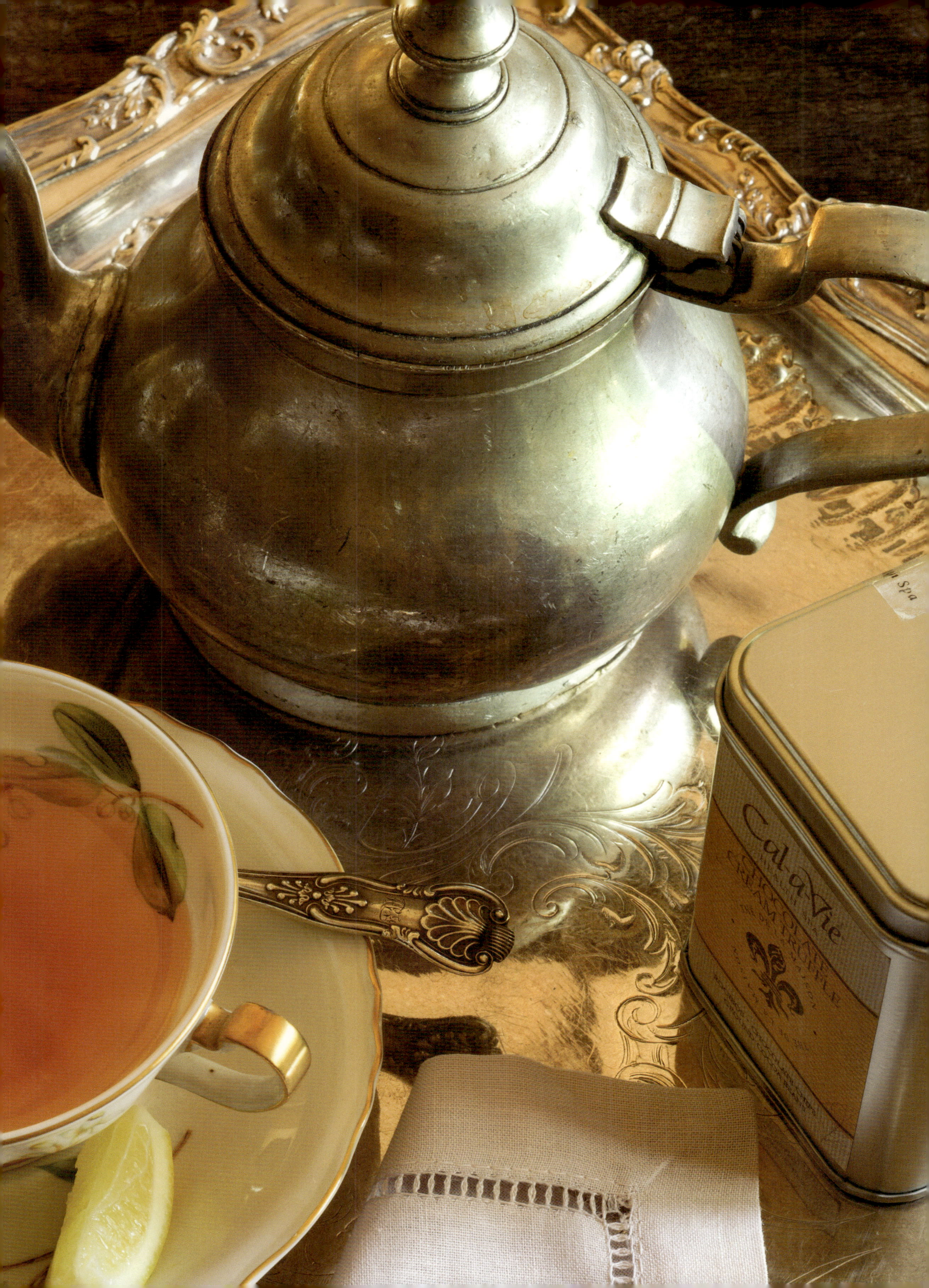
Cal-a-Vie
CHOCOLATE
CREAM TRUFFLE

DESSERT

CAL-A-VIE CARROT CAKE
WITH LEMON CURD

SERVES 32

This Cal-a-Vie dessert keeps the classic, timeless flavors of traditional carrot cake with a healthier spin. It includes plain Greek yogurt in place of butter and extra oil. The yogurt is a wonderful substitution, as it adds the perfect amount of moisture along with a boost of protein. This can be served as a light dessert or an accompaniment to a Sunday brunch.

CARROT CAKE

1½ cups gluten-free flour (we recommend Bob's Red Mill® brand)
1 teaspoon baking powder
1 teaspoon baking soda
¼ teaspoon allspice
¼ teaspoon ground cinnamon
¼ teaspoon ground nutmeg
1½ cups sugar
½ teaspoon sea salt
¾ cup plain Greek yogurt
¼ cup coconut oil (melt first if using solid coconut)
3 eggs
1½ cups grated carrots

Preheat the oven to 350°F. In a large bowl, combine the flour, baking powder, baking soda, allspice, cinnamon, nutmeg, sugar, and salt. Set aside.

Using a standing mixer with the paddle attachment, combine the yogurt and coconut oil, blending together for about 2 minutes. Gradually add the dry ingredients and mix until incorporated. Add the eggs one at a time and then gently add the carrots until mixed well. Grease a 9-inch cake pan with non-stick spray and pour in the batter. Bake for 30-40 minutes or until a toothpick comes out clean when inserted. Set aside to let cool.

LEMON CURD

3 egg yolks
⅓ cup sugar
⅓ cup fresh lemon juice

In a medium saucepan, add enough water to come about 1 inch up the side. Bring to a simmer over medium heat. In a small bowl, combine the egg yolks, sugar, and lemon juice. Place the bowl over the saucepan and whisk until the mixture is smooth and thickened (about 10 minutes). Set aside to cool.

Using a small biscuit cutter, cut cake into small squares and top each with a small amount of Lemon Curd.

NUTRITION PER SERVING	Cal	Fat	Protein	Carbs	Sugar	Fiber	Sod
	96	3g	2g	17g	12g	1g	90mg

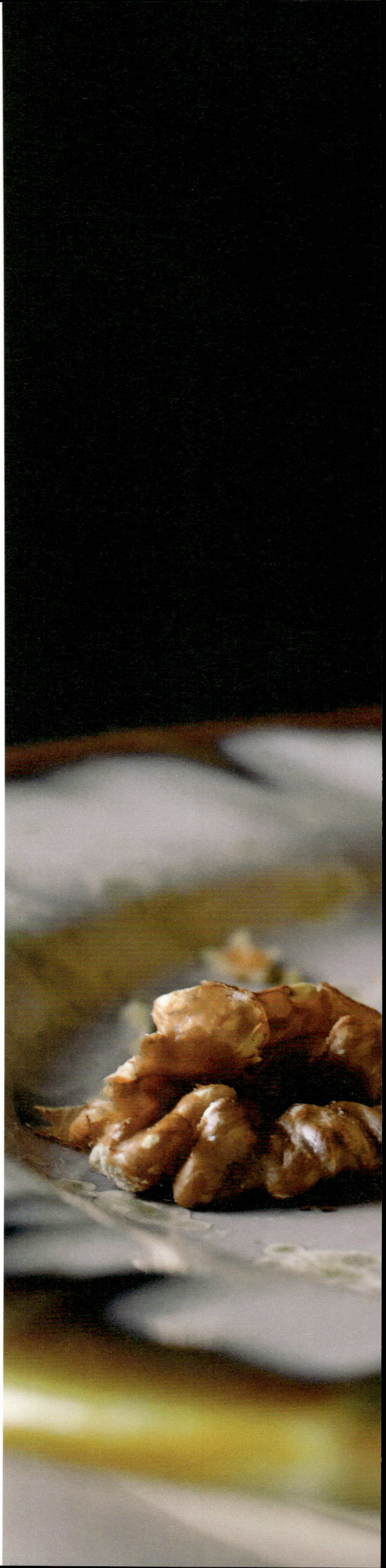

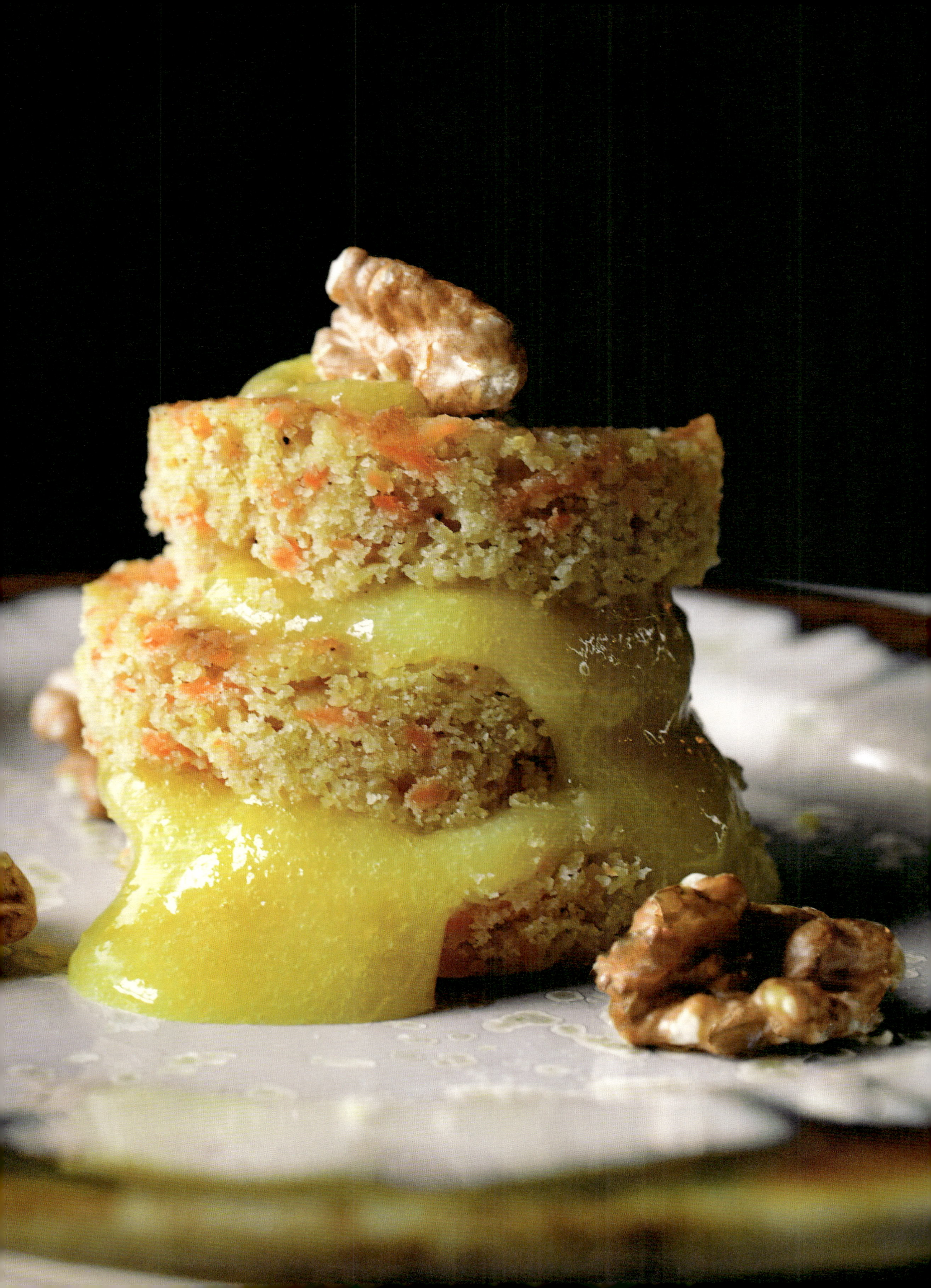

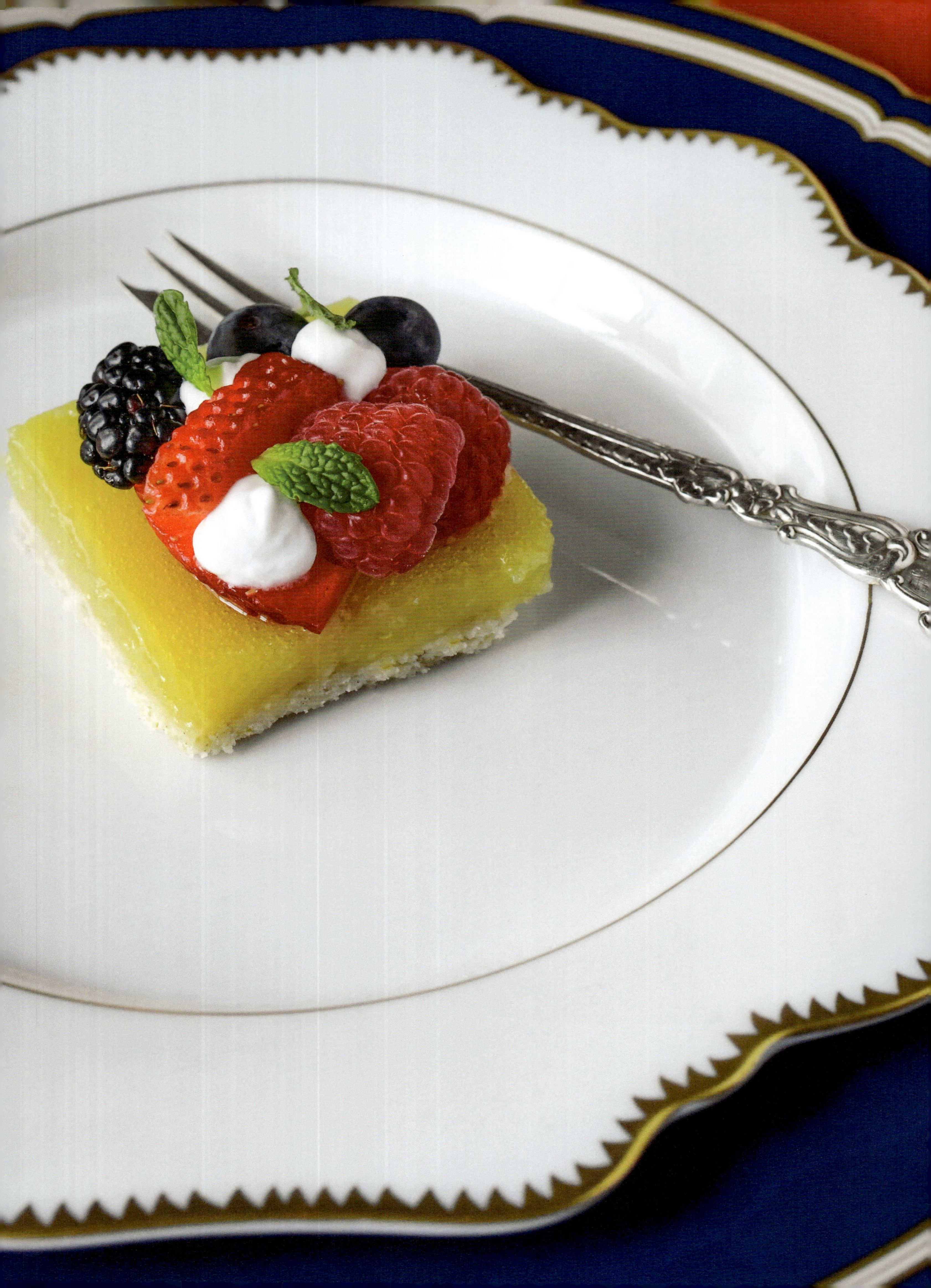

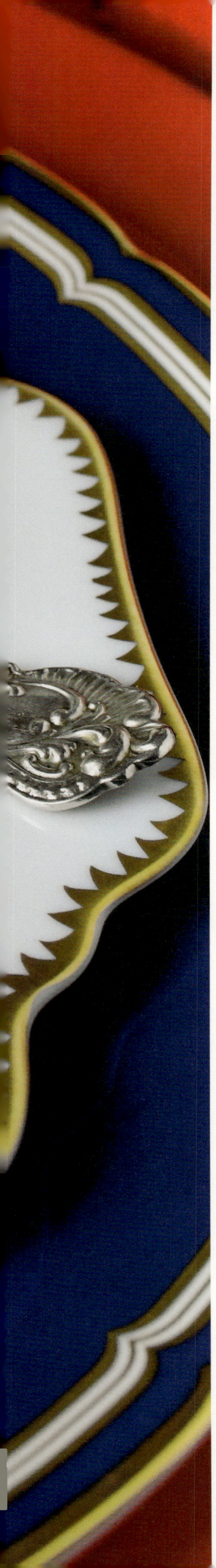

LEMON SQUARES
WITH WHIPPED COCONUT CREAM

36 SERVINGS

We love picking fresh lemons straight from the Meyer lemon trees growing on our property, and this dessert is best when served with our homemade Whipped Coconut Cream. It's easy, dairy-free, and vegan. Try to find coconut cream without the addition of guar gum, which inhibits whipping.

CRUST

2 cups Arrowhead Mills® flour

1 cup powdered sugar

1 teaspoon kosher or sea salt

2 lemons, zested

1 cup coconut oil
(melt first if using solid coconut)

Preheat the oven to 350°F. Line a 9 x 12-inch baking sheet with parchment paper and grease with non-stick cooking spray. In a large bowl, combine the flour, sugar, salt, lemon zest, and coconut oil. Press the crust down evenly to cover the bottom of the pan and bake for about 6 minutes. Remove from the oven and let cool.

LEMON CURD

1½ cups fresh lemon juice

2 cups unrefined cane sugar

4 eggs

2 egg yolks

1 tablespoon plus 1 teaspoon tapioca starch

pinch of kosher or sea salt

½ cup extra-virgin olive oil

Using a double boiler method, whisk the lemon juice, sugar, eggs, egg yolks, tapioca starch, and salt together until fully mixed and incorporated. Continue to whisk for 10-15 minutes, until the mixture is thick. Remove from the heat, stir in the olive oil, and strain the mixture through a fine-mesh sieve.

Pour the Lemon Curd over the cooled crust and return to the oven for 5 minutes. Remove and let cool, then place in the refrigerator so it will set firmly. Cut into 36 squares. Cover and store in the refrigerator.

WHIPPED COCONUT CREAM

1 13.5-ounce can organic full-fat coconut cream, chilled
(do NOT shake the can)

3 tablespoons powdered sugar

½ teaspoon vanilla extract

½ teaspoon cream of tartar

TIP: Save the coconut water at the bottom of the can. It can be used to make smoothies.

Open the can of coconut cream and spoon off the top cream, leaving the coconut water in the bottom. Using an electric mixer with the whip attachment, place the coconut cream, sugar, vanilla, and cream of tartar in the bowl and whip for 10 minutes or until the cream is thickened.

Garnish each Lemon Square with fresh fruit and a dollop of Whipped Coconut Cream.

NUTRITION PER SERVING	Cal	Fat	Protein	Carbs	Sugar	Fiber	Sod
	113	7g	1g	11g	5g	0g	46mg

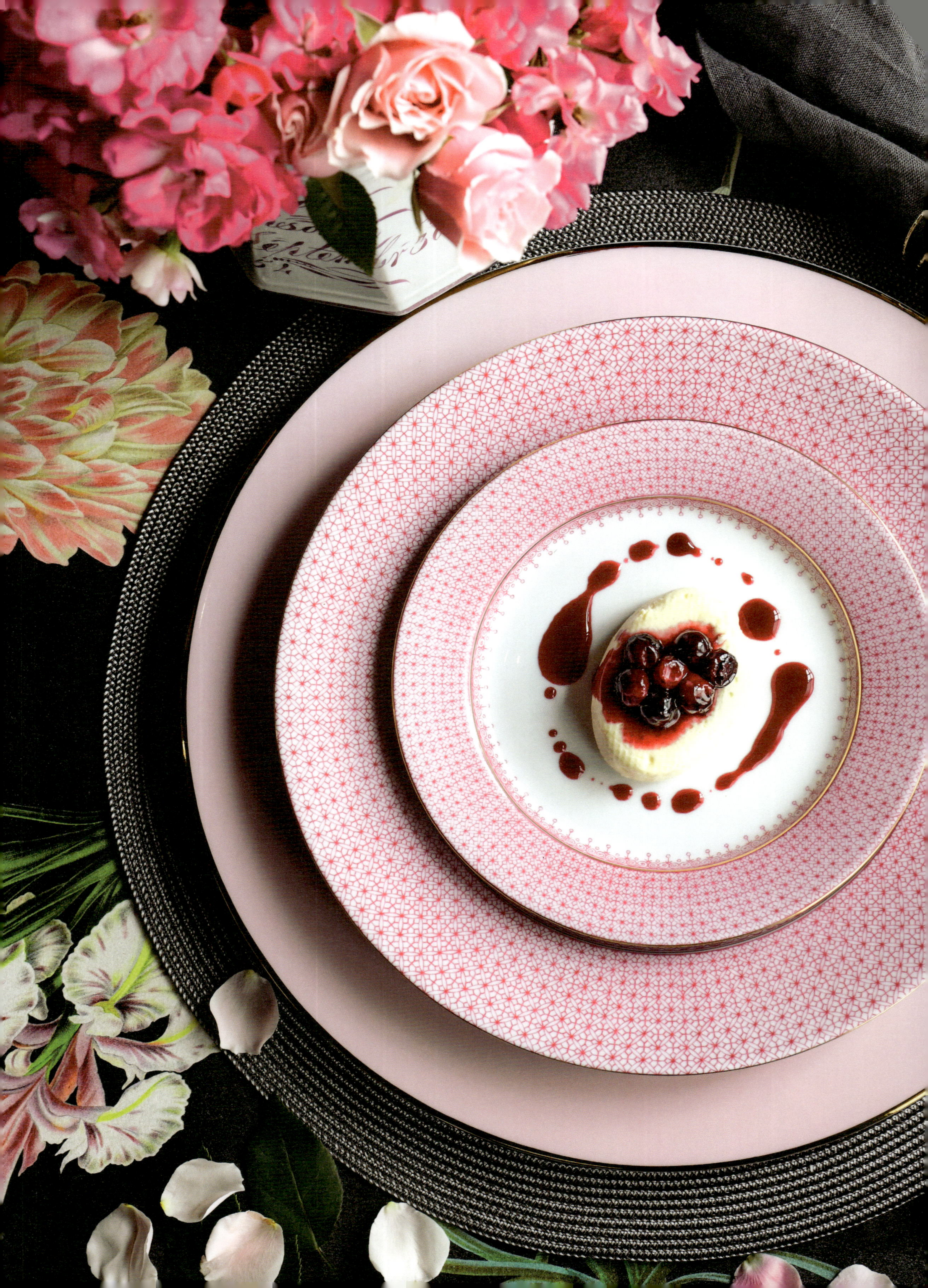

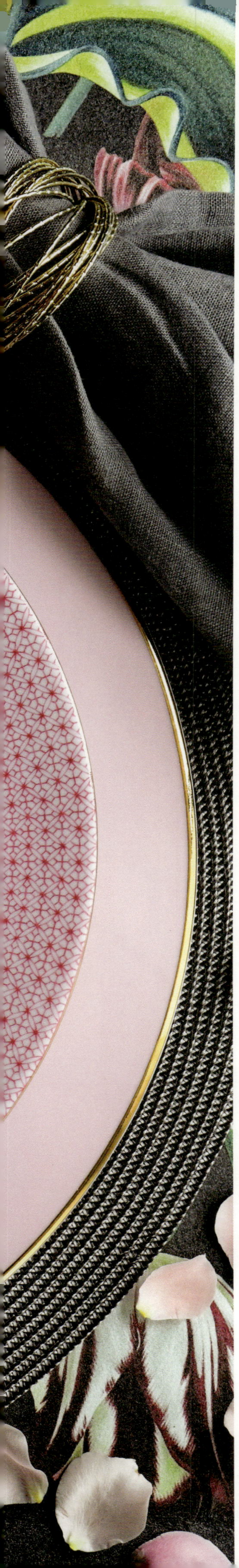

DESSERT

VANILLA CHEESECAKE
WITH BERRY COMPOTE

30 SERVINGS

Fat-free ingredients may save on calories, but you sacrifice a lot of texture and satiety. So we use real cream cheese and serve the proper Cal-a-Vie portion. To prepare the cheesecakes, we recommend using flex molds, which serve two purposes. First, they allow for pre-portioning, thus avoiding the temptation to serve yourself a bit too much of a good thing. And second, they allow for easy removal, so each cheesecake keeps its shape. Flex molds can be found at specialty kitchen stores or on the Internet. The Berry Compote adds some sweet tartness, and its beautiful splash of color is a deep-blue reminder of its high antioxidant content.

VANILLA CHEESECAKE

- 2½ pounds cream cheese (5 8-ounce packages), room temperature
- ½ cup honey
- 1 teaspoon fresh lemon zest
- 1 tablespoon fresh lemon juice
- ½ teaspoon kosher or sea salt
- 2 vanilla beans, split, and scraped
- 5 eggs
- ½ cup Greek yogurt, drained

Preheat the oven to 350°F. Prepare the flex molds by greasing with non-stick spray.

In a standing mixer with the paddle attachment, beat the cream cheese, honey, lemon zest, lemon juice, salt, and vanilla bean paste until fully incorporated. Scrape down the sides of the bowl often. With the mixer on low, add one egg at a time, mixing well before adding each additional egg. Gently fold in the yogurt. Pour the batter into the flex mold. Fill a larger pan with hot water that comes up halfway to the top of the flex pan and bake in the water bath for 20-25 minutes or until a toothpick comes out clean. Remove from the oven, let cool, and refrigerate to allow the cheesecakes to firm up.

BERRY COMPOTE

- 4 cups blueberries
- 1 cup organic refined cane sugar
- 2 tablespoons water
- 1 teaspoon fresh lemon juice

In a medium skillet over medium heat, mix the blueberries, sugar, and water. Allow to come to a boil and shake the pan occasionally until the berries begin to burst in 3-5 minutes. Remove from the heat, stir in the lemon juice, and set aside.

When ready to serve, carefully turn the mold upside down over a piece of parchment or wax paper and gently tug at the molds so the cheesecakes will release. Immediately turn the cheesecakes right side up. Top each cheesecake with a tablespoon of Berry Compote just before serving.

TIP: This recipe can be prepared in a 10-inch springform pan. Wrap the outside of the pan tightly with foil and bake for about an hour in a water bath. Turn off the oven and leave in for another 30 minutes. Refrigerate for at least 6 hours to allow the cheesecake to firm up.

NUTRITION PER SERVING	Cal	Fat	Protein	Carbs	Sugar	Fiber	Sod
	142	8g	2g	16g	15g	0g	105mg

VANILLA PANNA COTTA WITH CITRUS GELÉE

24 SERVINGS

This dessert is a creamy Italian classic with a Cal-a-Vie citrus twist. It works well for any occasion and can be prepared a day or two in advance. Greek yogurt and gelatin help give our panna cotta the texture it needs without adding extra fat. If you have trouble finding whole vanilla beans, you can also use wild vanilla bean powder, which is easy to find online and will last a long time.

VANILLA PANNA COTTA

2½ cups reduced fat milk, divided use

2½ teaspoons gelatin

½ cup honey

2 vanilla beans, scraped

1½ cups Greek yogurt

In a small, wide bowl, add ½ cup milk and sprinkle the gelatin evenly over it in a very thin layer. Do not stir. As the gelatin starts to activate, the dry spots from the gelatin will begin to fade away as it's absorbed. It will "bloom" in about 10 minutes.

In a medium saucepan over medium-high heat, combine the remaining 2 cups of milk, honey, and vanilla beans, and bring to a boil. Turn off the heat and stir in the gelatin-milk mixture.

Prepare an ice bath with a large bowl full of ice and a smaller bowl sitting on top of the ice. Pour the milk mixture into the bowl on top of the ice to cool it down. Once it is completely cool, whisk in the yogurt. Divide the mixture evenly into small ramekins or martini glasses. Refrigerate for 24 hours.

CITRUS GELÉE

¼ cup fresh lemon juice

2 teaspoons gelatin

¾ cup fresh orange juice

3 tablespoons honey

In a small, wide bowl, add the lemon juice and sprinkle the gelatin over it. Let sit for 10 minutes. In a small saucepan, heat the orange juice and honey to a boil, and turn off the heat. Prepare an ice bath with a large bowl full of ice and a smaller bowl sitting on top of the ice. Add the lemon juice and gelatin to the saucepan with the orange juice mixture, stirring to melt the gelatin. Pour the citrus mixture into the bowl on top of the ice to cool it down. Once it is completely cool, pour a very thin layer of gelée over the Vanilla Panna Cotta. The panna cotta should be completely set from the day before. Return to the refrigerator for 4-6 hours to set.

NUTRITION PER SERVING	Cal	Fat	Protein	Carbs	Sugar	Fiber	Sod
	129	3g	5g	22g	21g	0g	43mg

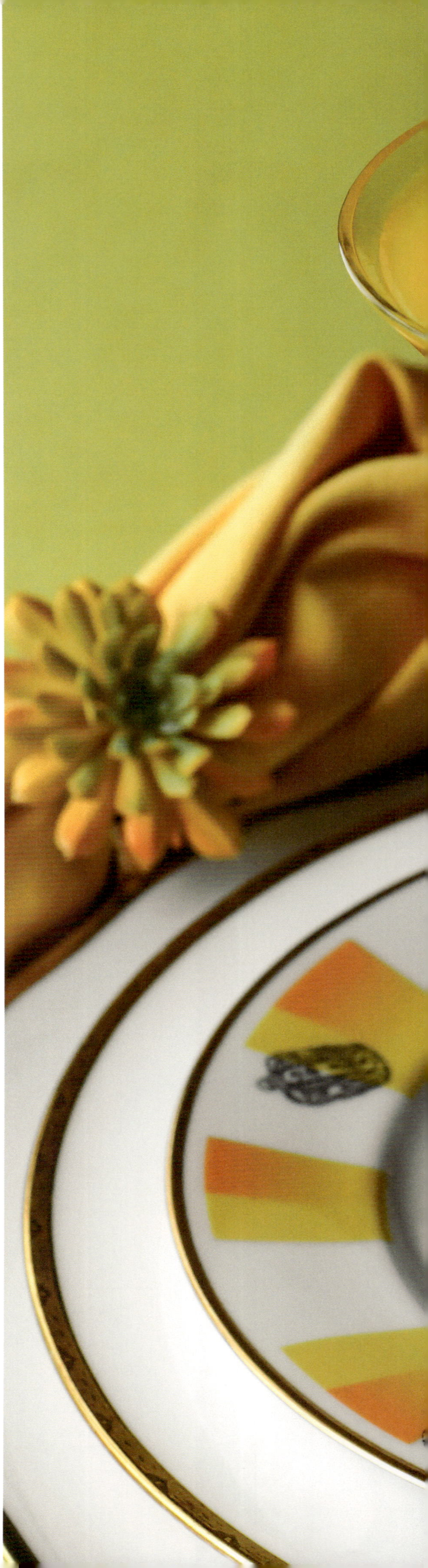

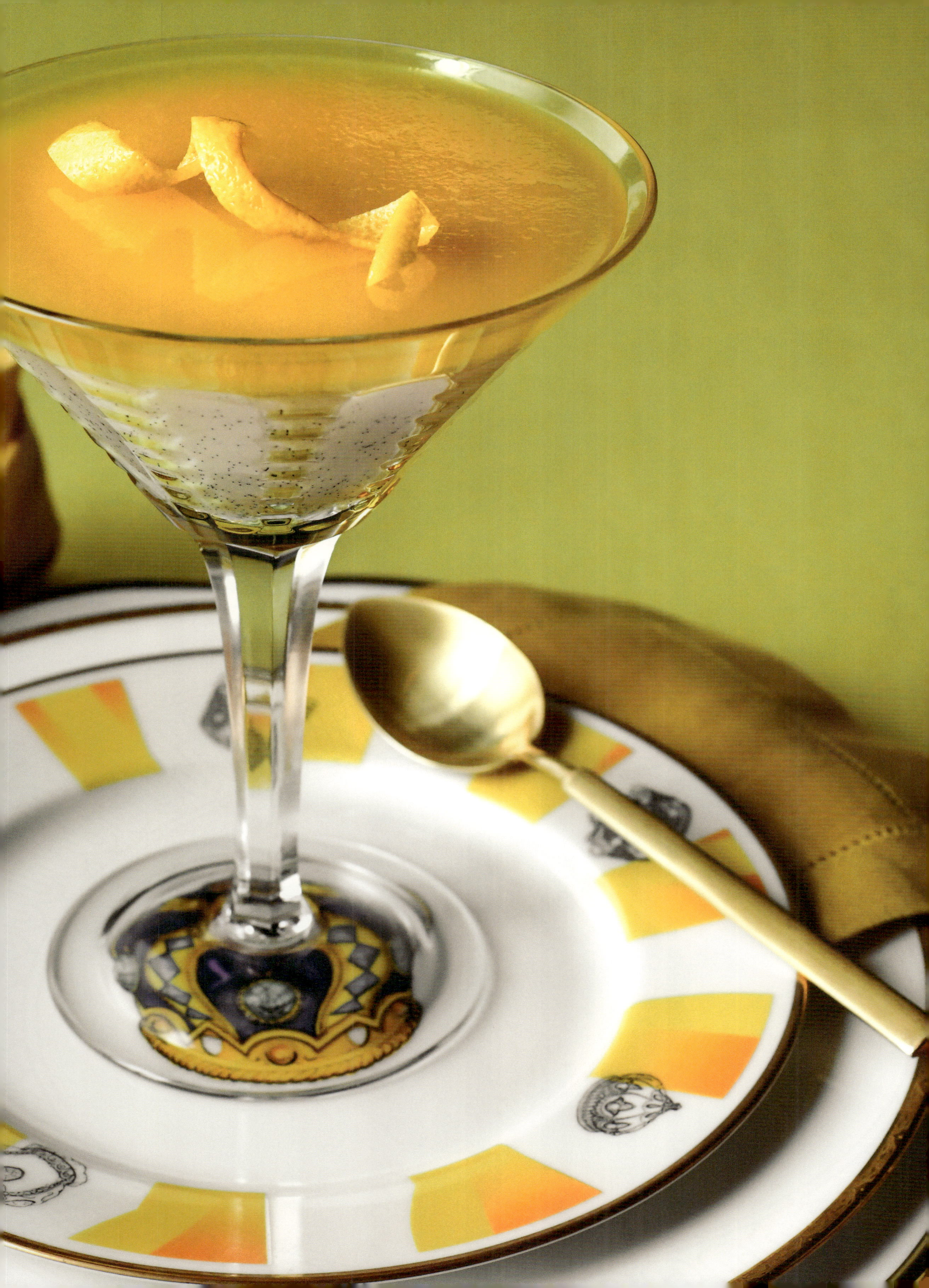

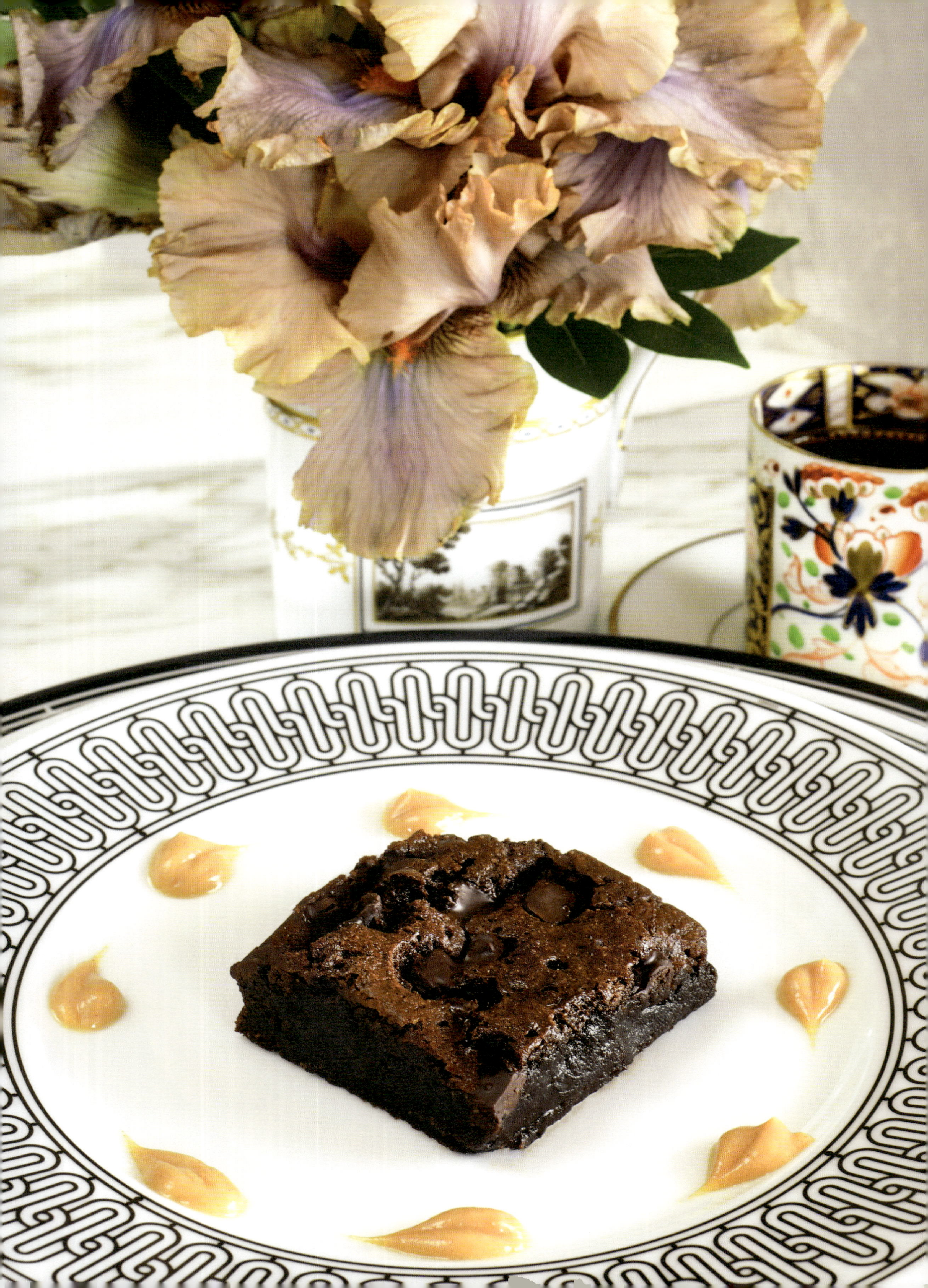

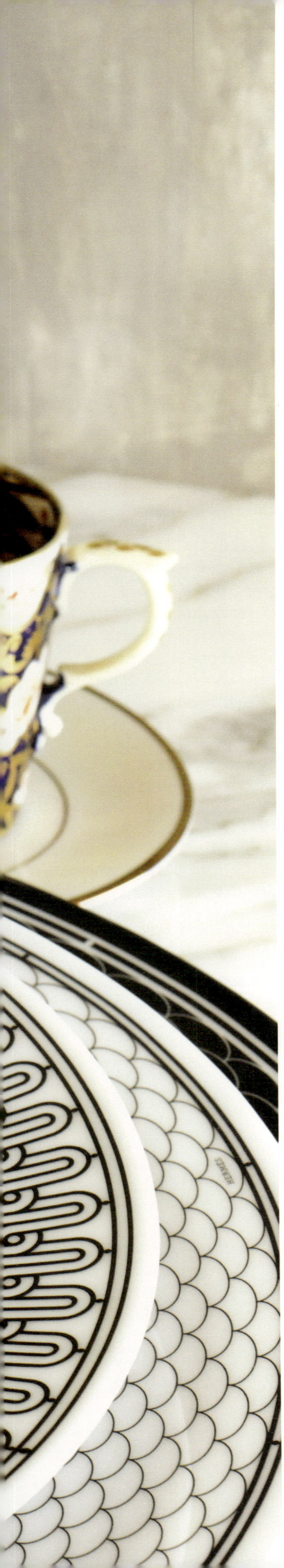

CHOCOLATE TORTE

32 SERVINGS

Cal-a-Vie's decadent chocolate torte is gluten-free and pairs wonderfully with our Vanilla Ice Cream (see the recipe on page 273) or fresh berries. For you chocolate lovers, this recipe will definitely hit the spot. Remember that a little goes a long way, though, so partake with a mindful, appreciative heart and enjoy every bite of this rich, satisfying dessert.

1 cup plus 1 tablespoon coconut sugar

½ cup natural almond meal

¼ cup plus 2½ teaspoons Arrowhead Mills® All Purpose Gluten-Free Flour

¾ teaspoon baking soda

¾ teaspoon pink Himalayan salt

1¾ cups semi-sweet chocolate chips, divided use (we recommend Enjoy Life® Dairy-Free and Soy-Free chips)

½ cup coconut oil

1½ tablespoons vanilla extract

3 large eggs

Preheat oven to 350°F. Line an 8 x 8-inch or 9 x 9-inch pan with parchment paper and lightly grease with non-stick spray.

In a large bowl, combine the coconut sugar, almond meal, flour, baking soda, and salt, and whisk well. Set aside.

In a medium metal bowl, heat 1¼ cups chocolate chips and coconut oil over a double boiler until melted, or melt in a glass bowl in the microwave. Be sure the chocolate doesn't burn. Remove from the heat once the chips are melted and stir to incorporate oil and chocolate. Add the vanilla extract and stir to combine. Once the chocolate mixture has cooled a bit, add the eggs one at a time and whisk well to combine.

Fold the wet ingredients into the dry ingredients until no pockets of the dry remain. Fold in remaining ½ cup of chocolate chips.

Spread the batter evenly into the prepared pan and bake for 10 minutes. Rotate the pan and bake for an additional 15-20 minutes. Check whether it's done by inserting a toothpick into the center of the cake, making sure it comes out clean.

Allow to cool in pan for 10 minutes. Cut into squares.

NUTRITION PER SERVING	Cal	Fat	Protein	Carbs	Sugar	Fiber	Sod
	116	7g	2g	13g	10g	1g	58mg

CHOCOLATE PEANUT BUTTER COOKIES

56 COOKIES

A tried-and-true chocolate peanut butter cookie is essential to your repertoire of confections. These cookies use three different sweeteners which add a unique sweetness. The agave and cane sugar give a light, sweet taste while the molasses brings in notes of a bold, almost smokey flavor. This combination will leave guests begging for your secret recipe to this classic cookie.

2½ cups Arrowhead Mills® All Purpose Gluten Free Flour

2 teaspoons baking soda

1 teaspoon kosher or sea salt

½ cup grapeseed oil

¾ cup agave

¾ cup unrefined cane sugar

1 teaspoon molasses

2 eggs

⅓ cup semi-sweet chocolate chips, gluten-free and soy-free

⅓ cup peanut butter chips

In a large bowl, combine the flour, baking soda, and salt. Set aside. In the bowl of a standing mixer, add the grapeseed oil, agave, cane sugar, and molasses. Using the paddle attachment, beat the mixture over low speed until fully combined (about 2 minutes). Raise the speed by one notch and add the eggs one at a time, mixing until completely combined. Lower the speed and add half of the dry ingredients. Mix until fully combined, and then add the other half.

Once completely mixed, add the chocolate and peanut butter chips and mix for another 30 seconds, until the chips are evenly incorporated. Place the batter in the refrigerator and chill for at least 2 hours.

When ready to bake, preheat the oven to 350°F. Line a sheet pan with parchment paper and grease with non-stick spray. Use a 1-ounce scoop per cookie, then flatten the cookie dough slightly with the palm of your hand or a wide spatula. Place in the oven on the middle rack and bake for 6-8 minutes, rotating halfway through, until the cookies are golden brown. Remove to a flat surface to cool and store in an airtight container.

NUTRITION PER SERVING	Cal 73	Fat 3g	Protein 1g	Carbs 12g	Sugar 7g	Fiber 1g	Sod 49mg

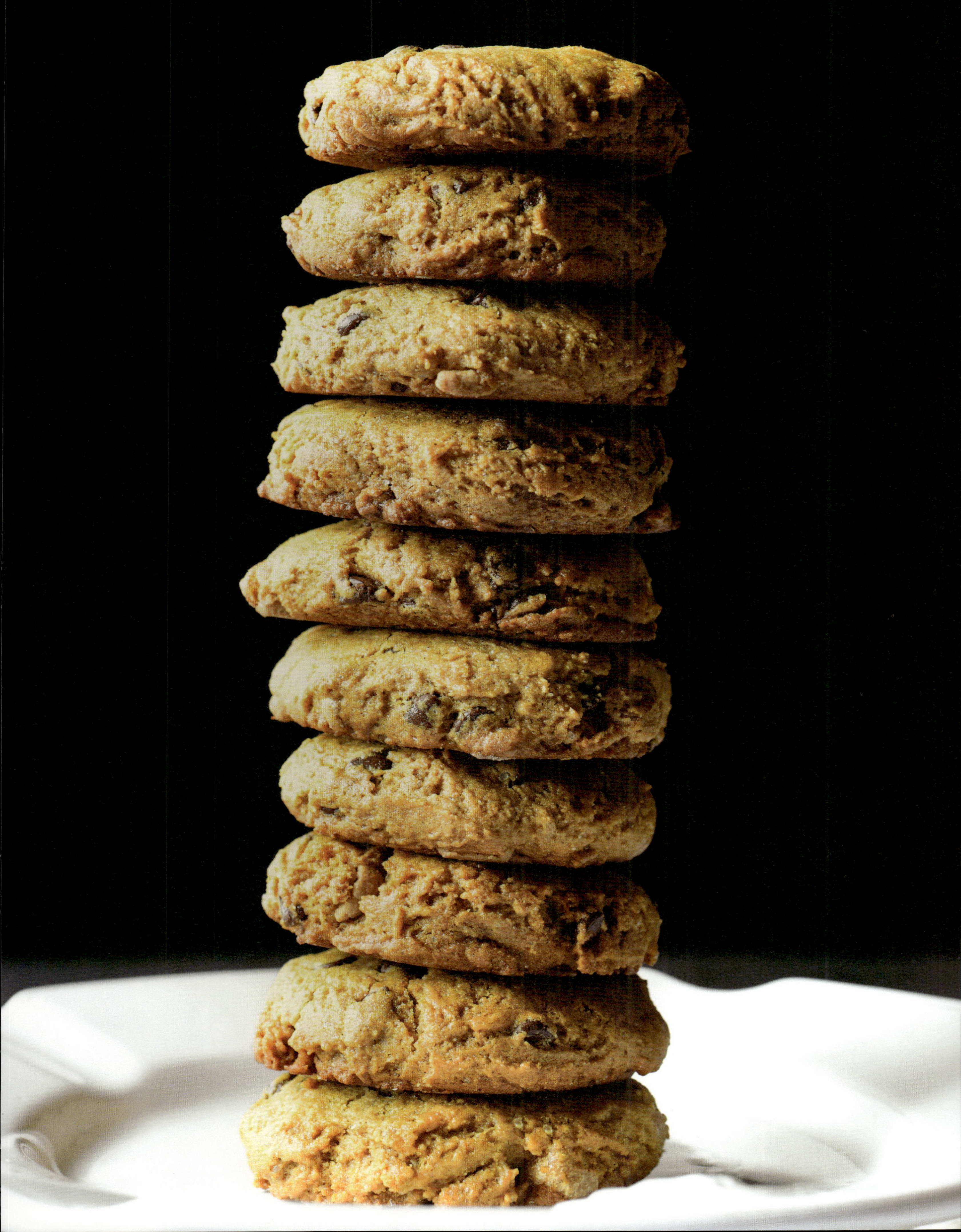

PEACH BLUEBERRY COBBLER

32 SERVINGS

This is the perfect dessert if you're dreaming of the fresh taste of peaches and blueberries, combined with warm hints of cinnamon and nutmeg, under a soft, golden biscuit topping. Peaches are sweeter when soft, so save your firm peaches for a low-glycemic snack and your softer peaches for this cobbler. Peaches are fantastic when they're in season and hit-or-miss when they're not, so substitute an in-season fruit if you plan on making this during non-summer months. This cobbler pairs beautifully with our Vanilla Ice Cream (see recipe on page 273) and fresh mint.

PEACH BLUEBERRY FILLING

3 cups peaches, diced
2 cups blueberries
2 tablespoons fresh lemon juice
¼ cup coconut oil
½ cup sugar
1 tablespoon all-purpose flour
½ teaspoon ground cinnamon
¼ teaspoon nutmeg
1 teaspoon vanilla extract

In a large bowl, add the peaches and blueberries and toss to combine. Stir in the lemon juice, coconut oil, sugar, flour, cinnamon, nutmeg, and vanilla. Mix well. Divide the fruit mixture among small ramekins. Set aside.

COBBLER CRUST

2 cups all-purpose flour
¼ cup sugar
2 teaspoons baking powder
½ teaspoon baking soda
½ teaspoon kosher or sea salt
½ cup coconut oil, chilled in the refrigerator for several hours
1 cup buttermilk
1 teaspoon lemon zest

Preheat the oven to 350°F. In a bowl, add the flour, sugar, baking powder, baking soda, and salt. Using a pastry cutter or two knives, cut in the coconut oil until it becomes crumbly. Add the buttermilk and lemon zest. Mix until a dough is formed. Place the dough ball on a lightly floured work surface. Roll out the dough, cut into small circles, and top the filled ramekins. Using a sharp knife, score each dough circle in the middle with an X. Bake for 15 minutes or until the dough is crisp and the filling is bubbling.

NUTRITION PER SERVING	Cal	Fat	Protein	Carbs	Sugar	Fiber	Sod
	73	4g	1g	10g	6g	1g	29mg

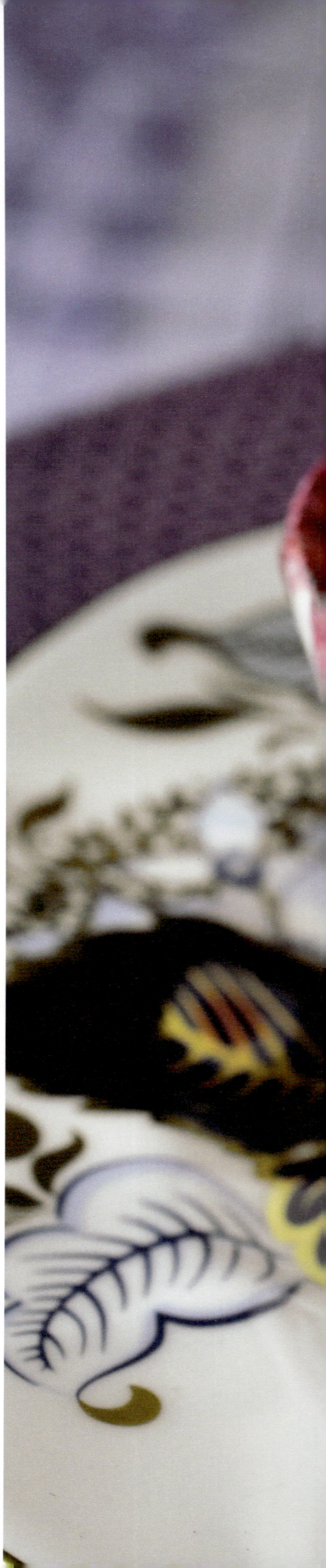

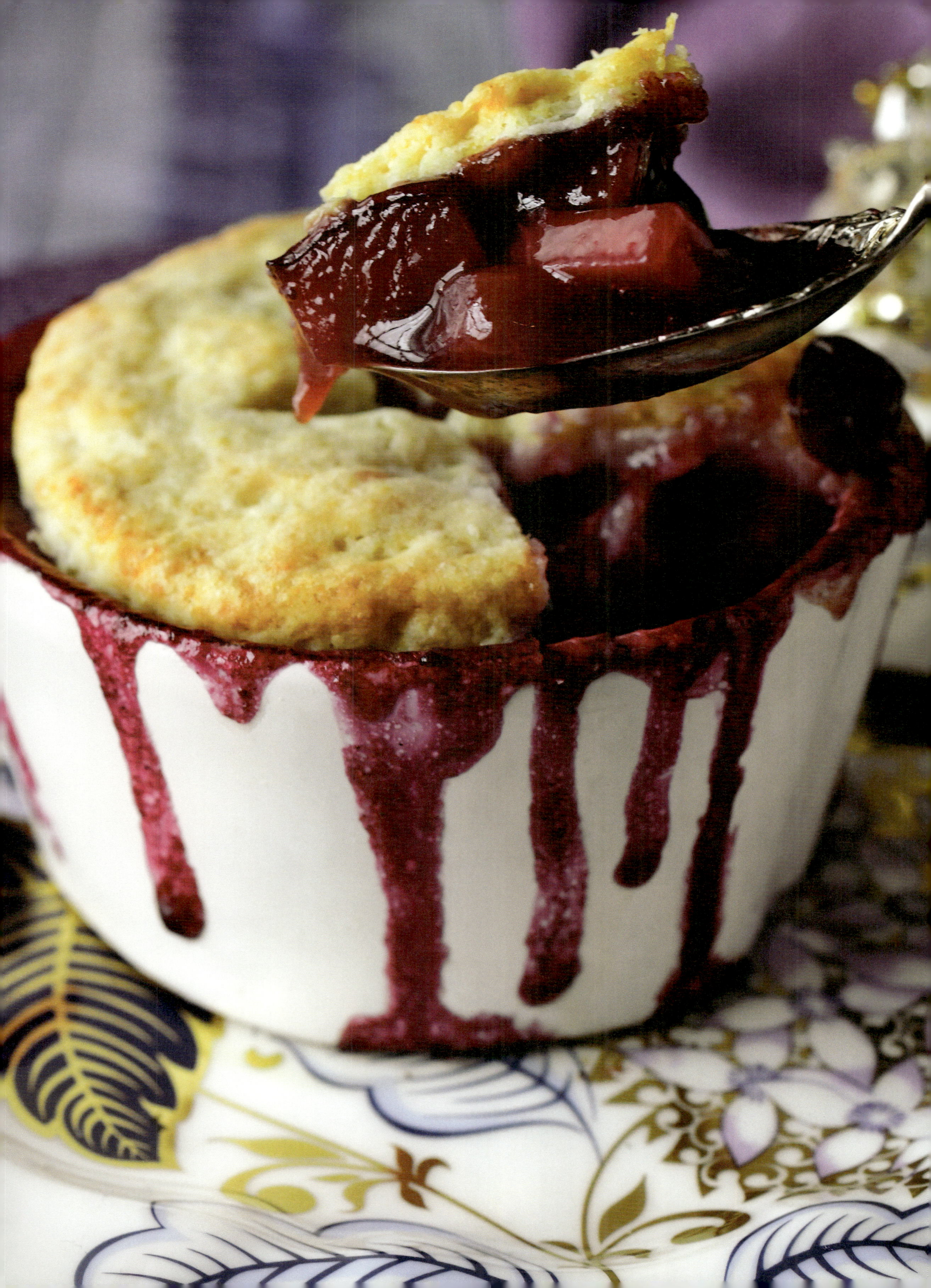

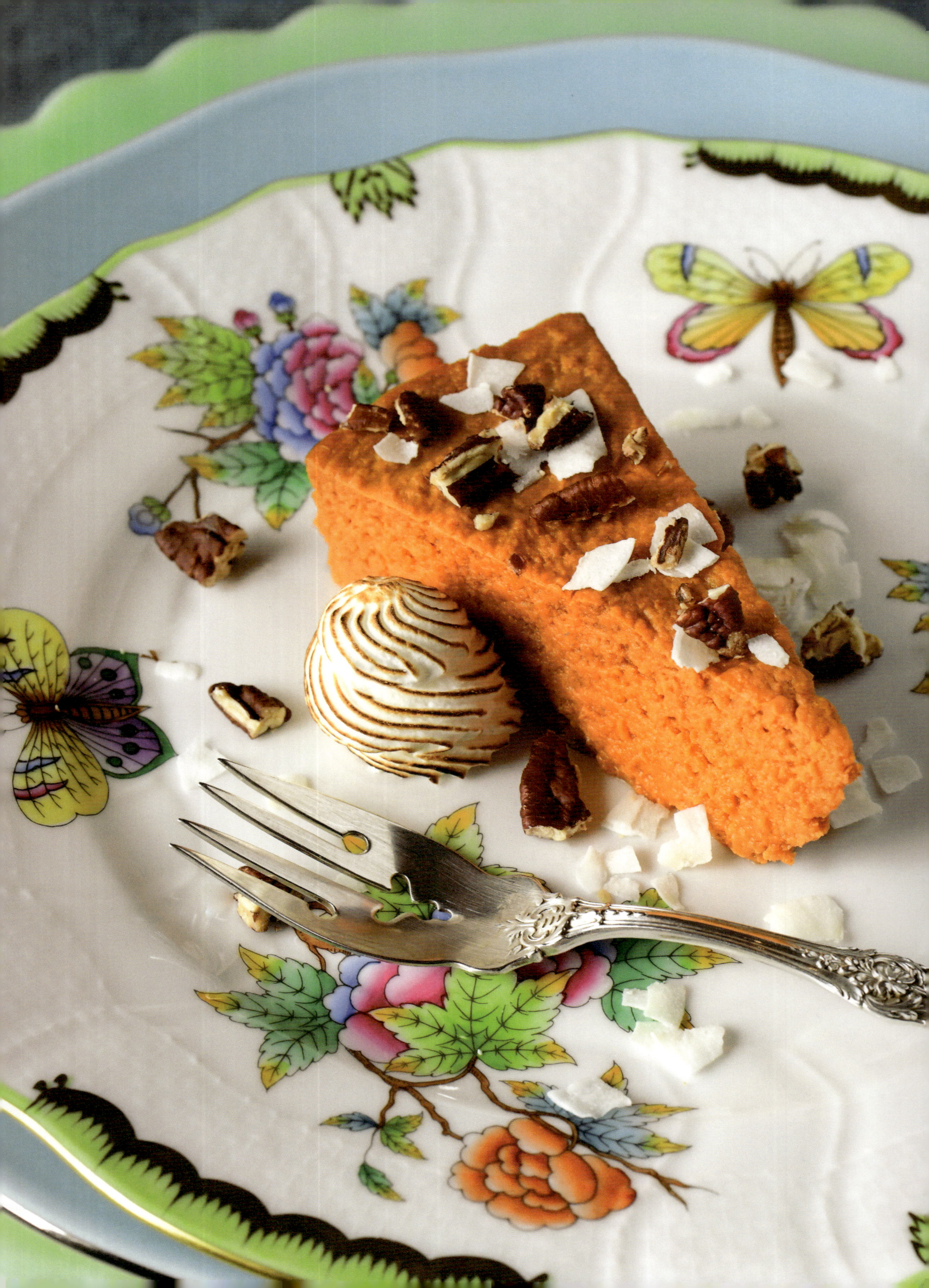

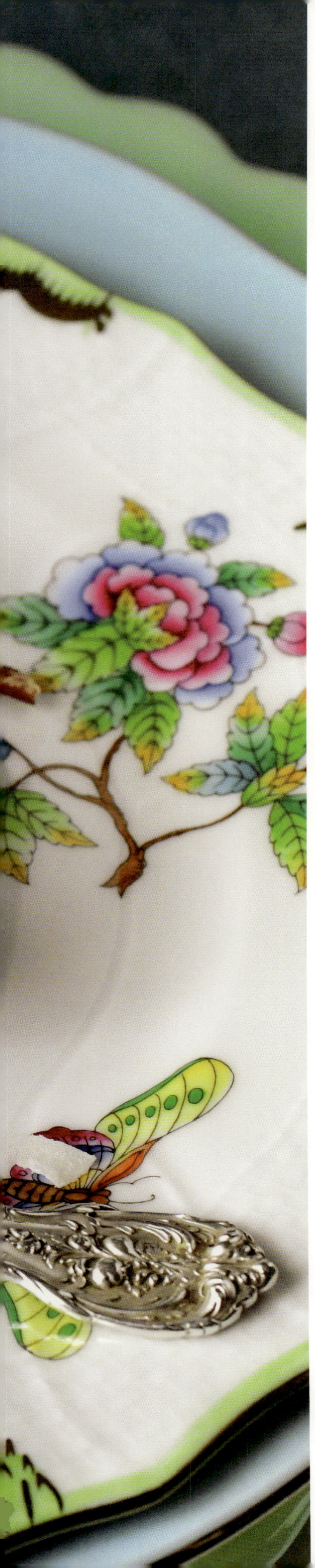

PUMPKIN COCONUT PIE
WITH WHIPPED COCONUT CREAM

30 SERVINGS

We love serving this dairy-free dessert during the holidays when pumpkins are in season. Pumpkins are a rich source of beta-carotene and other pro-vitamin-A carotenoids, which convert to vitamin A in the body. Did you know that to have pumpkins in time for Halloween you need to plant your seeds in June? It takes most pumpkins 90-120 days to go from seed to harvest. Makes you appreciate that farmers plan ahead.

PUMPKIN COCONUT PIE

1 15-ounce can pumpkin puree
1 cup coconut milk
½ teaspoon nutmeg
½ teaspoon ground cinnamon
¼ teaspoon cloves
½ teaspoon sea salt
¼ cup plus 2 tablespoons maple syrup
3 eggs

Preheat the oven to 350°F. In a medium saucepan over medium heat, bring the pumpkin puree to a simmer. Cook, stirring constantly for 3 minutes. Remove from the heat and add the coconut milk, nutmeg, cinnamon, cloves, and salt, and stir well. Allow mixture to cool, and blend in the maple syrup and eggs until smooth and completely incorporated. Pour into a pie dish greased with non-stick spray, and bake until the center jiggles slightly and a knife inserted in the middle comes out clean, about 30-45 minutes. Remove and allow to cool.

WHIPPED COCONUT CREAM

1 13.5-ounce can organic full-fat coconut cream, chilled (do NOT shake the can)
3 tablespoons powdered sugar
½ teaspoon vanilla extract
½ teaspoon cream of tartar

Open the can of coconut cream and spoon off the top cream, leaving the coconut water in the bottom. Using an electric mixer with the whip attachment, place the coconut cream, sugar, vanilla, and cream of tartar in the bowl and whip for 10 minutes or until the cream is thickened.

TIP: Garnish with toasted chopped pecans or walnuts and coconut flakes.

NUTRITION PER SERVING	Cal	Fat	Protein	Carbs	Sugar	Fiber	Sod
	30	2g	1g	4g	3g	1g	39mg

STRAWBERRY RHUBARB STREUSEL

16 SERVINGS

Rhubarb contains anthraquinones, which have laxative properties. Because of its tartness, rhubarb is generally used in desserts where it's cooked with sugar and often paired with fruit such as strawberries. Because of their high oxalic-acid content, the rhubarb leaves are not edible.

STRAWBERRY RHUBARB FILLING

2½ cups diced rhubarb

2½ cups strawberries, quartered

2 tablespoons coconut oil

½ cup agave

½ teaspoon ground cinnamon

2 teaspoons tapioca starch

In a bowl, combine the rhubarb, strawberries, coconut oil, agave, cinnamon, and tapioca starch, and mix well. Evenly divide the filling into 16 ramekins.

STREUSEL TOPPING

1½ cups brown rice cereal

1 cup organic whole wheat pastry flour

1 cup rolled oats

¼ cup agave

¼ teaspoon ground cinnamon

½ cup coconut oil

Preheat the oven to 375°F. In a food processor, add the brown rice cereal, pastry flour, rolled oats, agave, and cinnamon. Pulse until the mixture is mealy in texture. Add the coconut oil in small amounts while pulsing until the mixture forms little clumps. Chill the mixture for 15 minutes before spooning over the fruit filling in the ramekins. Bake for about 45 minutes or until the filling is bubbly and the topping is browned.

NUTRITION PER SERVING	Cal	Fat	Protein	Carbs	Sugar	Fiber	Sod
	108	5g	1g	17g	10g	2g	1mg

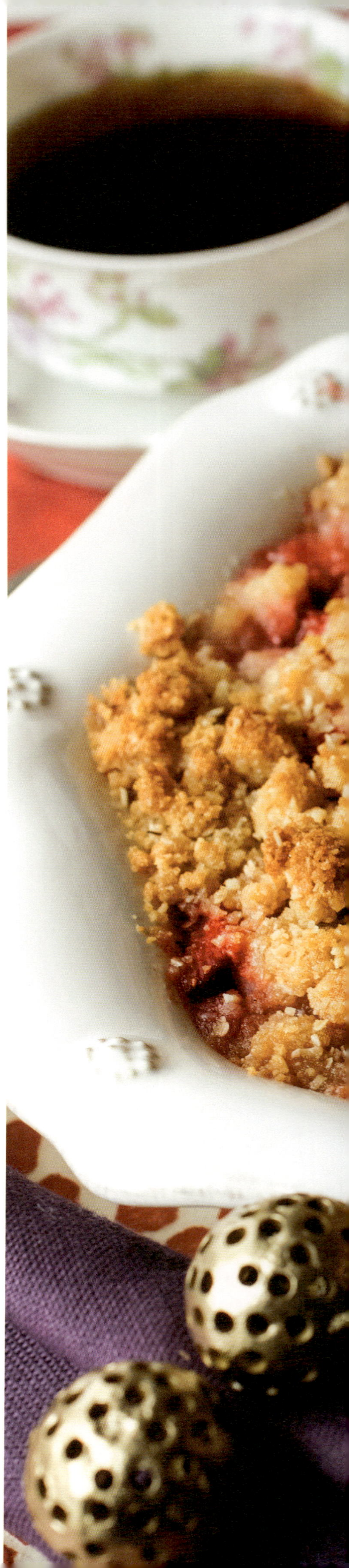

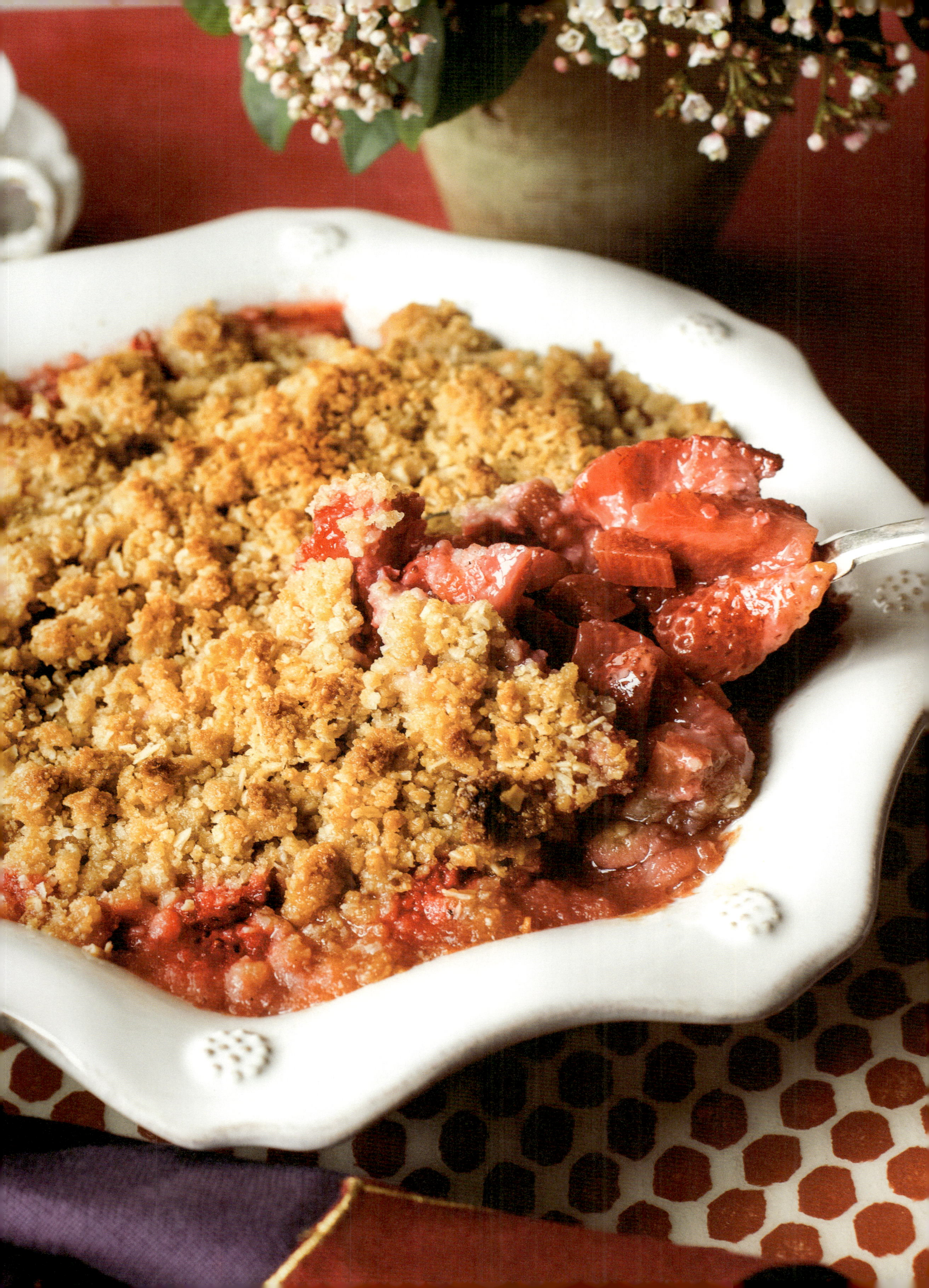

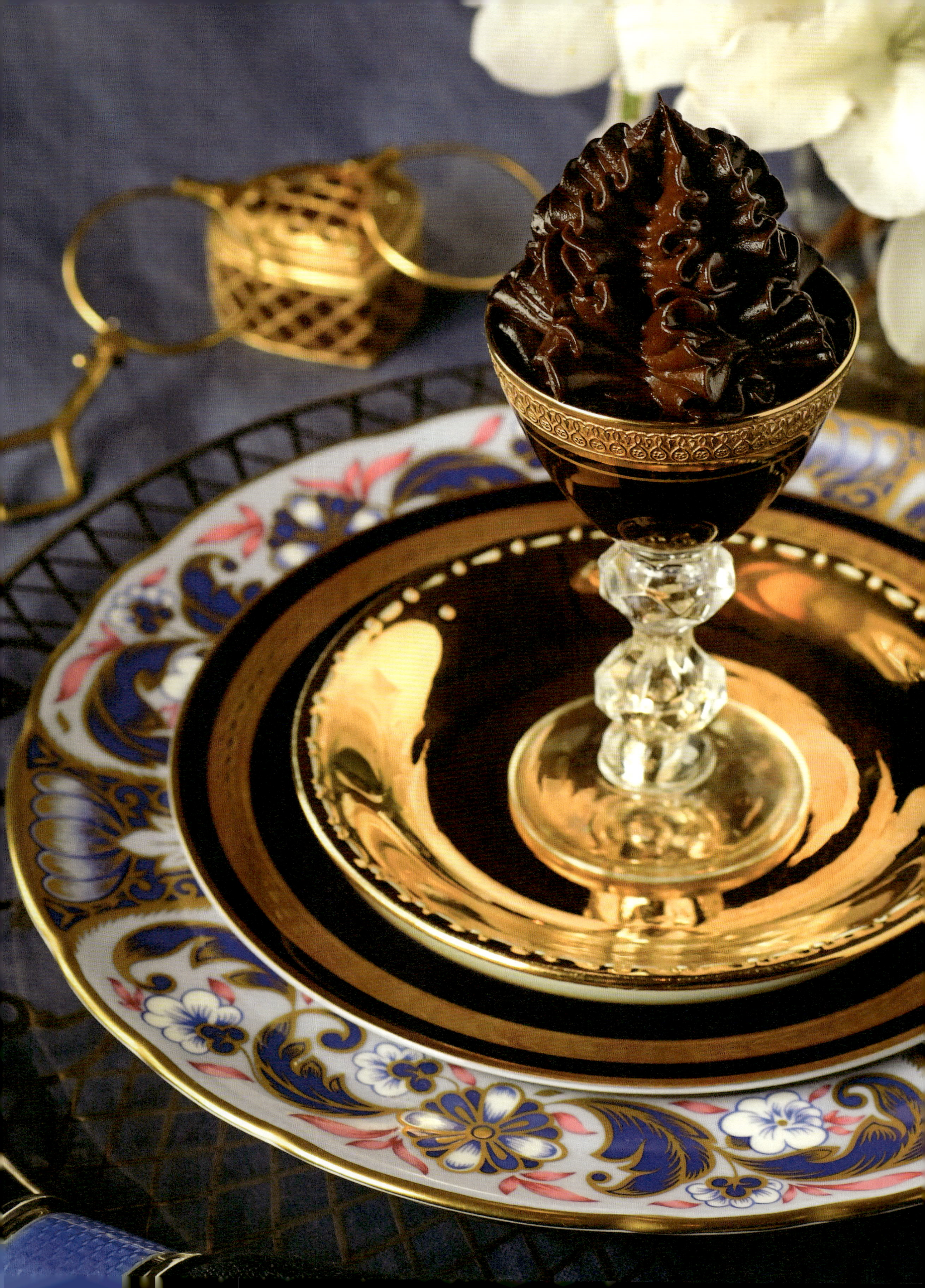

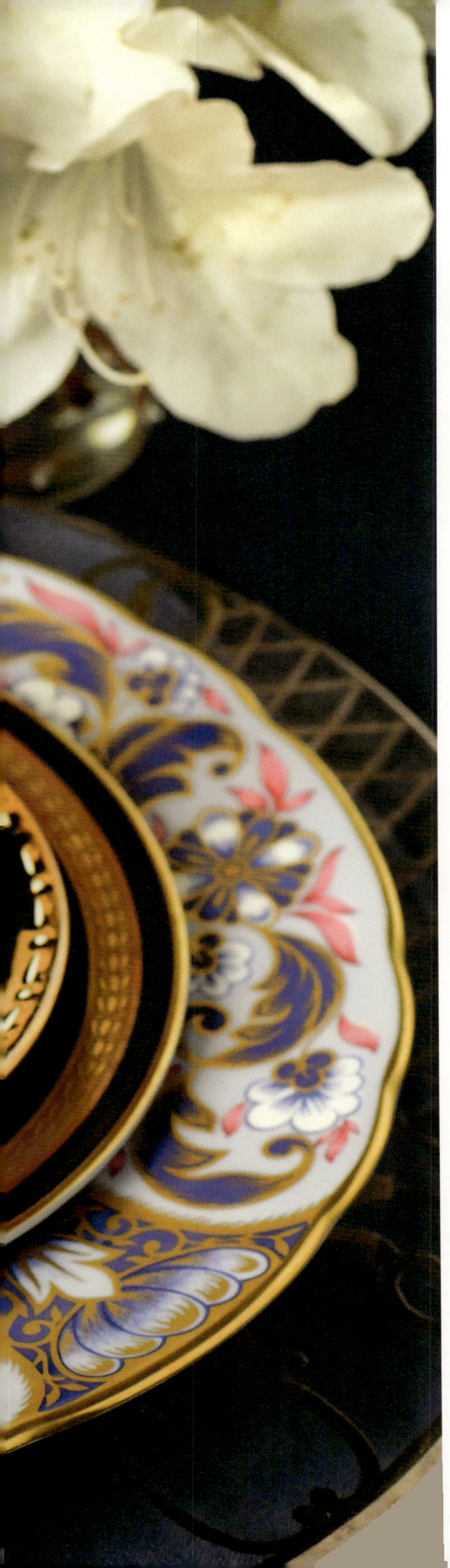

CHOCOLATE MOUSSE
WITH SALTED ALMONDS

SERVES 26

Adding a chocolate mousse to the menu has inspired our chef to create a deceptively delicious recipe. The secret ingredient is avocado, which is used as the base to give a creamy texture with a rich chocolate flavor for the ultimate decadent dessert. We love piping this into a beautiful mini-martini glass so you can have the proper amount without feeling deprived.

CHOCOLATE MOUSSE

2 medium avocados
1 cup dark cocoa powder
½ cup honey
½ cup maple syrup
¼ teaspoon ground cinnamon
1 tablespoon vanilla extract
1 tablespoon grapeseed oil
pinch of kosher salt

Combine all ingredients in a food processor, turn on, and let blend for 2 minutes. Scrape down the sides and blend for another minute. Chill for at least 4 hours before serving.

Note: Start with 1 and ½ avocados. If the mousse is too thin, add the other half.

SALTED ALMONDS (OPTIONAL GARNISH)

½ cup whole, raw almonds
¼ teaspoon kosher salt
1 teaspoon water

Preheat your oven to 350°F. In a small bowl, combine the almonds, salt, and water. Toss the almonds around until the salt and water have completely coated them. Place the almonds onto a small baking sheet and bake for about 7 minutes. Remove, let cool, and chop, then sprinkle on top.

NUTRITION PER SERVING	Cal	Fat	Protein	Carbs	Sugar	Fiber	Sod
	74	3g	1g	13g	9g	2g	7mg

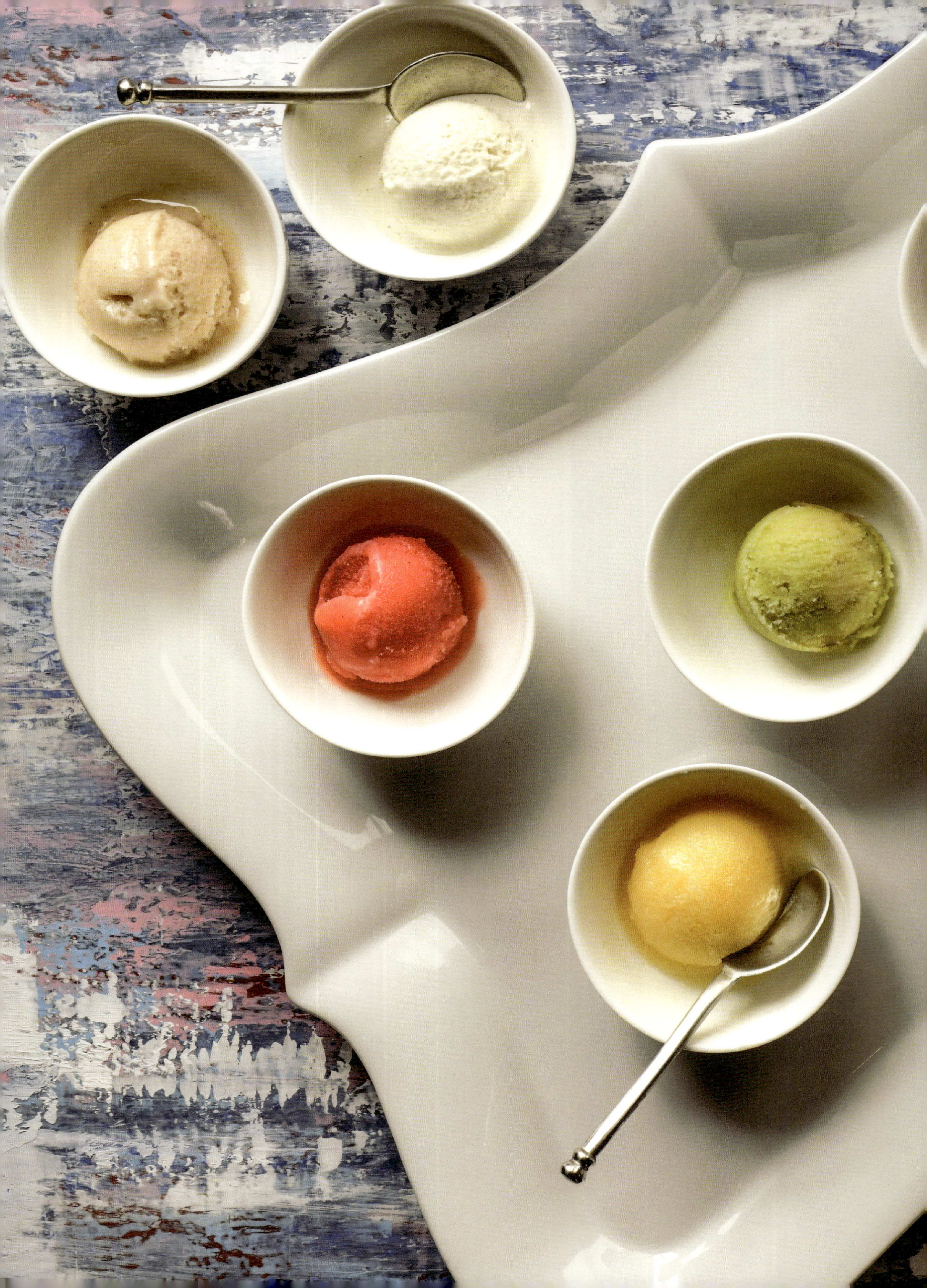

ICE CREAM AND SORBETS

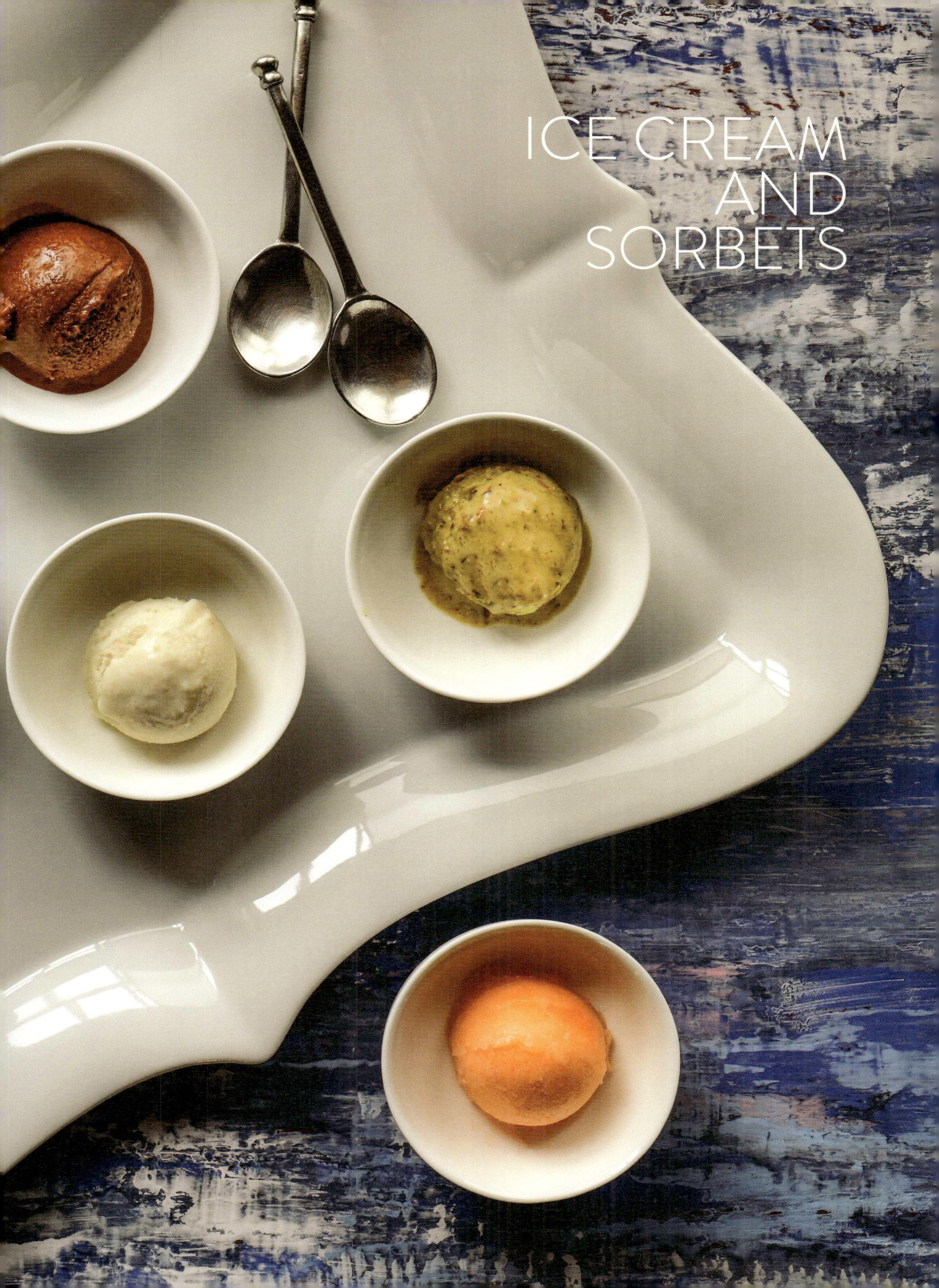

CHOCOLATE ICE CREAM

YIELDS 5 CUPS (40 SERVINGS)

Chocolate ice cream—too good to be true at a health spa, right? Nope. This recipe is just as simple as our Vanilla Ice Cream, but adds polyphenol-rich cocoa to create a decadent yet heart-healthy dessert.

4 cups soy milk

½ cup semi-sweet chocolate chips (we recommend using Sunspire® Grain Sweetened Chips)

¾ cup cocoa powder

1 cup agave

¼ teaspoon kosher or sea salt

½ teaspoon xanthan gum

½ teaspoon guar gum

In a blender, combine all the ingredients and mix on high. Once the ingredients are fully blended, churn in an ice cream maker to the manufacturer's specifications. When ready, remove and place in the freezer overnight.

NUTRITION PER SERVING	Cal 51	Fat 1g	Protein 1g	Carbs 10g	Sugar 8g	Fiber 1g	Sod 26mg

COCONUT VANILLA BEAN ICE CREAM

YIELDS 5 CUPS (40 SERVINGS)

Coconut milk is one of our favorite non-dairy milk alternatives, and it brings another layer of flavor to a traditional vanilla ice cream. Add a beautiful burst of color to this dessert by topping it with raspberries, mint, or dark chocolate chips.

Guar gum and xanthan gum are thickening agents in foods and medicine. Because they are gluten-free, they are often used as additives to replace wheat flour in baked goods. They also have been shown to reduce cholesterol and lower blood glucose levels. If you can't find them at your local health food store, they are available for order online. We recommend using Bob's Red Mill® brand.

4 cups coconut milk

1 cup agave

2 vanilla beans, scraped

3 tablespoons grapeseed oil

½ teaspoon xanthan gum

½ teaspoon guar gum

In a blender, combine all the ingredients and mix on high. Once the ingredients are fully blended, churn in an ice cream maker to the manufacturer's specifications. When ready, remove and place in the freezer overnight.

NUTRITION PER SERVING	Cal 66	Fat 4g	Protein 0g	Carbs 8g	Sugar 7g	Fiber 1g	Sod 3mg

GREEN TEA ICE CREAM

40 SERVINGS

Green Tea Ice Cream is perfect as a sweet, refreshing dessert after a traditional Japanese meal. The name is slightly deceptive, however, because the ice cream itself is not made from tea, but rather from matcha, a finely ground powder that comes from green tea leaves. By consuming the leaves as matcha instead of steeping them in water, you get a higher concentration of the cancer-fighting polyphenol epigallocatechin gallate (EGCG) that green tea is known for.

- 4 cups vanilla soy milk
- 3 tablespoons grapeseed oil
- 1 cup honey
- 2 tablespoons matcha powder
- juice of 2 lemons
- ½ teaspoon xanthan gum
- ½ teaspoon guar gum

Place the soy milk, grapeseed oil, honey, and matcha powder in a saucepan and bring to a boil. Reduce the heat to a simmer for 15 minutes. Remove from the heat and set aside for an hour. Blend in the lemon juice, xanthan gum, and guar gum. Set in the refrigerator for an hour and then churn in an ice cream maker to the manufacturer's specifications. When ready, remove and place in the freezer overnight.

NUTRITION PER SERVING	Cal 49	Fat 1g	Protein 1g	Carbs 9g	Sugar 8g	Fiber 0g	Sod 14mg

MELON SORBET

40 SERVINGS

Melon is considered a "Clean 15" fruit by the Environmental Working Group (www.ewg.org) because its thick skin minimizes pesticide exposure. But it's always best to wash your melons before you cut through them, as their skins are susceptible to mold contamination.

- 4½ cups cantaloupe, (about 3 pounds) peeled, seeded, and cut into chunks
- 2½ tablespoons honey
- ¾ cup unrefined cane sugar
- 2 tablespoons fresh lemon juice

In a blender, combine all the ingredients. Puree until completely smooth. Transfer to an ice cream maker and and churn according to the manufacturer's instructions. When ready, remove and place in the freezer overnight.

NUTRITION PER SERVING	Cal 25	Fat 0g	Protein 0g	Carbs 7g	Sugar 6g	Fiber 0g	Sod 3mg

STRAWBERRY SORBET

24 SERVINGS

Sweet delights don't get much simpler than this: a three-ingredient strawberry sorbet. This fresh and vibrant dessert not only tastes great, but also has numerous health benefits. Strawberries are rich in antioxidants and vitamin C. You can find them in peak season between April and June. Because strawberries tend to be sprayed with organophosphates, we recommend always buying the organic variety.

- 4 cups washed strawberries, tops removed
- ¾ cup honey
- 2 teaspoons fresh lemon juice

In a blender, add the strawberries, honey, and lemon juice. Puree on high for 1 minute. Using the back of a spoon, press through a fine mesh strainer. Transfer to an ice cream maker and churn according to the manufacturer's instructions. When ready, remove and place in the freezer overnight.

NUTRITION PER SERVING	Cal 38	Fat 0g	Protein 0g	Carbs 10g	Sugar 10g	Fiber 0g	Sod 1mg

MEYER LEMON SORBET

64 SERVINGS

This light and refreshing lemon sorbet tastes like summer. The key ingredient is the Meyer lemon juice. Unlike most conventional lemons, such as Lisbon or Eureka, Meyer lemons are rounder, smoother, and juicier, and their flavor is less acidic and much sweeter. You can find Meyer lemons in season from December through May.

- 4 cups fresh Meyer lemon juice
- 2 cups fresh orange juice
- 2 cups agave
- ½ teaspoon guar gum
- ½ teaspoon xanthan gum

In a blender, combine all the ingredients and mix on high. Once the ingredients are fully blended, churn in an ice cream maker according to the manufacturer's specifications. When ready, remove and place in the freezer overnight.

NUTRITION PER SERVING	Cal 36	Fat 0g	Protein 0g	Carbs 10g	Sugar 8g	Fiber 1g	Sod 1mg

PEANUT BUTTER ICE CREAM

40 SERVINGS

Peanut Butter Ice Cream is another amazingly delicious offering from our renowned collection of Cal-a-Vie frozen desserts. We make our peanut butter in-house on a weekly basis, and we do it the old-fashioned way: with a masticating juicer, using only freshly roasted peanuts.

- 4 cups soy milk
- 1½ cups peanut butter
- ¾ cup agave
- ¼ teaspoon kosher or sea salt
- ½ teaspoon xanthan gum
- ½ teaspoon guar gum

In a blender, combine the ingredients and blend on high. Once fully mixed, churn in an ice cream maker according to the manufacturer's specifications. When ready, remove and place in the freezer overnight.

NUTRITION PER SERVING	Cal 89	Fat 5g	Protein 0g	Carbs 16g	Sugar 13g	Fiber 1g	Sod 2mg

VANILLA ICE CREAM

40 SERVINGS

This healthy version of a classic tastes like the real deal—maybe even better. Our Cal-a-Vie ice cream is not only dairy-free, but also contains no refined sugars. A common sweetener you will find in many of our desserts is agave, which comes from the sap of the agave plant.

- 4 cups soy milk (or substitute almond or coconut milk)
- 1 cup agave
- 2 vanilla beans, scraped
- 3 tablespoons grapeseed oil
- ½ teaspoon xanthan gum
- ½ teaspoon guar gum
- 1 teaspoon ground cinnamon (optional)

In a blender, combine all the ingredients and mix on high. Once the ingredients are fully blended, churn in an ice cream maker according to the manufacturer's specifications. When ready, remove and place in the freezer overnight.

NUTRITION PER SERVING	Cal 47	Fat 1g	Protein 1g	Carbs 8g	Sugar 7g	Fiber 1g	Sod 13mg

PISTACHIO ICE CREAM

48 SERVINGS

The crunch of a toasted pistachio is a perfect reminder to slow down and savor the complex textures and flavors of one of life's little pleasures: pistachio ice cream. Ours is a delicious creamy dessert that actually sneaks in a number of health benefits. Pistachios contain a compound called oleanolic acid, which has been found to lower inflammation by inhibiting the production of leukotriene B. Reap the health benefits of pistachios by adding a mindful amount to your dessert.

- 4 cups soy milk
- 1 cup agave
- 2 cups pistachios, toasted and chopped, divided use
- 2 vanilla beans, scraped
- 3 tablespoons grapeseed oil
- ½ teaspoon xanthan gum
- ½ teaspoon guar gum

In a blender, combine the soy milk, agave, 1 cup toasted pistachios, vanilla, grapeseed oil, xanthan gum, and guar gum, and mix on high. Once the ingredients are fully blended, churn in an ice cream maker according to the manufacturer's specifications. Halfway through the churning, add the remaining cup of toasted pistachios. When ready, remove and place in the freezer overnight.

NUTRITION PER SERVING	Cal 69	Fat 4g	Protein 2g	Carbs 8g	Sugar 6g	Fiber 1g	Sod 11mg

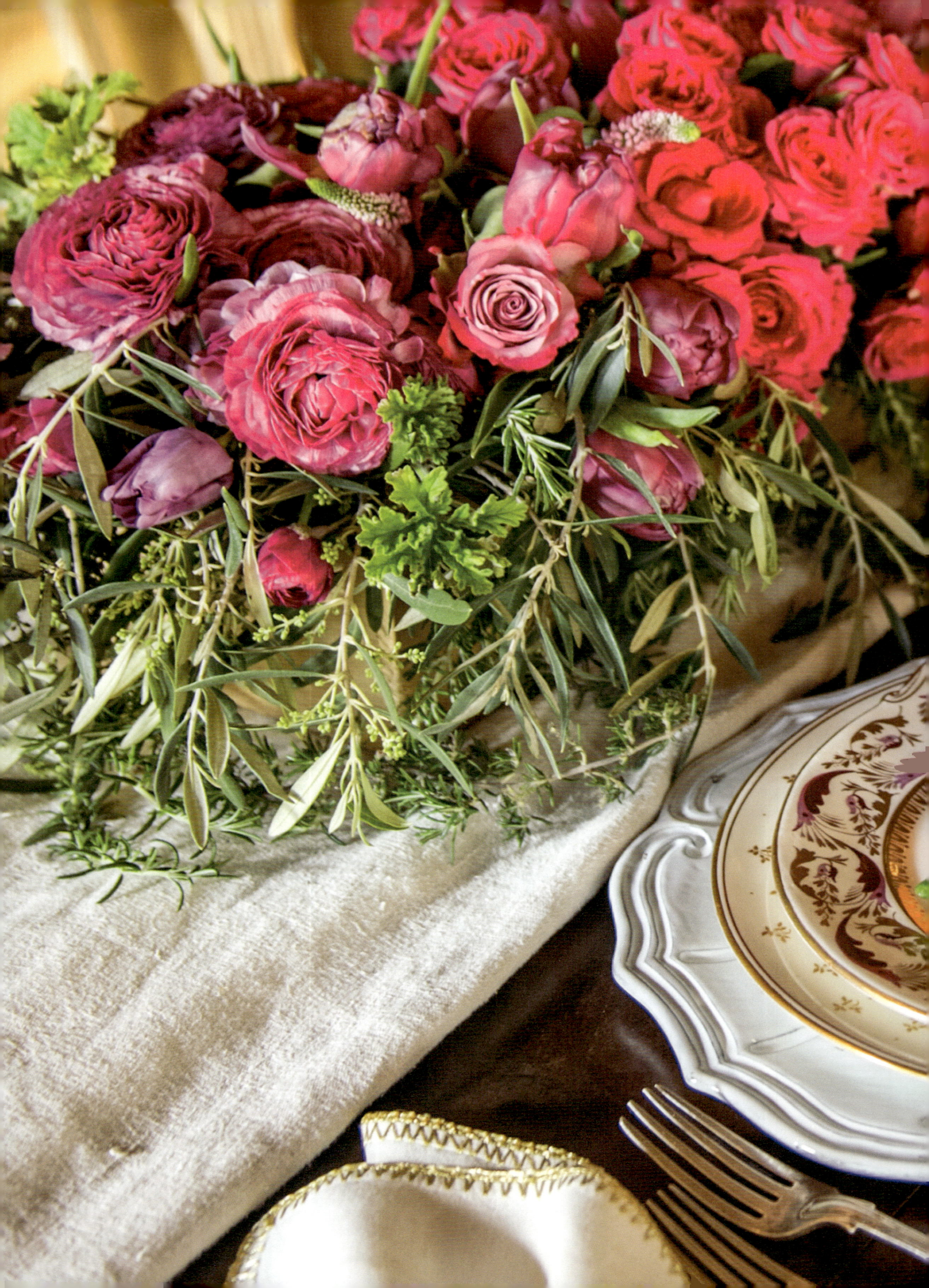

CAL-A-VIE HEALTH SPA

HEALTHY-COOKING ADVICE

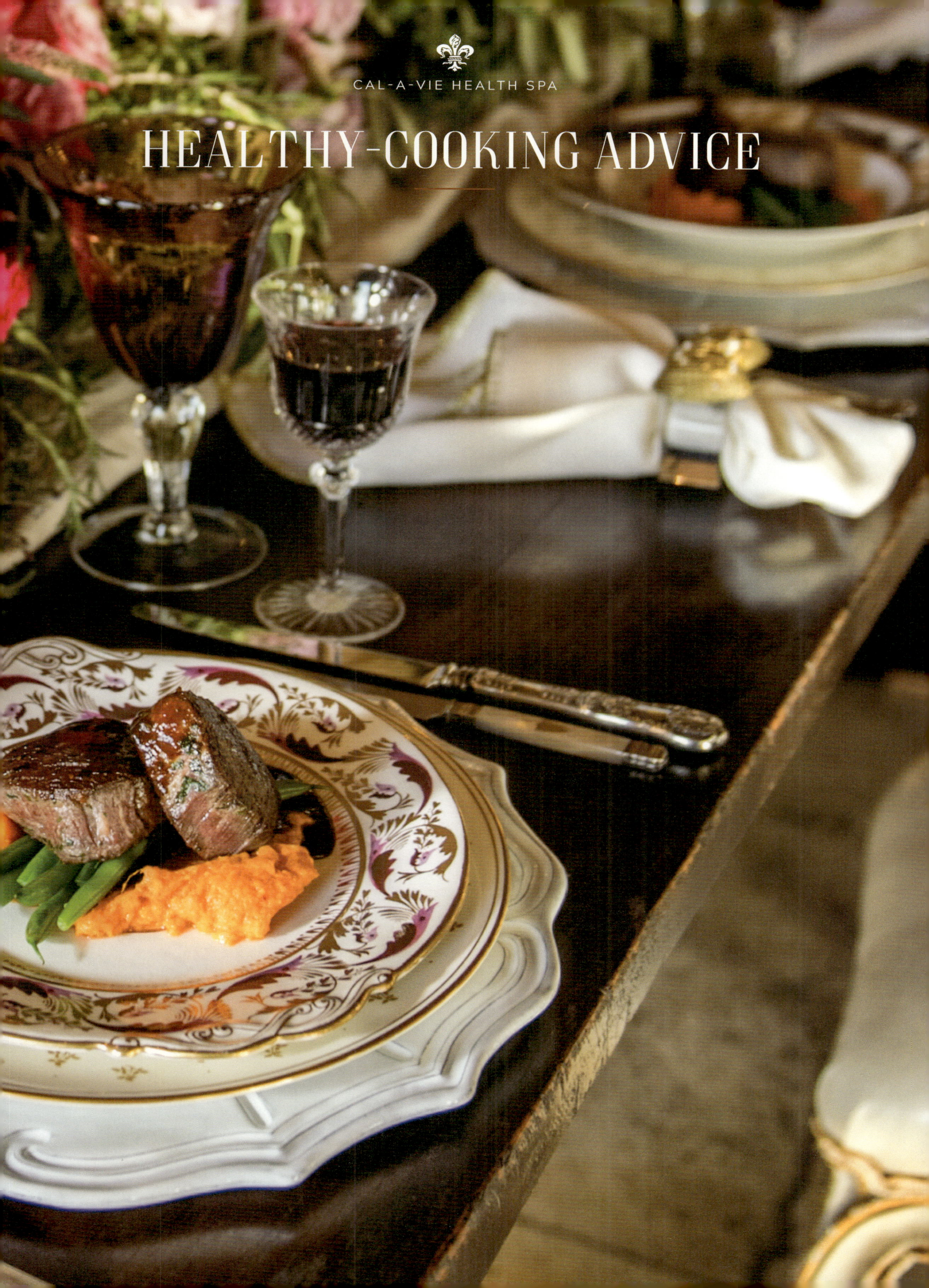

GO ORGANIC

AT CAL-A-VIE HEALTH SPA WE RECOMMEND USING ONLY ORGANIC FRUITS AND VEGETABLES THAT ARE GROWN WITHOUT USING CHEMICALS.

Organic foods generally have higher nutritional value. Conventional growers use pesticides to protect their crops from insects, and consuming high levels of pesticides can increase your risk of developing health issues. People with allergies to certain foods, chemicals, or preservatives often find their symptoms lessen or go away when they eat only organic. Of course, always thoroughly wash your vegetables and fruits before eating.

Every year, the Environmental Working Group (EWG) (www.ewg.org) publishes a list of the "Dirty Dozen" made up of the fruits and vegetables that have the highest amount of pesticides when grown conventionally versus organically. The EWG uses more than 40,000 samples for 47 different types of produce to create their list. Check their website annually for the latest items and choose organic when eating from this list.

2019 Dirty Dozen

1. Strawberries
2. Spinach
3. Kale
4. Nectarines
5. Apples
6. Grapes
7. Peaches
8. Cherries
9. Pears
10. Tomatoes
11. Celery
12. Potatoes

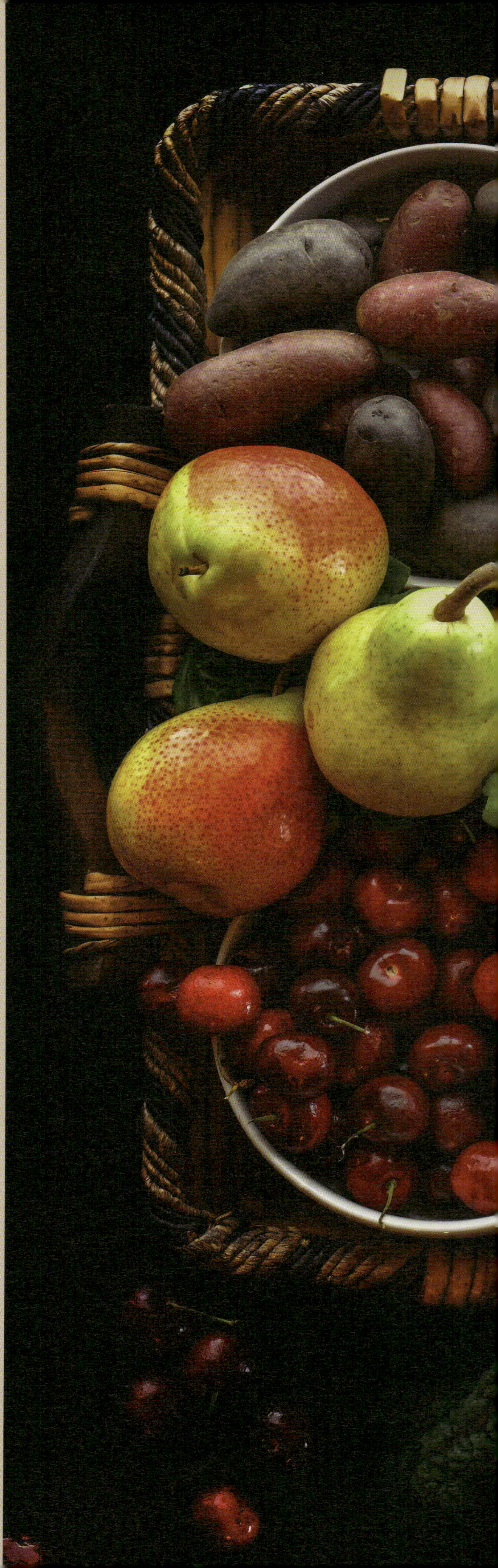

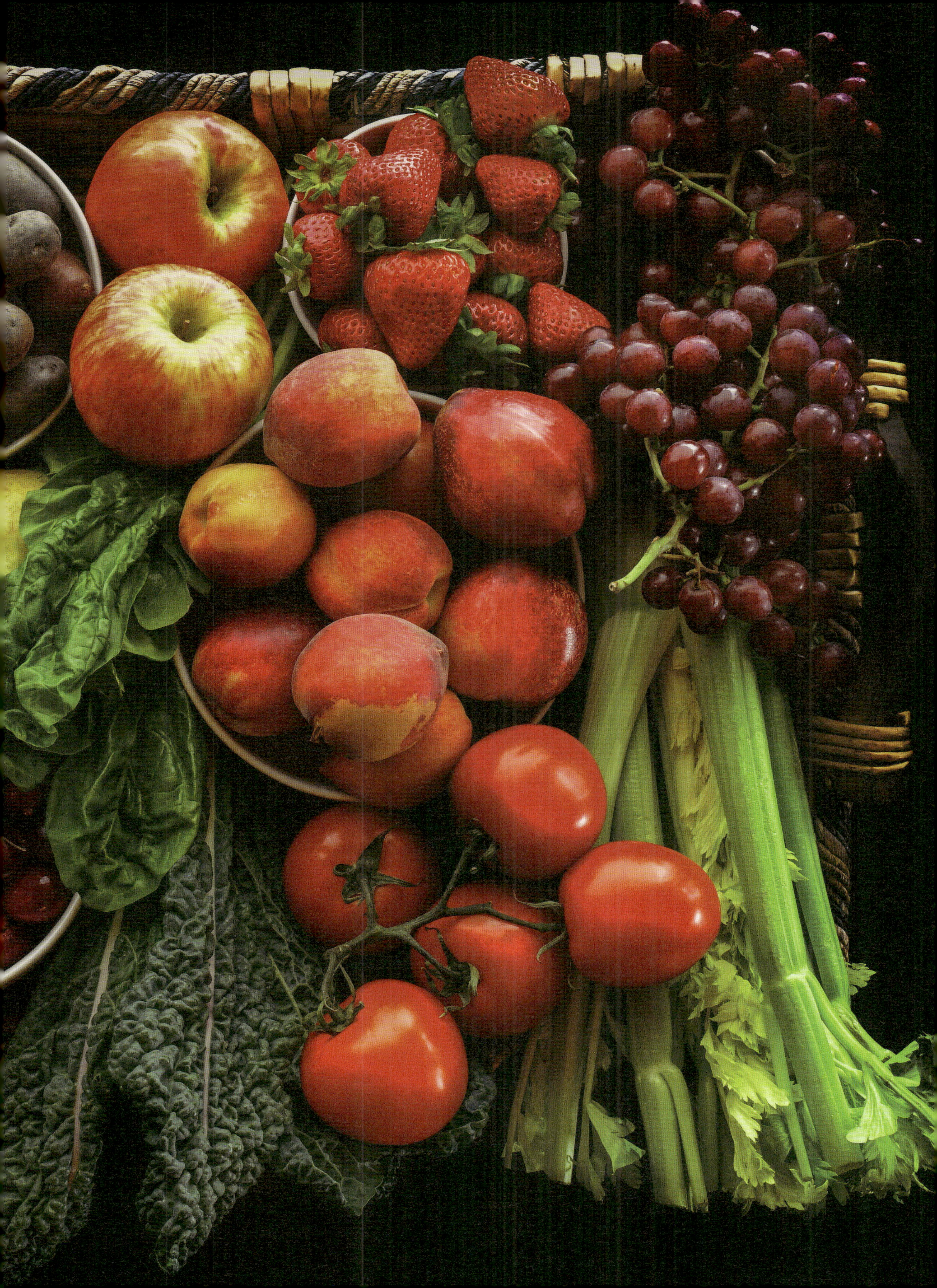

OILS

WE RECOMMEND USING THESE OILS AS MOST OF THEM DO NOT UNDERGO HEAVY PROCESSING.

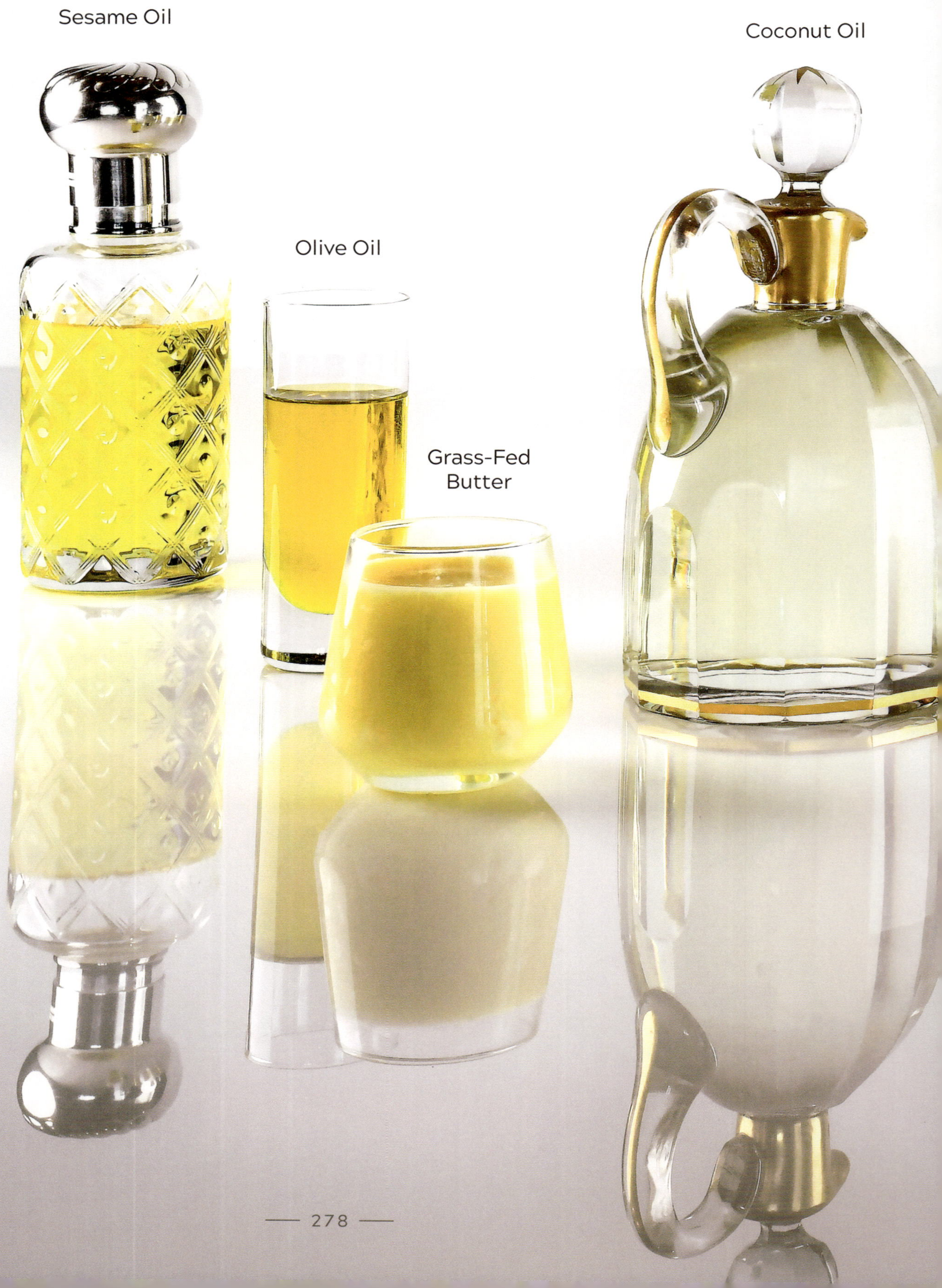

Grapeseed and coconut oil tend to tolerate more heat in the cooking process than more delicate oils like extra-virgin olive oil or flax oil (which never should be heated). Coconut oil can impart some flavor into your food unless you are using refined coconut oil, which has an even higher heat tolerance than virgin or extra-virgin coconut oil. Coconut oil is a plant-based saturated fat and can raise lipids in susceptible individuals, so moderation is key. On the flip side, coconut oil is a natural source of medium-chain triglycerides which are very easy to digest (especially if you don't have a gallbladder) and can help your body make ketones.

Like with any category of food, it's good to rotate oils so that you get a variety of fats in your diet. Remember that all oils are 100% fat! Use only the amount of oil you need when cooking so you can save your fat calories for other whole-food options such as olives, nuts, seeds, and avocados.

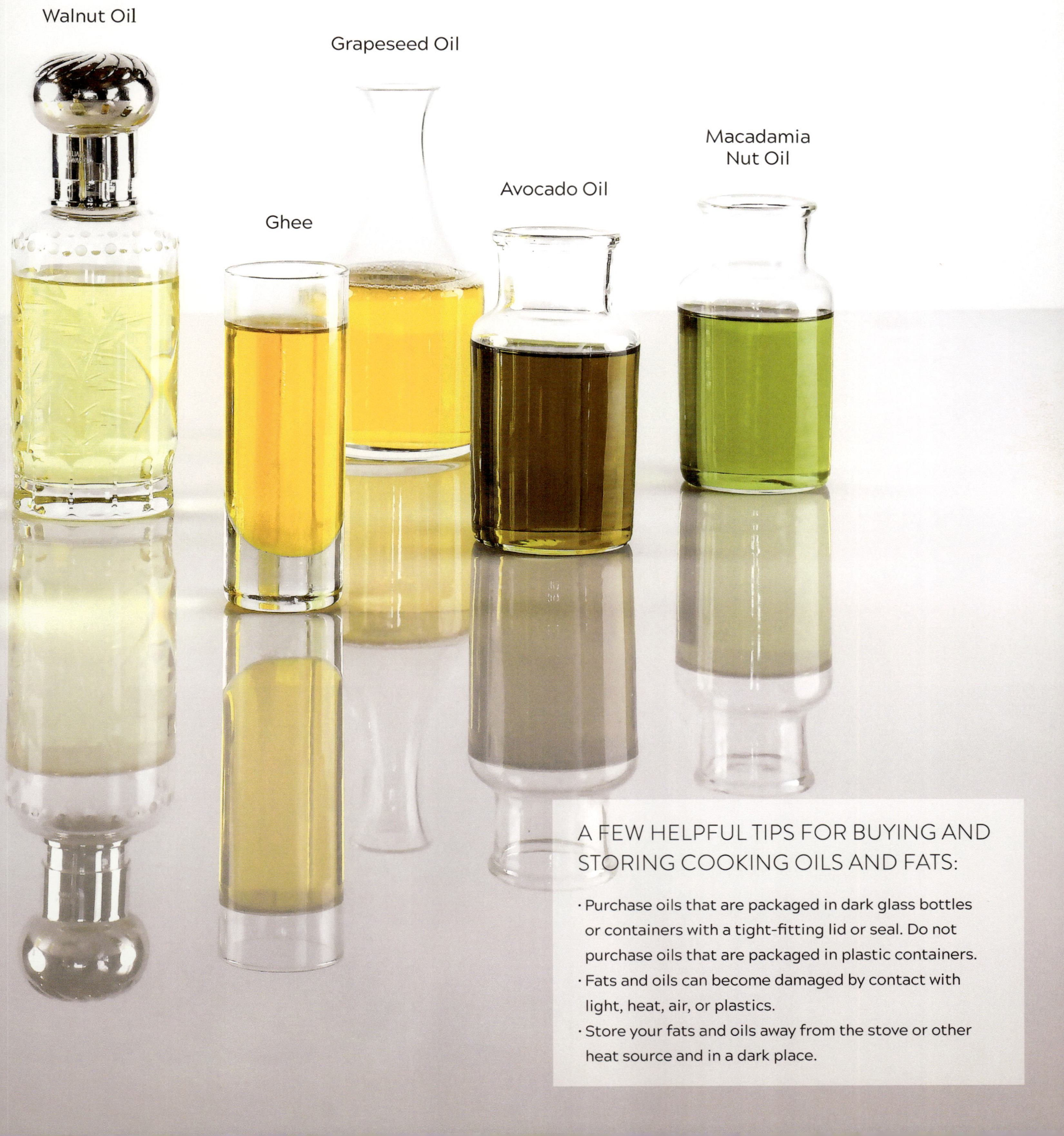

A FEW HELPFUL TIPS FOR BUYING AND STORING COOKING OILS AND FATS:

- Purchase oils that are packaged in dark glass bottles or containers with a tight-fitting lid or seal. Do not purchase oils that are packaged in plastic containers.
- Fats and oils can become damaged by contact with light, heat, air, or plastics.
- Store your fats and oils away from the stove or other heat source and in a dark place.

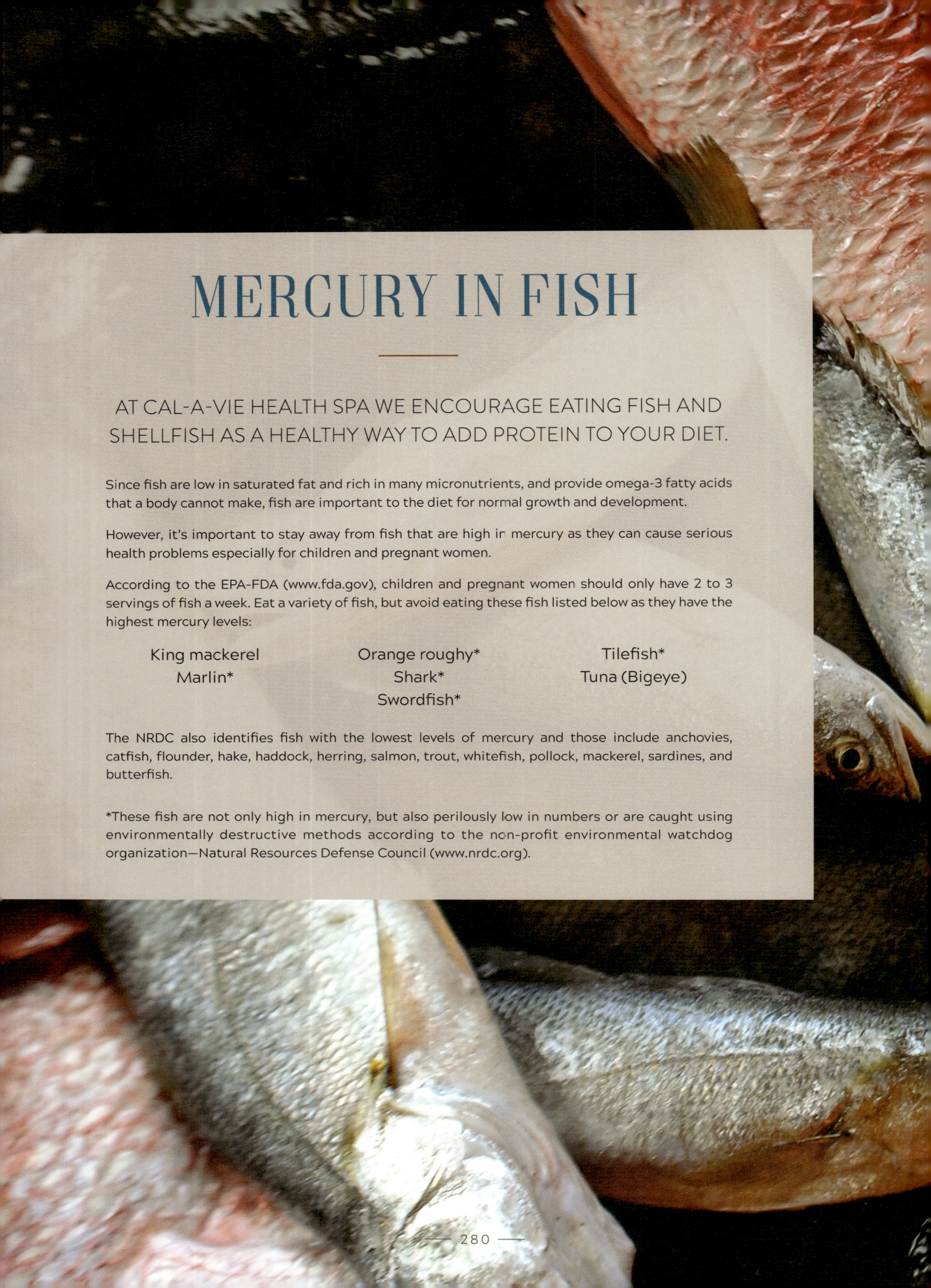

MERCURY IN FISH

AT CAL-A-VIE HEALTH SPA WE ENCOURAGE EATING FISH AND SHELLFISH AS A HEALTHY WAY TO ADD PROTEIN TO YOUR DIET.

Since fish are low in saturated fat and rich in many micronutrients, and provide omega-3 fatty acids that a body cannot make, fish are important to the diet for normal growth and development.

However, it's important to stay away from fish that are high in mercury as they can cause serious health problems especially for children and pregnant women.

According to the EPA-FDA (www.fda.gov), children and pregnant women should only have 2 to 3 servings of fish a week. Eat a variety of fish, but avoid eating these fish listed below as they have the highest mercury levels:

King mackerel
Marlin*
Orange roughy*
Shark*
Swordfish*
Tilefish*
Tuna (Bigeye)

The NRDC also identifies fish with the lowest levels of mercury and those include anchovies, catfish, flounder, hake, haddock, herring, salmon, trout, whitefish, pollock, mackerel, sardines, and butterfish.

*These fish are not only high in mercury, but also perilously low in numbers or are caught using environmentally destructive methods according to the non-profit environmental watchdog organization—Natural Resources Defense Council (www.nrdc.org).

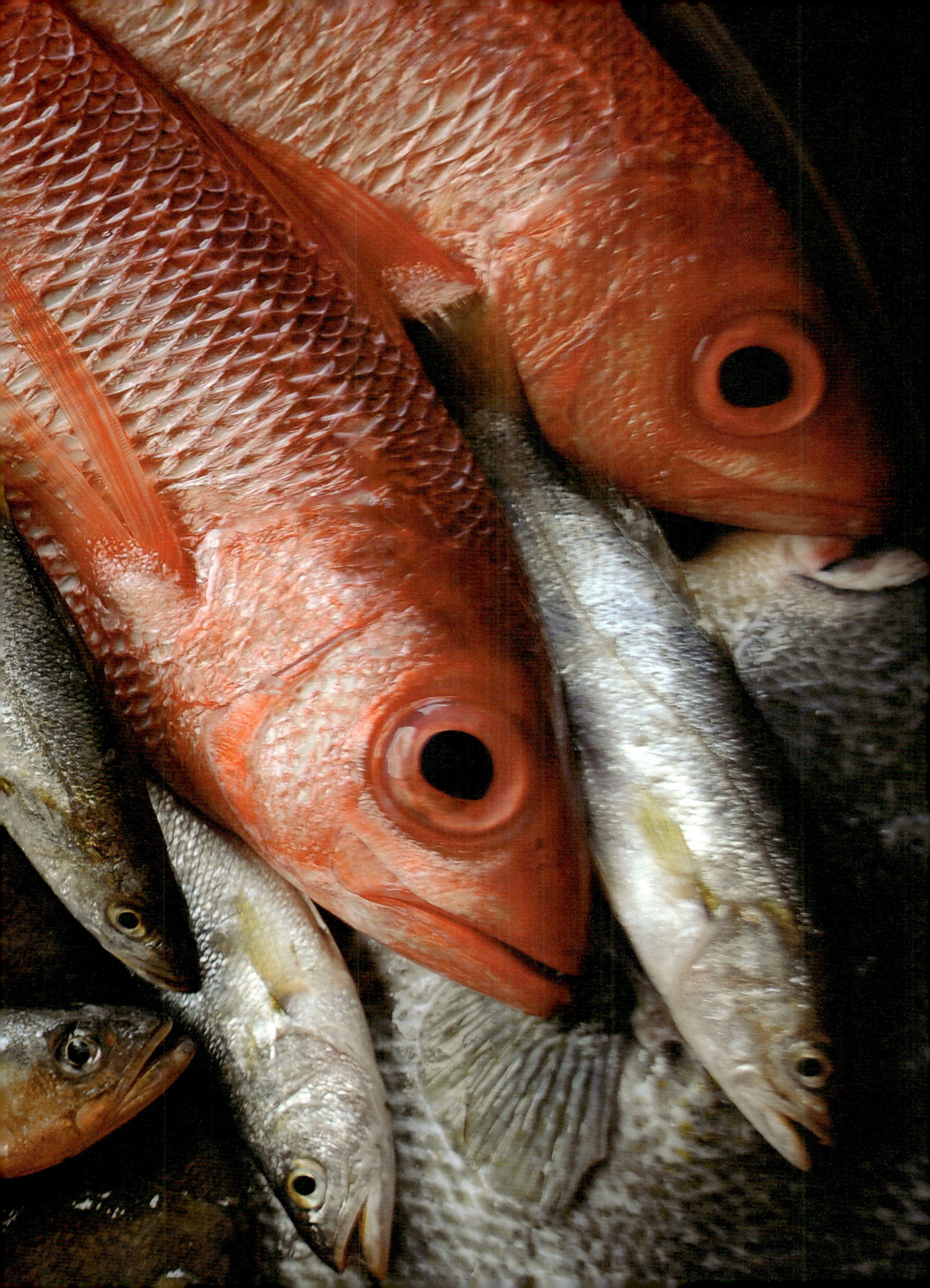

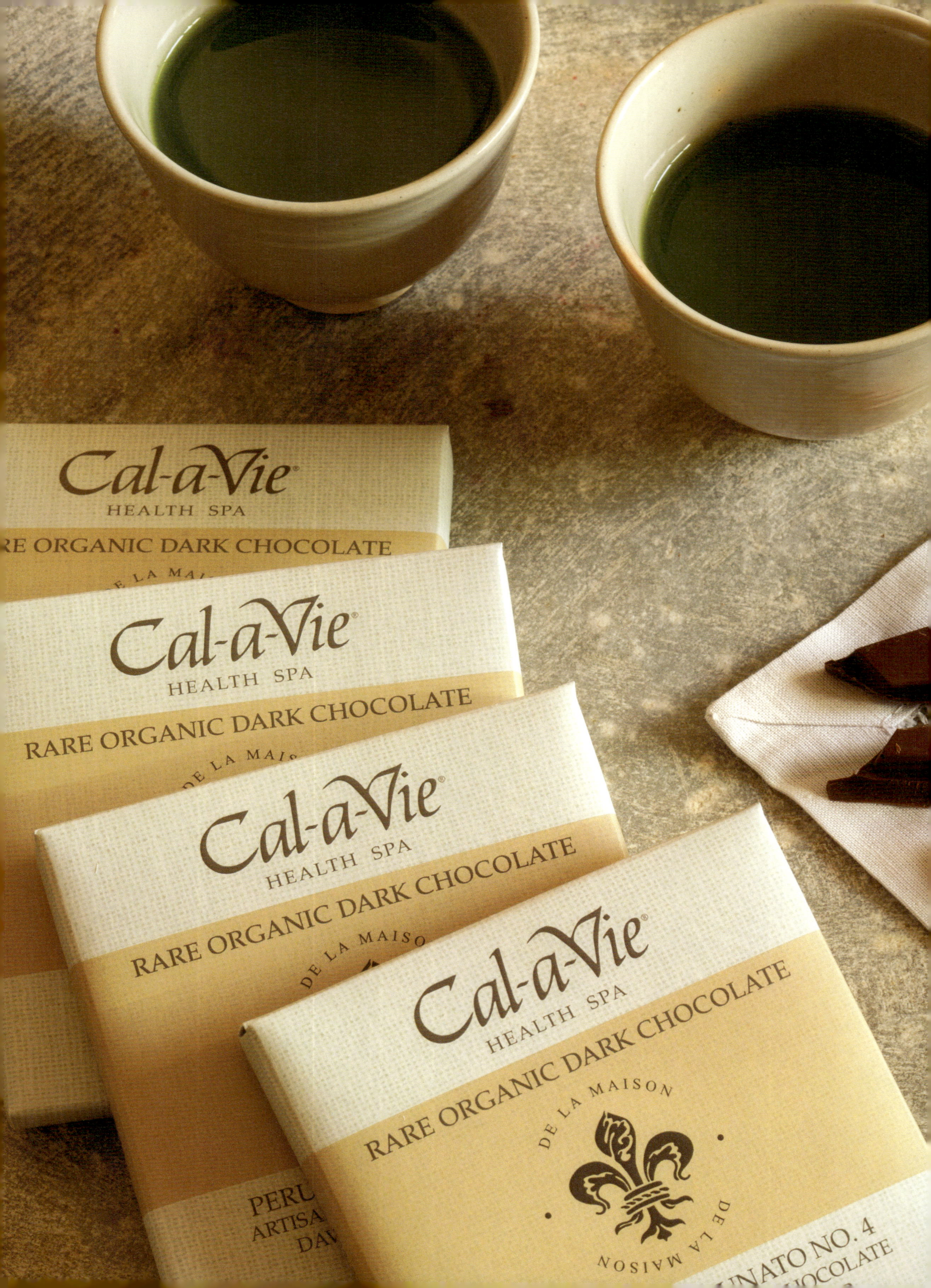
Cal-a-Vie
HEALTH SPA
RARE ORGANIC DARK CHOCOLATE
Cal-a-Vie
HEALTH SPA
RARE ORGANIC DARK CHOCOLATE
Cal-a-Vie
HEALTH SPA
RARE ORGANIC DARK CHOCOLATE
Cal-a-Vie
HEALTH SPA
RARE ORGANIC DARK CHOCOLATE
DE LA MAISON
DE LA MAISON

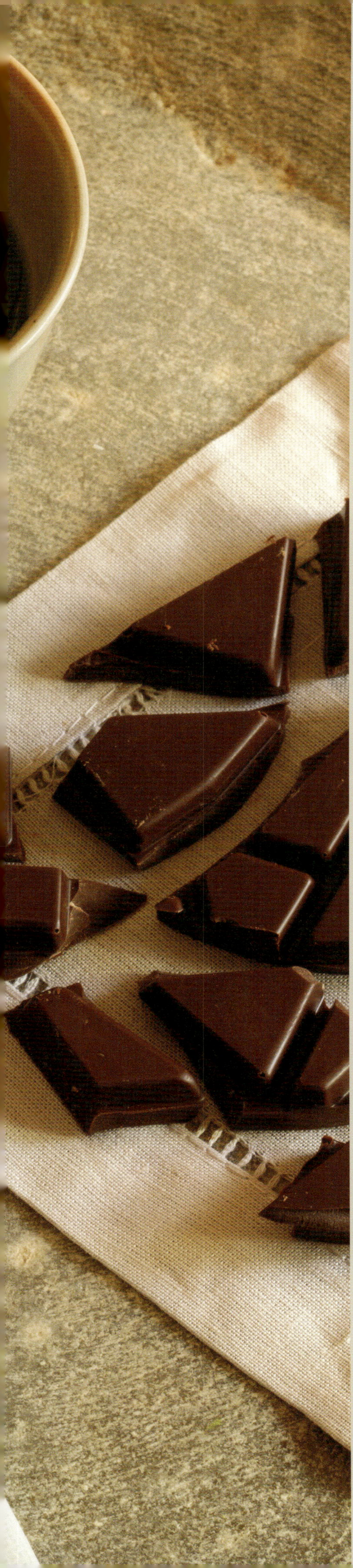

CHOCOLATE

CHOCOLATE IS RICH IN FLAVONOIDS WHICH OFFER NATURAL UV PROTECTION FOR YOUR SKIN FROM THE INSIDE OUT.

At Cal-a-Vie we search the world and research all varieties of chocolate to find the very best to share with our guests.

Chocolate also is a great vasodilator which can be very helpful for exercise performance and your love life! Selecting the right chocolate is all about quality and good portions. Rules of thumb: Select dark chocolate 70% and higher that has the best flavor profile for your taste buds. Stick to 1-2 thumb sizes at a given sitting, eaten mindfully. Cocoa butter is the natural fat found in chocolate that makes it so satiating, so a little goes a long way.

TEA

HEALTH BENEFITS OF GREEN TEA AND MATCHA:

Green tea has a high polyphenol content and has received a lot of positive attention in scientific research. It contains L-theanine, a brain-calming amino acid; chlorophyll, a pigment helpful in aiding in liver detox; and EGCG, a cancer-fighting antioxidant. EGCG is also a natural aromatase inhibitor, great for men and women who want to combat estrogen dominance.

Matcha is a form of green tea, originating from Japan, that is shade grown before harvest and ground into a fine powder. We recommend drinking matcha or green tea as part of a healthy diet. If you are sensitive to caffeine, choose decaffeinated versions of green tea that use the CO_2 method of decaffeination to avoid any added contamination. For cardiac benefits, consider drinking 4-6 cups of green tea a day.

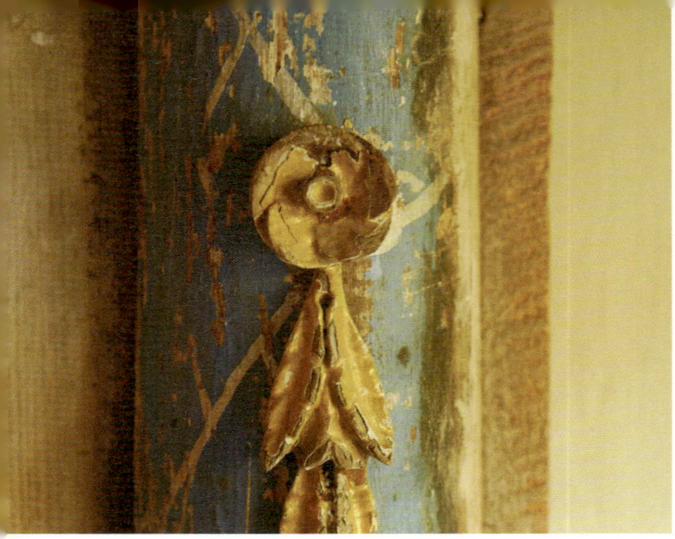
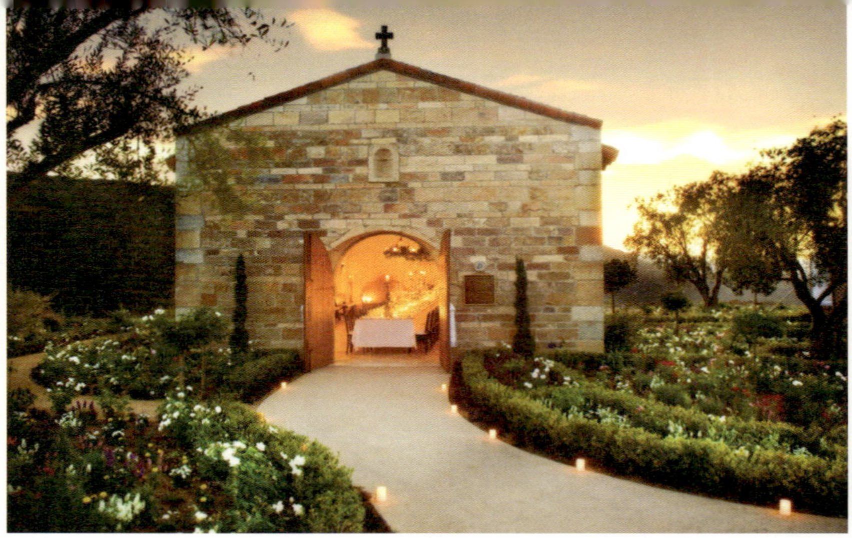
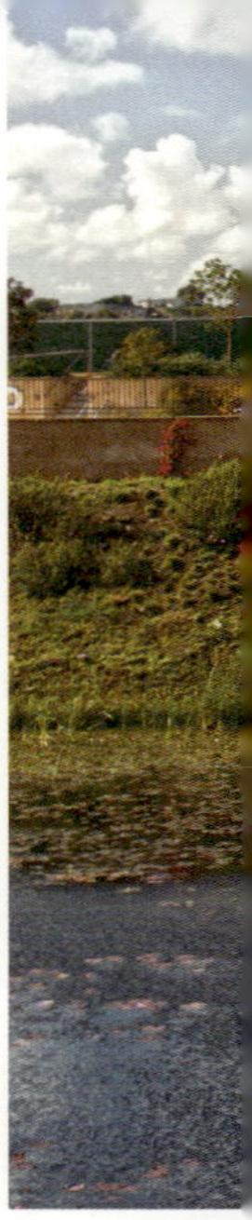
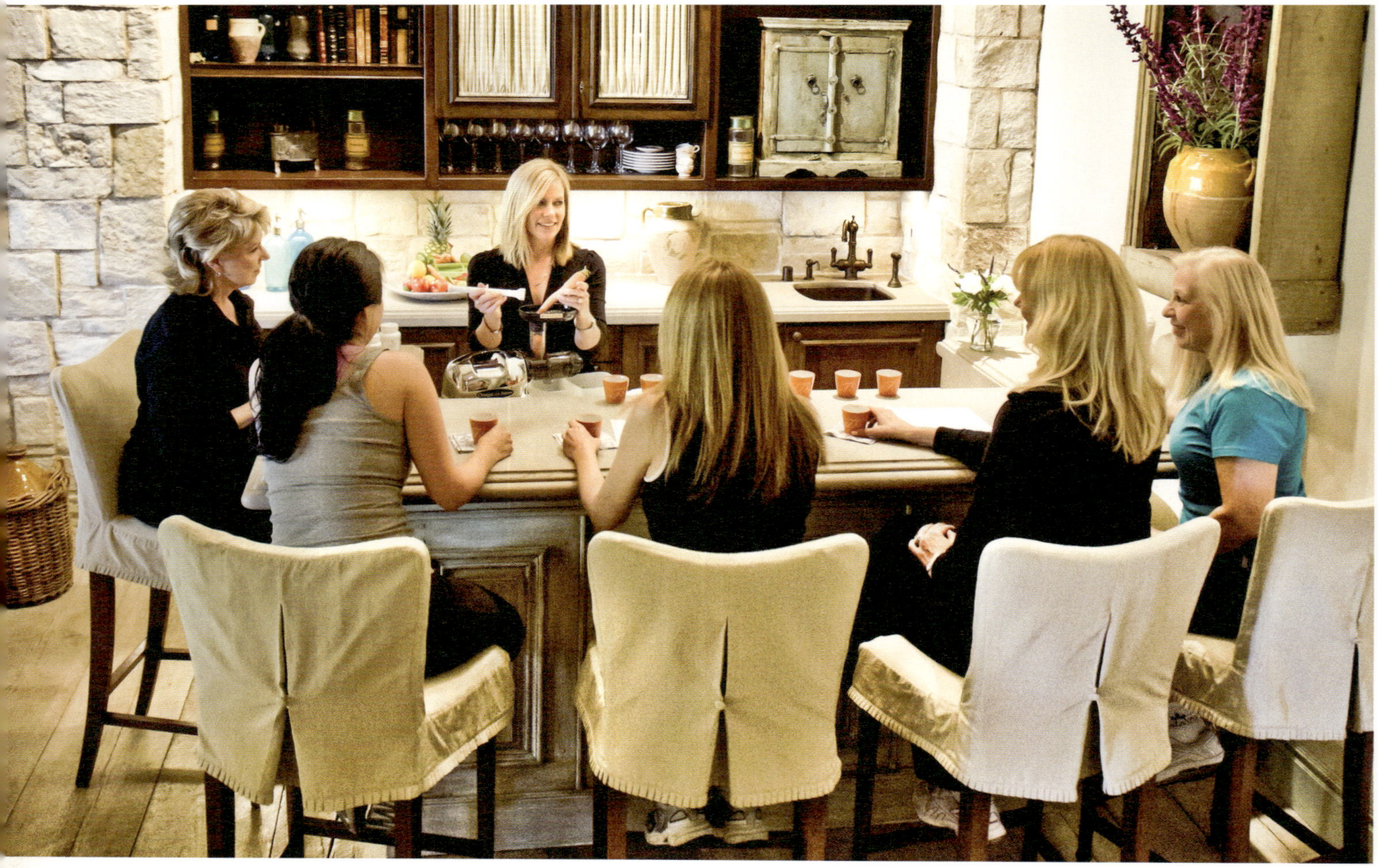
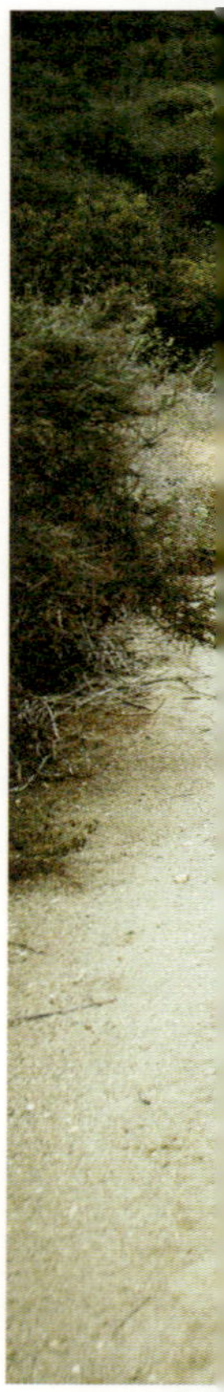
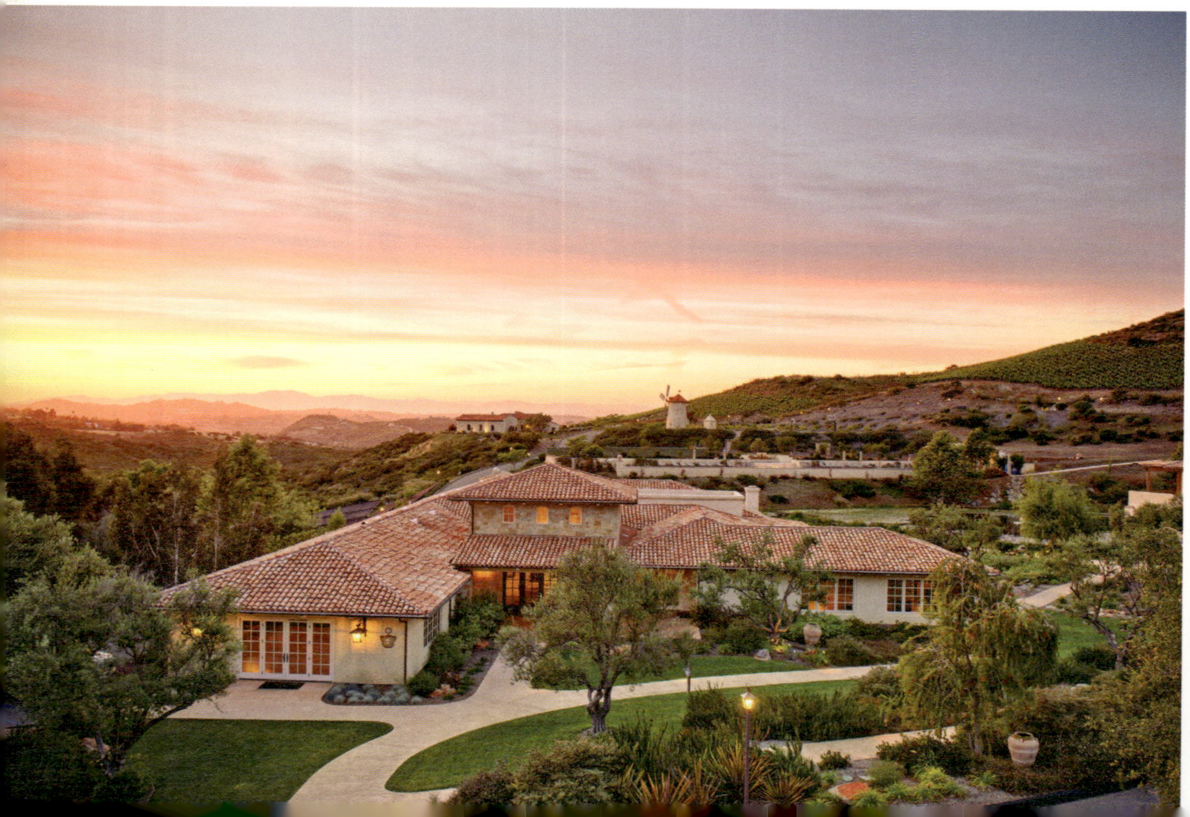
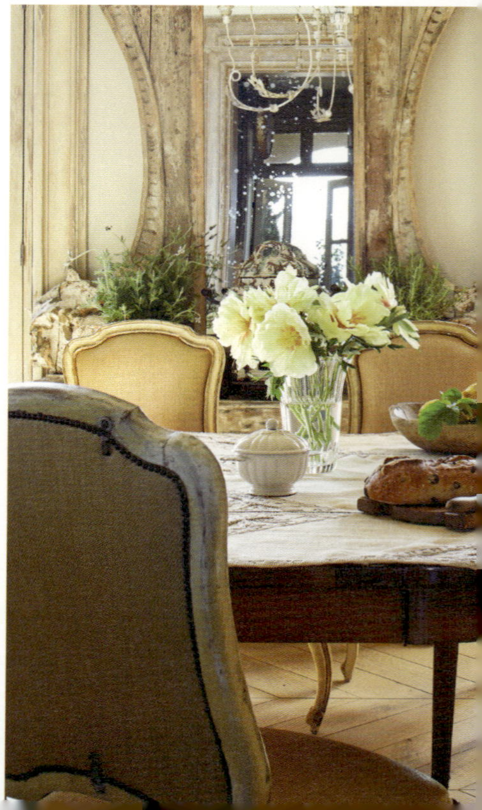

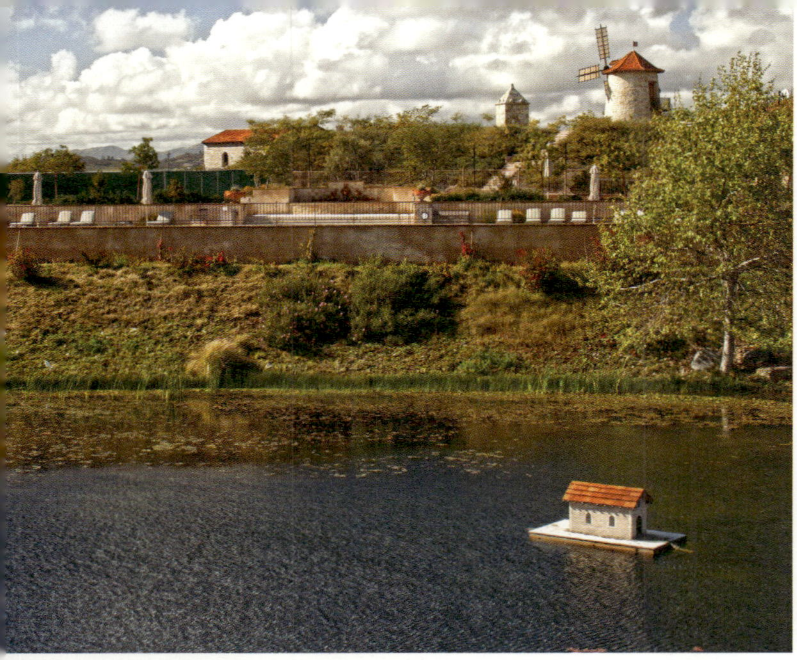

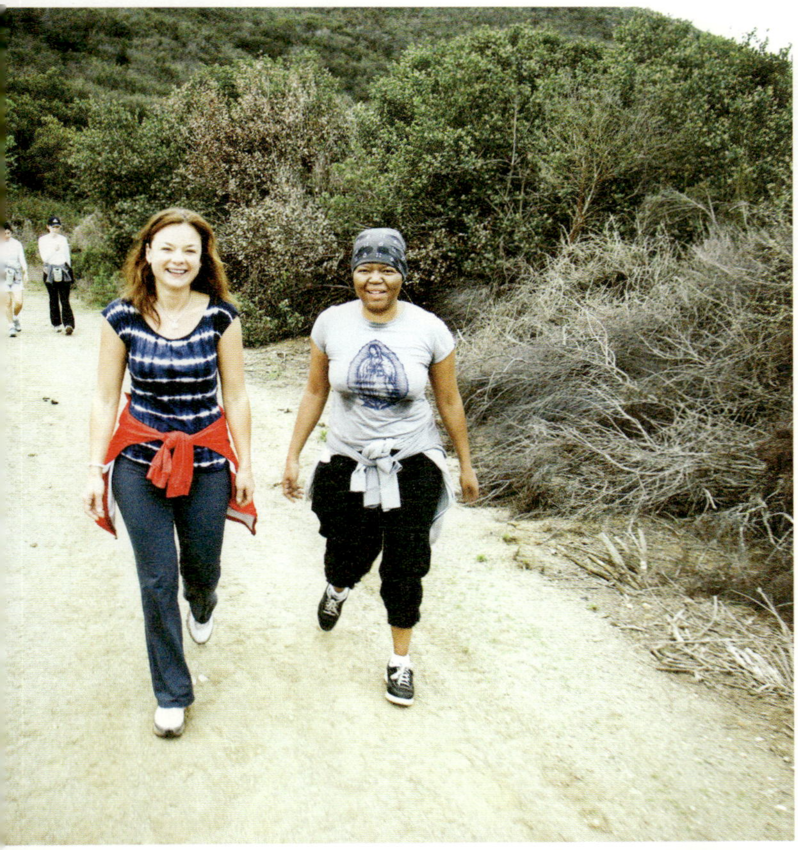

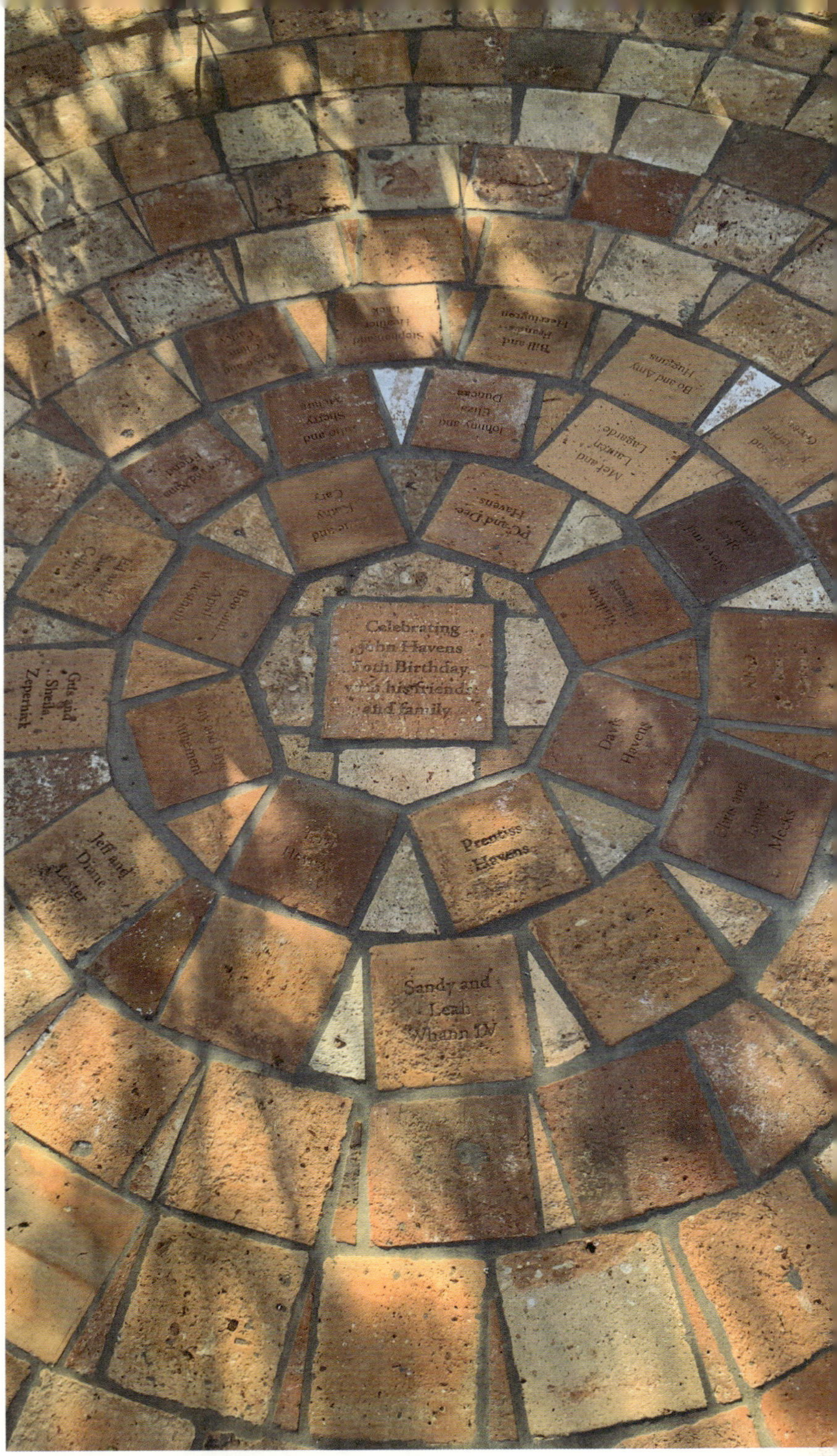
Prentiss
Havens
Sandy and
Leah
Whann IV

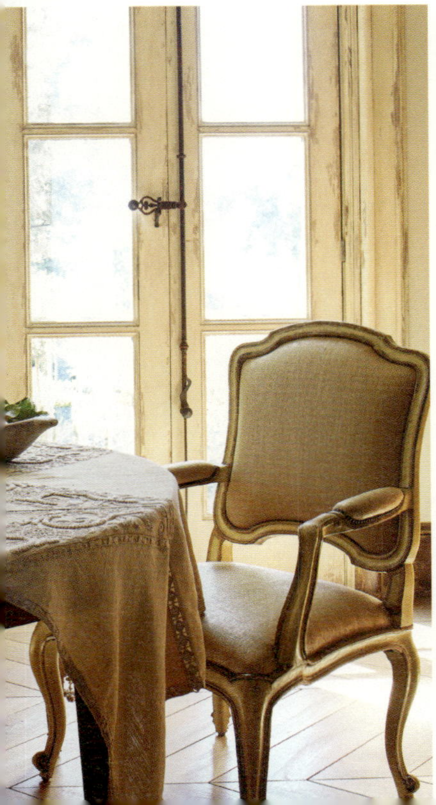

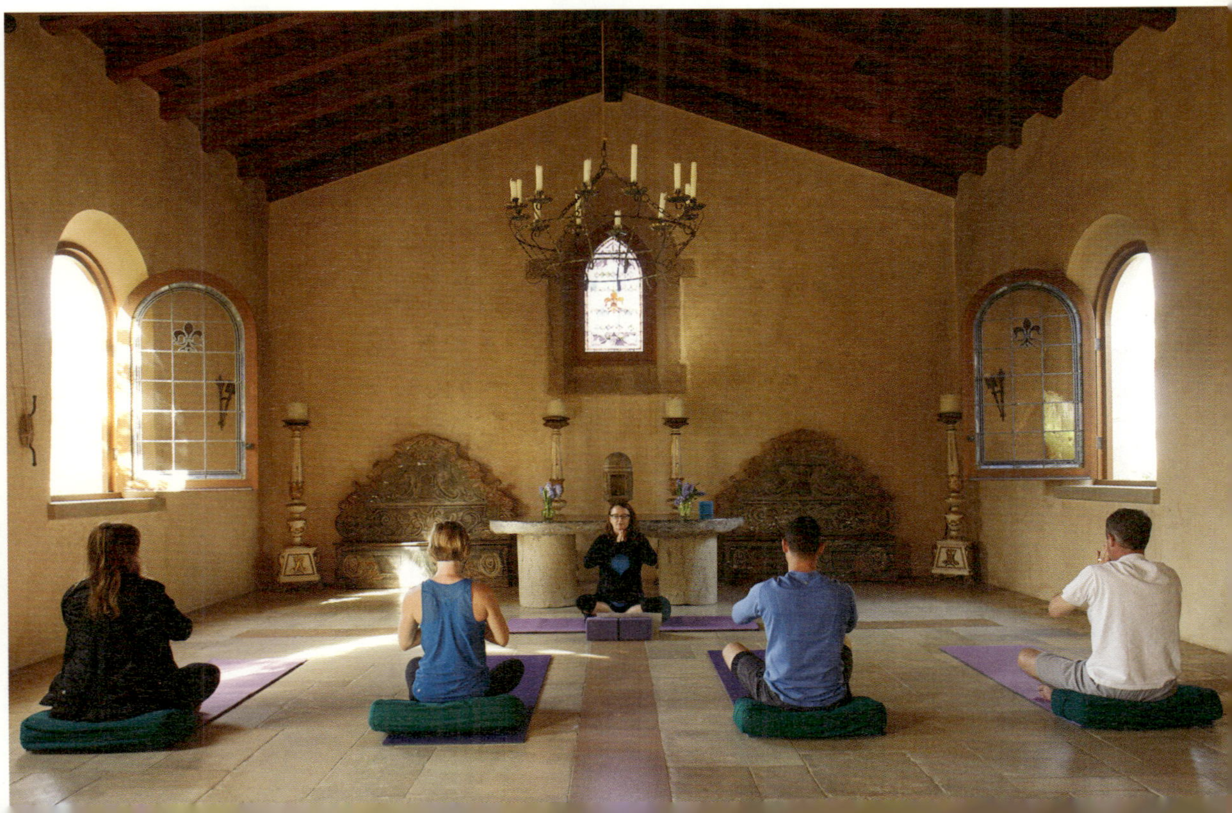

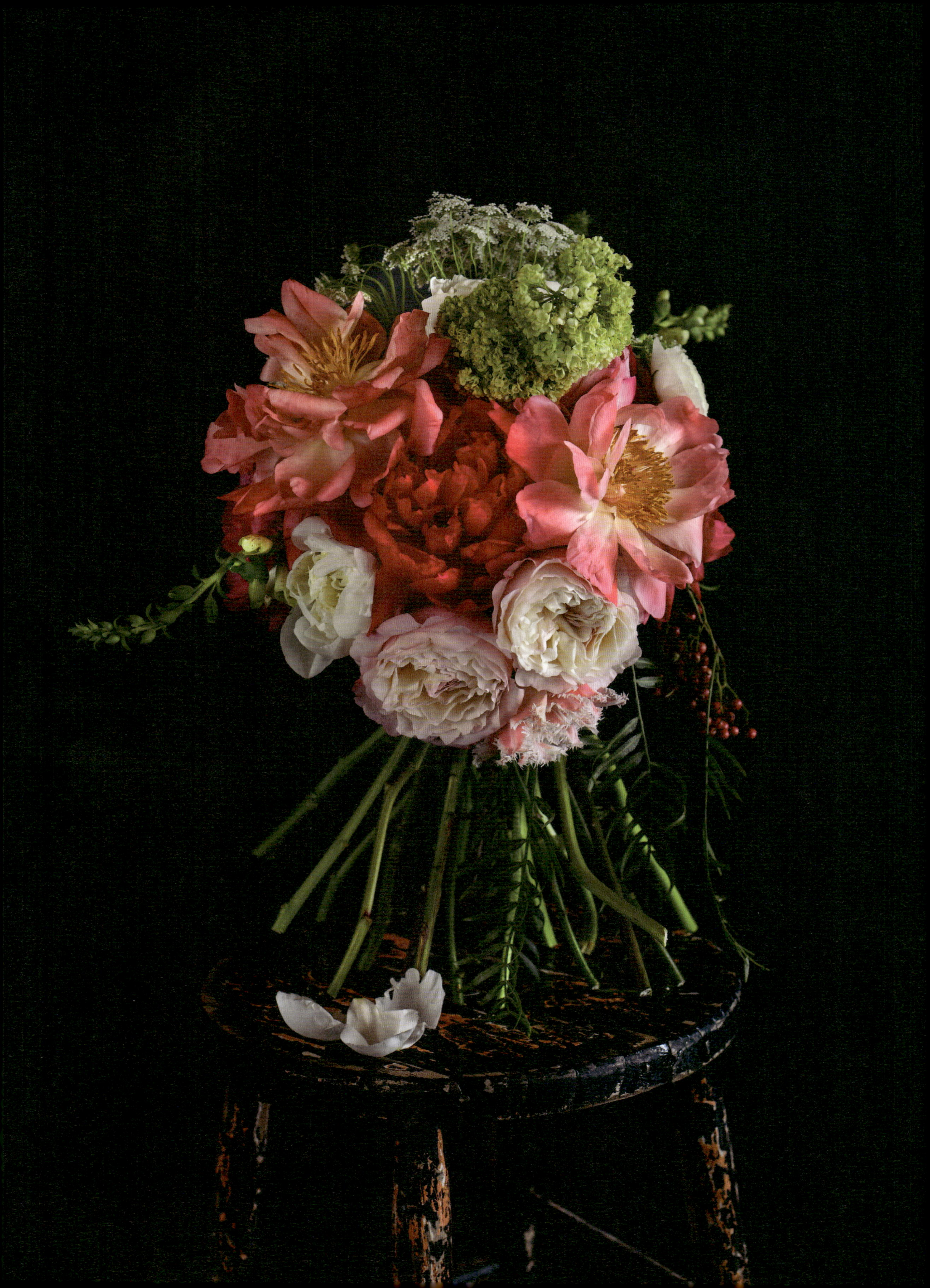

ACKNOWLEDGMENTS

A PROJECT LIKE THIS COOKBOOK DOESN'T HAPPEN ACCIDENTALLY.

It relies on the time, effort, skills, and creativity of dozens of people. Without their contributions and commitment, none of this would have been possible. So we would like to acknowledge the talented team of friends, family, and professionals whose help has been invaluable:

- I have to start by thanking **Roni Atnipp** and **Elise DeSilva**. From reading early drafts to giving me advice on the cover to spending every day with me on photo shoots, they were as important to this book getting done as I was. Definitely the proverbial "I couldn't have done it without you" fits here perfectly. Putting together a book is much harder than I thought. None of this would be possible without this dynamic duo.

- I am eternally grateful to my husband, **John**, who taught me how to think big. He helped me know that I could tackle big, huge projects no matter how much other work I had going on. I truly don't know where I would be if I didn't have his love and support through all of the crazy ideas I come up with.

- I am indebted to my children, **Prentiss, Davis,** and **Mallette,** who had to listen to me speak about all aspects of the cookbook 24/7. Whether it was discussing photo shoots, treasure hunts for place settings, or ideas for book sales, they did not complain one bit about my obsessive topic of conversation.

- I am thankful for my mom, **Faye,** who is an amazing cook. She instilled a love of food in me that I have passed to my daughter. I didn't say I loved to cook, but I definitely love to check out recipes and interesting food presentations from her, always trying to experiment in the kitchen at home. She belonged to a gourmet club that prepared dinners from around the world, inspiring me to try different cuisines and appreciate them. I now am an official foodie thanks to her, and my daughter will not go to a restaurant without looking up the menu first to see if it is worthy.

- Businesses and homes around the country are a more beautiful place thanks to **Laurie Steichen** and **Kara Childress**, two amazing Interior Decorators that I admire so much. Their incredible style ideas have catapulted Cal-a-Vie and my home to new heights. Both have contributed to designs that were done 10 years ago. Not a day goes by that I don't ogle in the beauty of the decoration. They are still as fresh today as they were 10 years ago.

- Without the incredible eye and experience of **Max Kim-Bee, Anne Watson** and **Debra Smail,** this book would be pure facts. They transformed each of their respective photographs to new levels. Their skill and creativity catapulted the book to new heights. I drool over every picture and want to look at them over and over again.

- **Carolyn Englefield,** editor of *Veranda*, for helping me realize I could actually put together a cookbook that contained more than just recipes. Your great advice was to make the book have a feeling! I hope I achieved that.

- To all our **staff** who helped contribute to the cookbook by being their incredible selves each day. Their enthusiasm for life spills over into their jobs, making every guest at Cal-a-Vie Health Spa want to come back. Whether they directly or indirectly helped on the cookbook, we couldn't have done it without you.

- **Curtis Cooke** for his sheer dedication to wanting to provide delicious, clean, organic recipes each day to our guests and for working hard to complete our cookbook.

- **May Tom** and **Gina Worful** for their commitment and enthusiasm in helping our guests live nutritionally better and healthier lives. They provided the nutrition breakdown and information on all our recipes which help the home cook prepare meals the Cal-a-Vie way.

- **Karin Lamon** and her mom, **Iris Jensen.** Iris did the large flower arrangement on the cover. Her floral abilities continue to amaze me. She is 90 years old and still creative as ever. Karen got her creativity from her mom and puts together the most inviting place settings. Her table scape classes at Cal-a-Vie are a highlight of the day. Of course, we don't mind mentioning she serves champagne if you attend.

- **Pam Kuhl-Linscomb** and **Dan Linscomb** are the owners of Kuhl-Linscomb. They didn't realize when they agreed to let us borrow china for the photo shoots that it would involve days of looking and selecting hundreds of pieces and then itemizing each one. We shot 100 photos of food—which meant 100 different place settings—and with the help of Pam and Dan, we have elegant pictures with tantalizing food placed perfectly on the plates. When I realized that we didn't have what was needed for the photos, they cheerfully obliged, showing a level of service that is unmatched by anyone, anywhere. We will be eternally grateful for all of their help.

- Also from Kuhl-Linscomb was **Shelby Balmer**, whose fantastic taste helped us put together all the fabulous place settings. If you're looking for a go-to home design adviser, look no further.

- **Jane Scott Hodges** of Leontine Linens, who graciously offered the gorgeous monogrammed linens that elevated the place settings to 5-star status.

- **Ellie Tagdishi** at Plush Home, who provided unique items for our place settings and whose sense of style made for one-of-a-kind displays.

- **Leslie Sinclair** of Segreto Finishes. We needed many different backgrounds for our photography shoots, and I remembered she had done a number of samples for me to choose from for my walls. She was happy to provide the backdrops of fabulous Venetian plaster that gave the pictures the depth we needed. I thought we could get by with just a few, but soon realized we needed more—a lot more. Thanks so much for being there for us.

- **Laurie Moran** for volunteering the samples she used while decorating her house. **Jenny Elkins** for providing on-point theme salt and pepper shakers.

- Thanks to **Kameron Kraft** whose flower design work I admire. I love the romantic feel of her arrangements as well as her attention to detail. She finds the most unusual flowers that are in fabulous uncommon colors.

- **Linda Gayle White, Estelle Racusin,** and **Susan Thompson** for their talents and time in helping to edit the book.

- **Martha Britton** for helping us get all of our promotions in order. I asked her to help arrange some book signings—and had to call her off because she booked so many! What a dynamo!

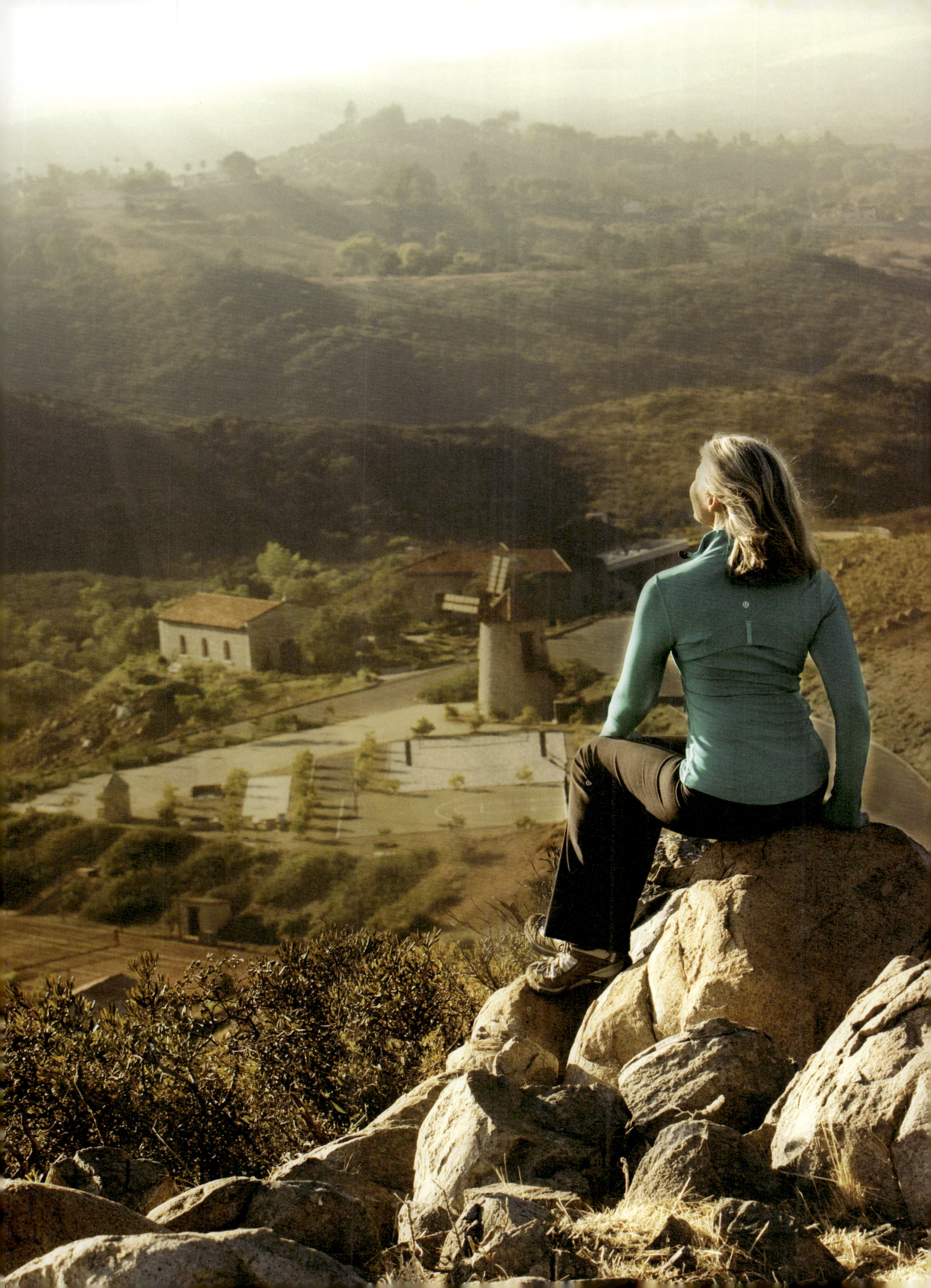

VISTA VALLEY COUNTRY CLUB

Cal-a-Vie Health Spa is excited that we also own the property right next door, Vista Valley Country Club. Nestled in a tranquil valley, the golf course offers stunning views of the Southern California landscape, impeccable course conditions, unmatched playability, and superlative golf shop service. Designed by Ted Robinson Sr., Vista Valley Country Club was established as a par-72 golf course. This 18-Hole Championship layout is renowned for its dramatic elevation changes, undulating fairways, and fast greens. Vista Valley provides a range of tees suitable for any handicap and an extensive practice range and short game areas. So, if you think you might get tired of hiking, boxing, or lifting, you can take a few hours off and go play this gorgeous golf course.

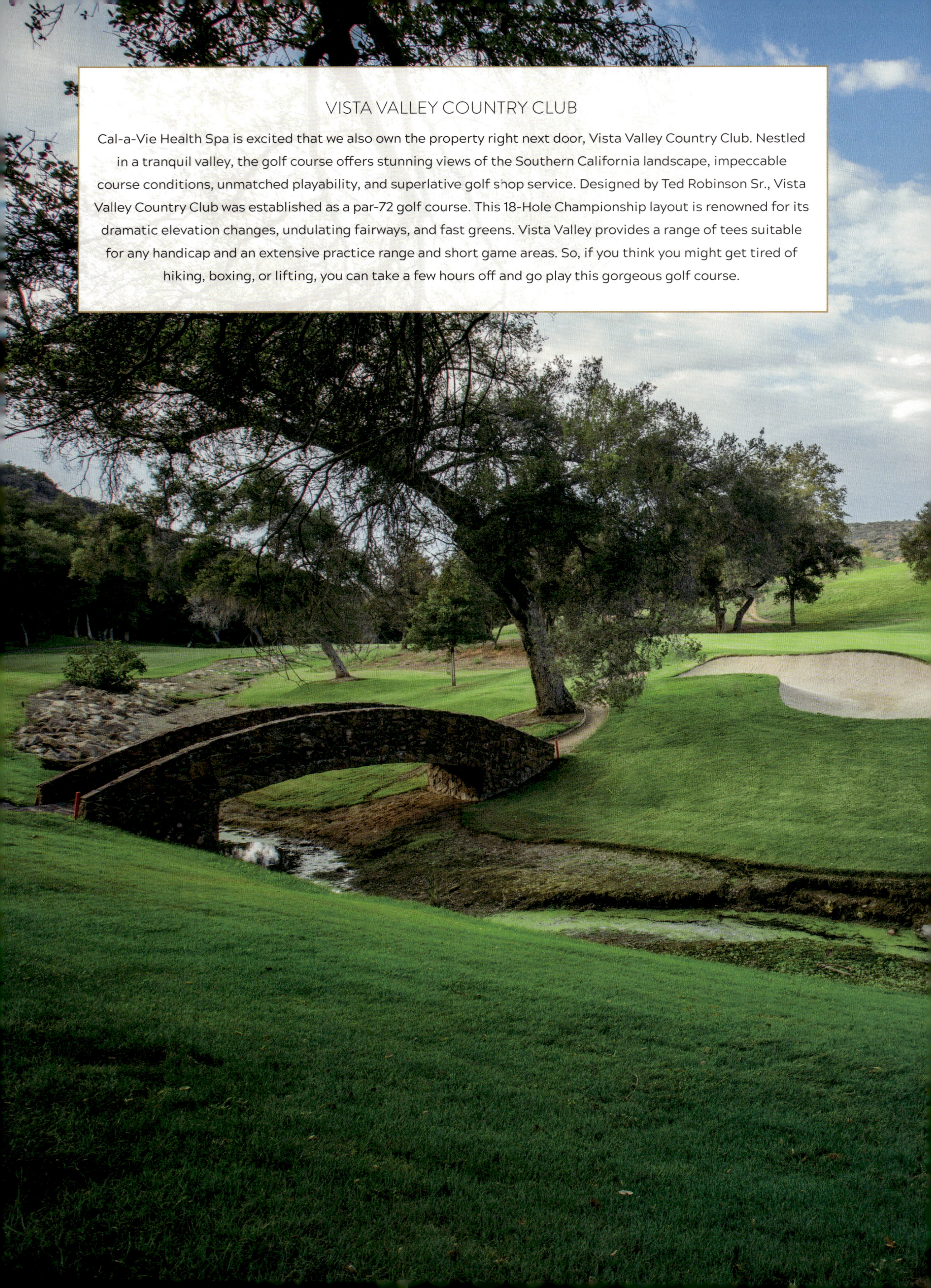

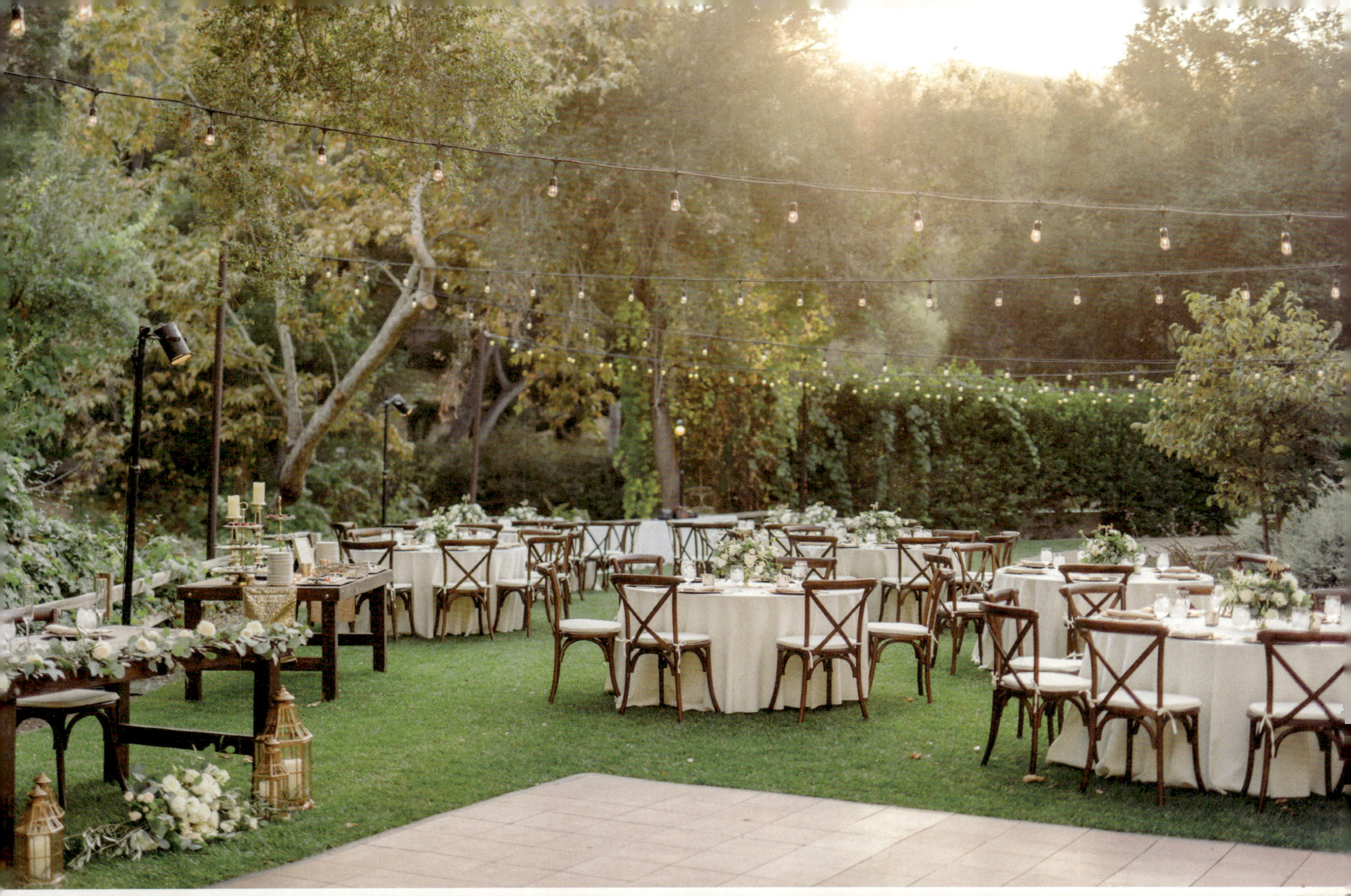
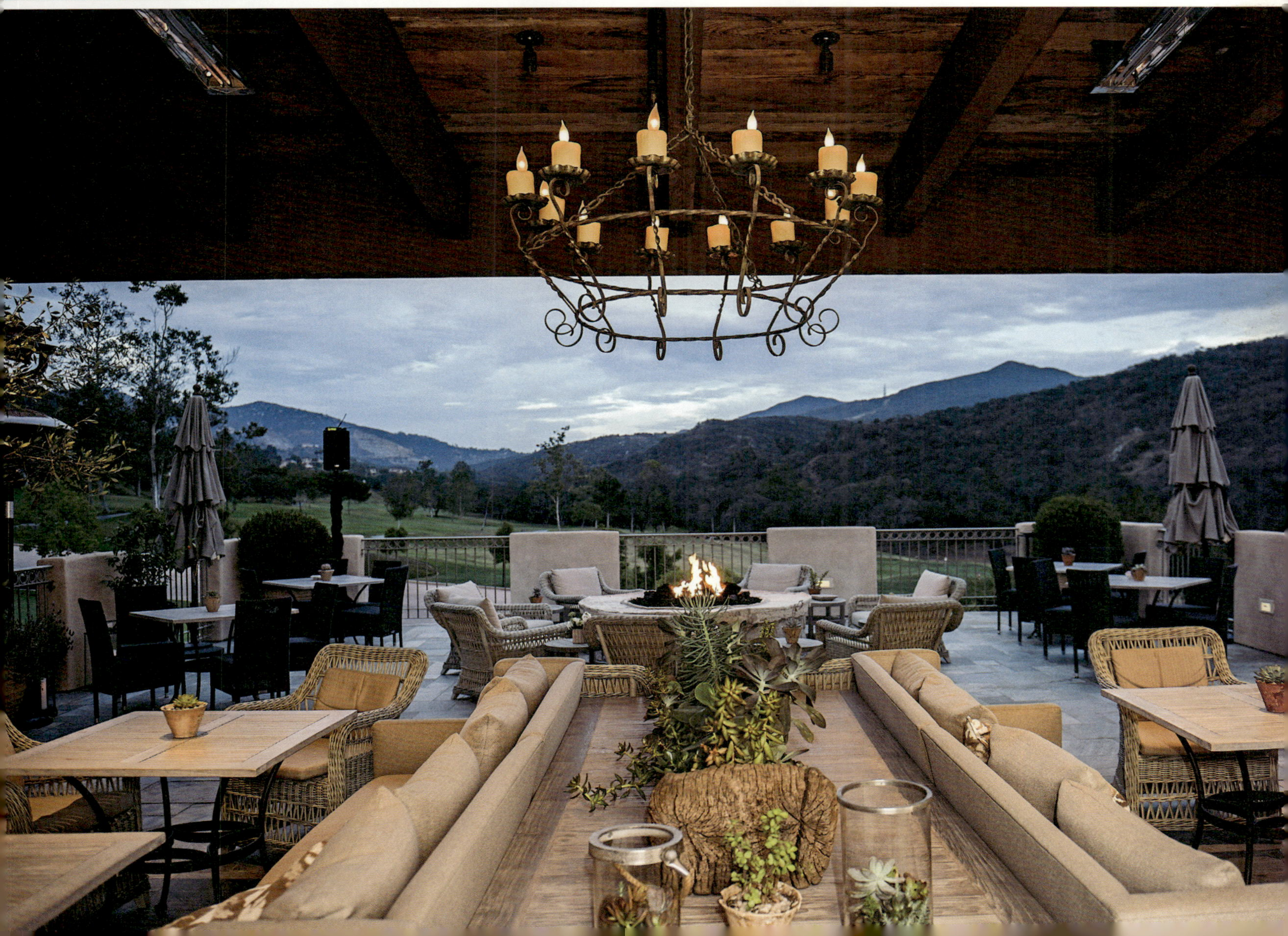

Thank You

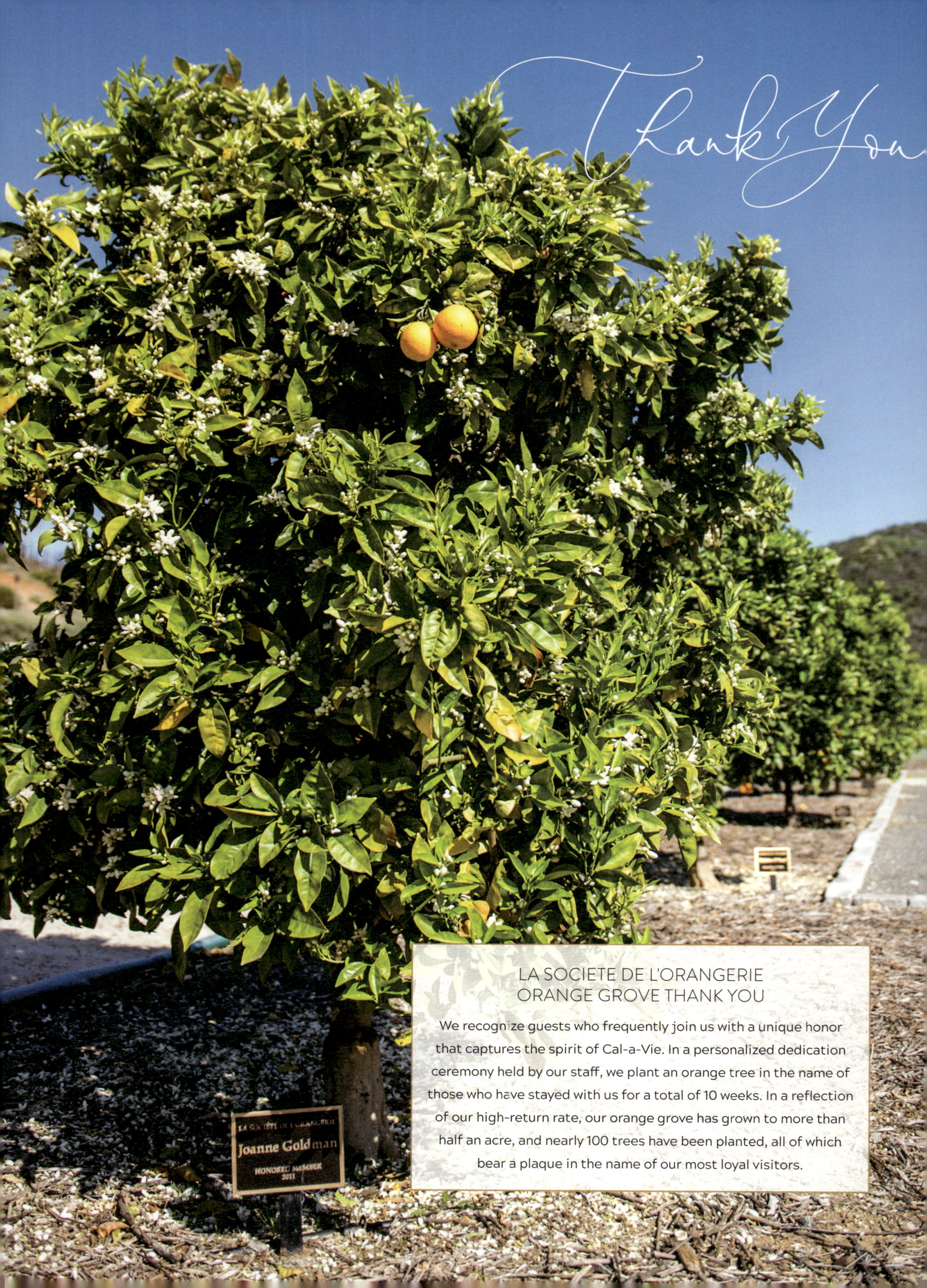

LA SOCIETE DE L'ORANGERIE
ORANGE GROVE THANK YOU

We recognize guests who frequently join us with a unique honor that captures the spirit of Cal-a-Vie. In a personalized dedication ceremony held by our staff, we plant an orange tree in the name of those who have stayed with us for a total of 10 weeks. In a reflection of our high-return rate, our orange grove has grown to more than half an acre, and nearly 100 trees have been planted, all of which bear a plaque in the name of our most loyal visitors.

Our photographs are beautiful and spectacular thanks to the help of several stores and lots of our friends who loaned us their fabulous treasures.

Below you will find a reference guide so you can purchase them at these retailers. The items without a notation are from the personal collections of our home and those of our friends. Thank you for trusting us with them during the weeks of photography.

KUHL-LINSCOMB
THE DESIGN AND LIFESTYLE STORE

K Kuhl-Linscomb is a designer-owned lifestyle store in Houston, Texas. They offer well-designed products in a campus of repurposed mid-century buildings that sprawls nearly two city blocks. Their 100,000 square feet of showroom space offer niche and coveted items in departments that include apothecary, men's and women's fashion, tabletop, bedding, furniture, and gifts. Kuhl-Linscomb carries products in every price point, countless styles, and options in every category.
www.kuhl-linscomb.com

LEONTINE

L Founded in New Orleans in 1996 by Jane Scott Hodges, Leontine Linens is preserving and reinventing the classic art form of beautiful linens and infusing it with a modern twist. Leontine Linens are admired around the world for their luxurious, unique, custom embroidery, but are also designed for the modern family. The linens are machine washable and can be ironed.
www.leontinelinens.com

PLUSH HOME

P Plush Home is a one-stop shop for some of the best linens in Houston. Plush Home carries sheets, blankets, and pillows from around the world as well as tabletop items, candles, and other fabulous gift items for the home.
713.522.5230

APPETIZERS

Pages 55-56: Towers of Classic Meatballs with Marinara Sauce and Parmesan Polenta
- Deshoulieres Arcades dessert plate in grey and gold K
- Bernardaud Limoges bread and butter plate in the Elysee pattern K

Page 62: Artichoke and Olive Tapenade
- Herend dessert plate in the Songbird Chickadee pattern K

Page 65: Baba Ganoush
- Deborah Rhodes runner in Washed Fringe mustard color K

Page 66: Cashew Stuffed Mushrooms
- Razor Clam tray in mint color K
- Astier de Villatte panorama cup in Empire K

Page 69: Buffalo Cauliflower
- F. Dommatin Paris antique monogrammed compote dish
- Gorham 1876 antique sterling silver spoon in the Versailles pattern
- F. Dommatin Paris antique monogrammed gold-rimmed luncheon plate
- Minton Cilogan Collamore antique dinner plate with gold rim dated England 1872
- Pier One gold charger

Page 70: Roasted Brussel Sprouts with Peanut Chili Vinaigrette
- Vagabond House jam server plates K
- Reed & Barton Francis the First antique silver forks

Pages 72-73: Tomato Broccoli Flatbread
- Juliska tidbit plates in Forest Walk pattern—Friendship, Gratitude, and Love K
- Saro LIfestyle cocktail napkins K

Page 77: Watermelon, Cucumber, and Tomato Skewers
- Vagabond House olive cheese picks in pewter K
- Annieglass Edgey cheese slab K

SOUPS

Pages 78-80: Chilled Avocado Soup
- Juliska votives in berry and thread pattern K
- Hermès scarf

Pages 82-83: Broccoli Soup
- Tizo teardrop crystal bowl K
- Woodbury spoon in copper K

Page 85: Bloody Mary Gazpacho
- Assortment of antique tea cups–Roman China, Prince Rainier & Grace Kelly of Monaco, Paris Dommartin, Haviland
- Roman China antique vase

Page 86: Carrot Coconut Soup
- Juliska ramekin in Acanthus pattern in white wash K
- Juliska cocktail plate in Acanthus pattern in white with gold K
- Limoges, antique plate marked France
- Juliska dinner plate charger in Emerson pattern K

Page 89: Garden Pumpkin Soup
- Astier de Villatte Paris Emilie cup in white K
- Woodbury Simon Pearce dinner spoon in burnished-copper finish K
- Vietri tray in white K
- Tabac de StrasBourg antique French vase

Page 90: Golden Lentil Soup
- Boheme soup bowl in blue and yellow K
- H & M gray linen napkin
- Kim Seybert patina napkin ring in gold and silver K

Page 94: Parsnip-Apple Soup
- Juliska soup tureen in forest pewter pattern K

Pages 96-98: Roasted Cauliflower Soup with Curry Oil
- Moser Pebbles shot glasses in topaz, edlor, rosalin, aquamarine, beryl, Alex colors K

SALADS

Pages 100-102: Fennel, Carrot, Apple, and Bibb Lettuce Salad with Green Goddess Dressing
- Michael Aram Palace dinner plate, salad plate, bowl K
- William Yeoward crystal glass K

Page 104: Arugula with Strawberry and Vanilla Champagne Vinaigrette
- Hermès pink scarf
- R.H. May & Co. Royal Gallery 1994 gold charger made in Indonesia
- Rosenthal Versace Les Reves Byzantins Dreams pink dinner and salad plates K
- M. Redon Limoges France antique pink and gold-rimmed dinner plate

Page 107: Asian Chicken Salad
- Arte Italica Merletto canape plate K
- Blue Pheasant Nolan bread plate K
- Vietri Bellezza Canape plate in aqua K

Page 109: Green and Yellow Bean Salad
- Reed & Barton crystal Soho condiment set K

Page 113: Peach Salad
- Astier de Villatte La Tropicale Fermee Par Jose plate K
- Lee Jofa fabric K
- Vagabond House napkin ring K

Page 115: Petite Arugula Salad with Pear and Candied Walnuts
- H&M pink and green fabric
- Reed & Barton Francis™ 1st sterling silver luncheon fork K
- SCM brushed aluminum charger in graphite K
- Juliska Firenze Medici dessert plate in silver/gold K

Page 116: Roasted Beet Salad with Toasted Hazelnuts
- Jaune de Chrome Aguirre gold Finition dinner plate K

Page 119: Spiced Poached Pear Salad
- Lee Jofa table cloth
- Annieglass Mod cake stand and round plate in gold K

Page 120: Texas Caviar
- R.H. May & Co. Royal Galley 1994 gold rimmed plate–made in Indonesia

Pages 122-123: Vinaigrettes
- Juliska mini vase trio in clear K

MEAT

Page 128: Pork Tenderloin with Honey Mustard, Parsnip Mash, and Savoy Cabbage
- Mottahedeh Vista Allegre Tobacco Leaf service plate K
- Leontine Linens L

Pages 131-132: Beef Tenderloin with Red Wine Demi-Glace, Mashed Sweet Potatoes, and Green Beans
- Royal Crown Derby Aves dish in gold K

Page 135: Bison Lasagna Rolls with Basil Pesto and Toasted Garlic
- L'Objet Perlee gold charger and dessert plate K
- Bernardaud Aux Rois Flannelle dinner K
- Leontine Linens L
- Reed & Barton Francis™ the First sterling silver K

Page 139: Roasted Lamb Loin Chops with Beluga Lentil Ragu and King Trumpet Mushrooms
- Hermès Balcons du Guadalquivi presentation plate K
- Leontine Linens L

Page 142: Roasted Rack of Lamb
- Hermès Sabliers square plate K

SEAFOOD

Page 145: Herb Shrimp
- Juliska Puro Dappled dessert plate in cobalt K

Page 147: Lobster Curry with Baby Carrots, Beech Mushrooms, Snap Peas, and Coconut Cilantro Rice
- Herend Fishscale dinner plate K
- Leontine Linens L
- Royal Limoges Mark Grey dinner plate K
- Herend Fishscale dessert bowl K

Pages 154-155: Seared Branzino
- Anna Weatherley Designs Annas Palette charger in aqua green K
- Leotine Linens L

Page 155: Shrimp Taco Bowl
- Royale Limoges Recamerie Roseraie dinner plate K
- Anna Weatherley Designs, pink charger K

Pages 159-160: King Salmon
- Anna Weatherley Designs, hand painted in Hungary, exotic butterfly dinner and dessert plates K
- Anna Weatherley Designs, made in Portugal, Anna's Palette charger in green K

Page 164: Loup de Mer with Thai Chili Glaze Vinaigrette
- Saladmaster saute pan

Page 167: Roasted Ora King Salmon
- Arlberg platter and plates in the Wave pattern, color pearl P
- Garnier Thiesbaut fabric from France

Page 170: Sea Bass Veracruz with Wild Rice and Broccolini
- Hermès Mosaique Au24 square plates in platinum P

POULTRY

Pages 174-175: Herb Chicken with Calypso Beans
- Royal Crown Derby Ashbourne dinner plate K
- Herdmar silverware Vintage pattern in gold K

Page 176: Cornish Game Hens with Grilled Zucchini, Roasted Tomatoes, and Chimichurri
- Match tray K
- Osteia white tray K

Pages 179-180: Duck Breast with Spaghetti Squash, Olive Golden-Raisin Relish, and Spiced Yogurt

- Anna Weatherly Designs scalloped charger in indigo blue K
- Mottahedeh Chinoise blue dinner plate K
- Meissen No. 41 Noble blue dinner plate K

Page 183: Grilled Chicken Kebabs

- Victorian Royal Doulton Burslem antique pitcher marked Norfolk Road no 2516/2
- Beatrice Ball heart bowl K
- Schott Zwiesel hand blown martini glass

Page 186: CAV Pizza Three Ways

- Colonial Casting Company, Meridian, Conn. antique pewter dish

Page 190: Turkey Burgers on Homemade Wheat Buns

- Lifestyle wood cake stand in natural K

SIDES

Pages 194-199

Swiss Chard - Merci No. 7 deep plate in ocre/brown K

Spaghetti Squash - FMA dip bowl in poppy K

Parsnip Mash and Cipollini Onions - Merci No. 7 deep plate in blue/grey K

Celery Root Mash - Battuto bronze glaze cup K

Roasted Roots - Vietri Lastra condiment bowl in gray K

Carrot Sunchoke Hash - dip bowl in cobalt K

Black Barley - Vietri Lastra condiment bowl in aqua K

- Displayed on a Bar Keepers tray and Chilewich Bean table mat in azalea

SNACKS AND SMOOTHIES

Pages 206-207: Red Pepper Hummus, Carrot Hummus, and Traditional Hummus with Baked Pita Chips

- Deborah Rhodes Grass Patchwork Daisy placemat K
- Juliska Quinta Hugo pinch bowls and tray K

Page 209: CAV popcorn

- Haviland Limoges Sheraton K

Pages 214-216: Hot Salsa, Medium Salsa, and Salsa Verde with Homemade Corn Chips

- Blue Pheasant Dinnolan Nolan pasta bowl in black and cream K
- Jan Barboglio Madre goblet, bowl with iron base and bowl K

BREADS AND BREAKFAST

Pages 220-222: Broccoli Frittata with Broccoli Balsamic Salad

- Jaune de Chrome porcelain tortoise dinner plate K

Page 224-226: Eggs Benedict Towers

- Arte Italica Merletto dinner plate in antique K
- Haviland & Co. Limoges

Page 230: Huevos Rancheros

- Jaune de Chrome Tango Spirale dinner plate K
- Artifact Trading Company placemat K

Page 234: Waffles with Strawberry Sauce and Maple Syrup

- Astier de Villatte Etoile dinner plate K

Page 236: Steel Cut Oatmeal with Fruit Compote

- Vine Gold by Royal Crown Derby coffee cup and saucer
- Sunny Vale by Castleton bowl and plate
- Chappel white and gold plates

Pages 239-243: Muffins

- Imperial Crown Austria china, Haviland & Co. 1890 Tuscan china England, Royal Tuscan, Duchess Fox Hunt

DESSERTS

Page 248: Cal-a-Vie Carrot Cake with Lemon Curd

- Allison Evans ceramics plate K

Page 253: Vanilla Cheesecake with Berry Compote

- Bangle Design napkin ring K
- Mottahedeh Lace service plate in pink K
- Anna Weatherley Designs pink charger K
- Deborah Rhodes of New York two-tone Indonesian placemat K
- Antique pink pitcher marked "John and June Thompson married September 30, 1854"

Page 254: Vanilla Panna Cotta with Citrus Gelée

- Neiman Marcus Mardis Gras design plates
- Herdmar gold spoon K
- Minton Gilman Collamore Co. antique plate
- SFerra cocktail napkin K
- Herend china Gwendolyn charger K
- William Yeoward yellow martini crystal glass
- Deborah Rhodes Design napkin ring K

Page 257: Chocolate Torte

- Hermes H Deco plates K

Page 258: Chocolate Peanut Butter Cookies

- Osteir plate K

Page 260: Peach Blueberry Cobbler

- Royal Crown Derby Seasons Accent dinner plate in midwinter blue K
- Mottahedeh Lace service plate in plum K
- Vietri Lastra condiment cup in white K

Page 263: Pumpkin Coconut Pie

- Queen Victoria Herend dinner plate K
- Moser milk glass charger in Gigi in jade K
- Chappel blue plate K
- Reed & Barton Francis the First dessert fork K

Page 264: Strawberry Rhubarb Streusel

- Terrafina Ceramics Dot Poppy plate K
- Match silver charger in Gaelic pattern K
- Juliska ceramic scallop pasta white dish K
- Haviland & Co. antique china tea cup and saucer by Koch Braunstein

Page 267: Chocolate Mousse with Salted Almonds

- Royal Crown Derby Blue Camellias dinner plate K

Pages 269-273: Ice Cream and Sorbets

- Match Italian Pewter small ball spoon K
- MIY Cups K

OBSERVATORY

Cal-a-Vie guests can stargaze—literally—from our two-story observatory, which sits atop a remote hill overlooking the grounds. Taking it easy on one of the 26 chairs that came from the original Houston Astrodome, you can marvel at the wonders of space on either a state-of-the-art telescope or on eight large-screen television screens. It is truly a celestial experience that is at once calming and breathtaking.

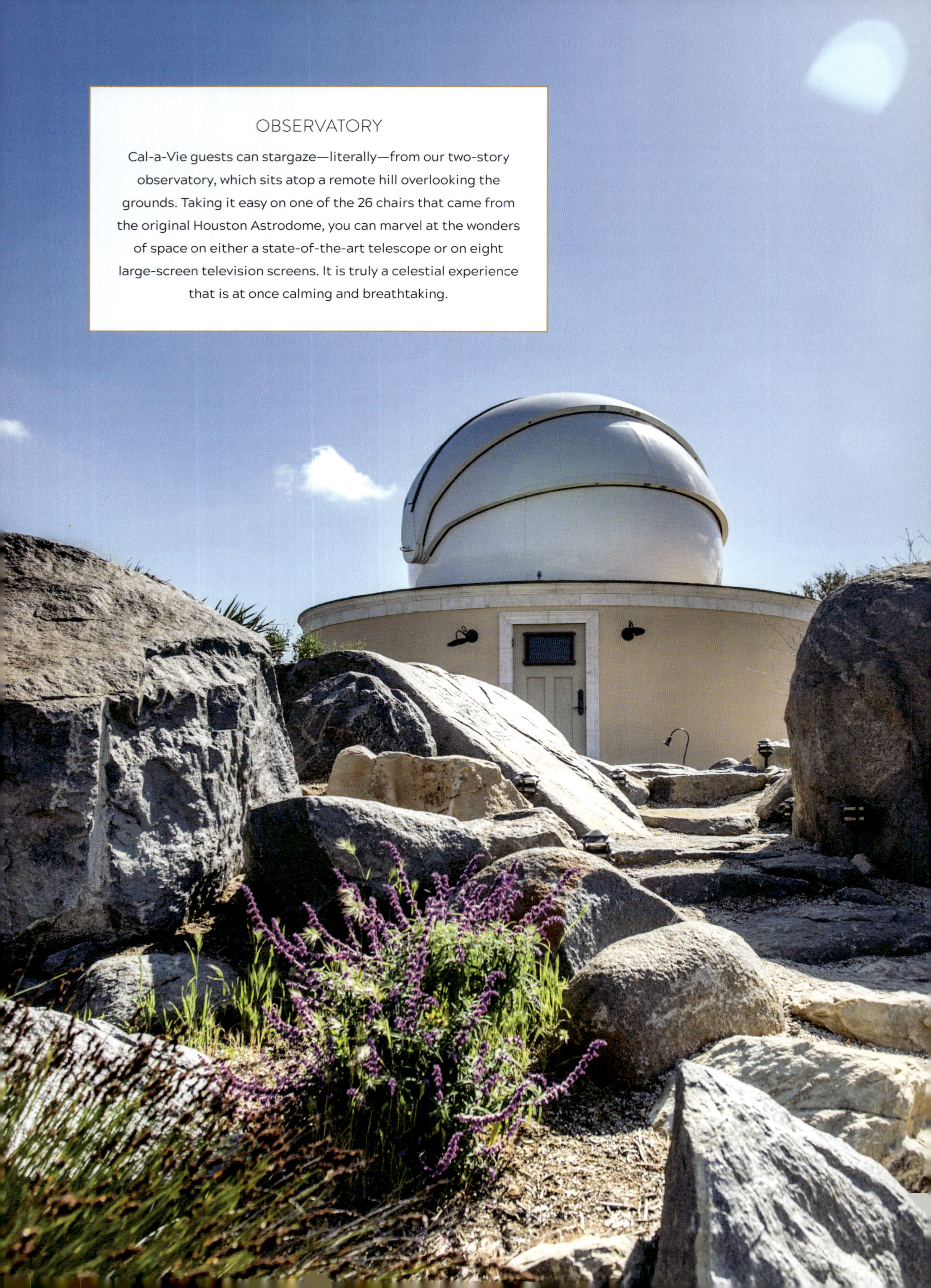

INDEX

A

Almond butter
  Banana Almond Smoothie, 203
  Coconut Almond Protein Bars, 218, *219*
Almond flour: Coconut Almond Protein Bars, 218, *219*
Almond milk
  Banana Almond Smoothie, 203
  Blackberry Lemon Smoothie, 202
  Peach Maple Smoothie, 203
Almonds
  Almond Coleslaw, 192
  Arugula with Strawberries and Vanilla Champagne Vinaigrette, 104, *105*
  Chocolate Mousse with Salted Almonds, *266*, 267
Ancho chili peppers: Romesco Sauce, 167
Appetizers
  Artichoke and Olive Tapenade, *88*, 89
  Baba Ganoush, 64, *64-65*
  Buffalo Cauliflower, 68, *68-69*
  Cashew-Stuffed Mushrooms, *66*, 67
  Caviar Salmon Cucumber Crudités, *60*, 60-61, *61*
  Poached Shrimp with Persimmon Salsa, 58, *59*
  Roasted Brussels Sprouts with Peanut Chili Vinaigrette, *70*, 71
  Tomato Broccoli Flatbread, *72-73*, 74
  Towers of Classic Meatballs with Marinara Sauce and Parmesan Polenta, 56-57
  Watermelon, Cucumber, and Tomato Skewers with Vanilla-Honey Gastrique, 78, *79*
Apples
  Apple Spice Muffins, 240
  Fennel, Carrot, Apple, and Bibb Lettuce Salad with Green Goddess Dressing, 102, *103*
  Kale Salad with Persian Cucumbers, Salted Pepitas, and Whole Grain Mustard Vinaigrette, 110, *111*
  Parsnip-Apple Soup, 94, *95*
Árbol chili peppers
  Hot Salsa, 216
  Huevos Rancheros, *229*, 230
Arrowhead Mills® flour: Lemon Squares with Whipped Coconut Cream, *250*, 251
Artichoke and Olive Tapenade, *88*, 89
Arugula
  Arugula with Strawberries and Vanilla Champagne Vinaigrette, 104, *105*
  Petite Arugula Salad with Pears and Candied Walnuts, *114*, 115
Asian Chicken Salad, *106*, 107
Asparagus, Lemon-Garlic Shrimp with Sautéed, *162-163*, 164
Avocado
  Chilled Avocado Soup with Roasted Corn Salsa, 80
  Petite Arugula Salad with Pears and Candied Walnuts, *114*, 115
  Texas Caviar, 120, *121*

B

Baba Ganoush, 64, *64-65*
Baked Pita Chips, 207
Baked Wonton Strips, 107
Balsamic Vinaigrette, 124
  Peach Salad with Spinach, Toasted Pecans, and White Balsamic Vinaigrette, *112*, 113
Balsamic vinegar
  Grapefruit Vinaigrette, 124
  Orange Vinaigrette, 125
  Peanut Chili Vinaigrette, 71
  Red Wine Honey Sauce, 140
  Roasted Beet Salad with Toasted Hazelnuts and Citrus Vinaigrette, 116, *117*
  Tomato Broccoli Flatbread, *72-73*, 74
  White Balsamic Vinaigrette, 124
Bamboo skewers
  Grilled Chicken Kebabs with Garlic Flatbread, Tzatziki Sauce, and Greek Salad, *182*, 183-185
  Watermelon Cucumber Tomato Skewers, 76, *77*
Banyuls Vinaigrette, 119
Barbecue Spiced Snack Nuts and Marinated Olives, *210*, 211

* *Italic* indicates photographs

Basil
  Basil Pesto, 135
  Green Curry Paste, 147
  Heirloom Tomato Provençal, 174
  Herb Mayonnaise, 192
  Marinara and Turkey Sausage Pizza, 189
  Marinara Sauce, 135
  Texas Caviar, 120, *121*
  Towers of Classic Meatballs with Marinara Sauce and Parmesan Polenta, 56-57
Basil Pesto, 135, 174
  Bison Lasagna Rolls with Basil Pesto and Toasted Garlic, *134*, 135
BBQ Chicken and Pesto Pizza, 188
Beans. *See* Black beans; Calypso beans; Garbanzo beans; Green beans
Beef. *See also* Ground beef
  Beef Tenderloin with Red Wine Demi-Glace Mashed Sweet Potatoes and Green Beans, 132-133
Beef stock: Red Wine Demi-Glace, 133
Beets, Roasted, Salad with Toasted Hazelnuts and Citrus Vinaigrette, 116, *117*
Bell peppers. *See* Green bell peppers; Red bell peppers; Yellow bell peppers
Beluga Lentil Ragu, 139
Beverages. *See* Smoothies
Bison Lasagna Rolls with Basil Pesto and Toasted Garlic, *134*, 135-136
Black Barley, 197
Black Beans, 156
Black-eyed peas
  Kale and Veggie Soup, 92, *93*
  Texas Caviar, 120, *121*
Blanched Carrots and Peas, 148
Bloody Mary Gazpacho, 84, *85*
Blue cheese: Buffalo Cauliflower, 68, *68-69*
Bolognese sauce: Bison Lasagna Rolls with Basil Pesto and Toasted Garlic, *134*, 135
Branzino, Seared, with Chanterelle Mushroom Puree and Roasted Brussels Sprouts, 152, *153*
Bread. *See* Flatbread; Muffins
Breakfast
  Apple Spice Muffins, 240
  Broccoli Frittata with Broccoli Balsamic Salad, *221*, 222-223
  Carrot Apple Muffins, 241
  Coconut Pistachio Muffins, 243
  Eggs Benedict Towers, *224*, 225-226
  Huevos Rancheros, *228-229*, 230
  Lemon Blueberry Muffins, 242
  Lemon Poppyseed Muffins, 242
  Macadamia Chocolate Muffins, 241
  Pancakes with Blueberry Compote, *231*, 232, *333*
  Steel-Cut Oatmeal with Fruit Compote, 236, *237*
  Strawberry Lemon Muffins, 243
  Waffles with Strawberry Sauce and Maple Syrup, 234, *235*
  Welcome Banana Muffins, *238*, 239
  Zucchini Muffins, 240
Breese, Drew, 17
Broccoli
  Broccoli Frittata with Broccoli Balsamic Salad, *221*, 222-223
  Broccoli Soup with Parmesan Crisps, *82*, 83
  Loup de Mer with Thai Chili Glaze Vinaigrette and Roasted Broccoli, 164, *165*
  Roasted Cherry Tomatoes and Broccoli, *72-73*, 74
  Broccolini, 170
  Frittata with Broccoli Balsamic Salad, *221*, 222-223
  Sea Bass Veracruz with Wild Rice, *169*, 170
Brown rice pasta: Bison Lasagna Rolls with Basil Pesto and Toasted Garlic, 136
Brussels sprouts
  Roasted Brussels Sprouts with Peanut Chili Vinaigrette, *70*, 71
  Seared Branzino with Chanterelle Mushroom Puree and Roasted Brussels Sprouts, 152, *153*
Buffalo Cauliflower, 68, *68-69*
Burgers, Turkey, on Homemade Wheat Buns with Sweet Potato Fries and Almond Coleslaw, 190, *191*, 192

Buttermilk
Avocado Soup, 80
Peach Blueberry Cobbler, 260, *261*
Butternut squash: Kale and Veggie Soup, 92, *93*

C

Cabbage
Almond Coleslaw, 192
Asian Chicken Salad, *106*, 107
Pork Tenderloin with Honey Mustard, Parsnip Mash, and Savoy Cabbage, 128, *129*
Cal-a-Vie Carrot Cake with Lemon Curd, 248, *249*
Cal-a-Vie Health Spa, 32
beauty treatments and spa therapies at, 45
cooking philosophy at, 20-23
dining room at, *17*
Dirty Dozen and, 276
dream weddings at, 46, *47, 48, 49, 50*
encouragement of seafood in diet, 280
end of stay at, 51-52
fitness at, 42, *43, 44*
French Chapel at, 34, *34*
general philosophy at, 28
maintaining passion for life at, 31
making decisions on, 12, 14, 17
nutritionists at, 24, 26
oils recommended by, 278-279
orange grove thank you for guests at, 284
staff at, *29*
wine at, 37, 38, *38, 39, 40, 41, 42*
Cal-a-Vie Pizza Three Ways, 186, *187*
Cal-a-Vie Popcorn, *208*, 209
Cal-a-Vie Traditional Hummus, 206
Calypso Beans, 174
Candied Walnuts, 115
Cantaloupe: Melon Sorbet, 271
Capers
Caviar Salmon Cucumber Crudités, *60*, 60-61, *61*
Veracruz Sauce, 170
Carrots
Almond Coleslaw, 192
Asian Chicken Salad, *106*, 107
Blanched Carrots and Peas, 148
Bolognese Sauce, 135
Carrot Apple Muffins, 241
Carrot Coconut Soup, 86, *86-87*
Carrot Hummus, 206
Carrot Sunchoke Hash, 197
Fennel, Carrot, Apple, and Bibb Lettuce Salad with Green Goddess Dressing, 102, *103*
Kale and Veggie Soup, 92, *93*
Red Wine Demi-Glace, 133
Roasted Roots, 196
Cashews
Asian Chicken Salad, *106*, 107
Cashew-Stuffed Mushrooms, *66*, 67
Fennel, Carrot, Apple, and Bibb Lettuce Salad with Green Goddess Dressing, 102
Green Goddess Dressing, 102
Cauliflower
Buffalo Cauliflower, 68, *68-69*
Roasted Cauliflower Soup with Curry Oil, *96-97*, 98
Caviar, grades of, 61
Caviar Salmon Cucumber Crudités, *60*, 60-61, *61*
Celery
Broccoli Soup with Parmesan Crisps, *82*, 83
Buffalo Cauliflower, 68, *68-69*
Celery Root Mash, 196
Red Wine Demi-Glace, 133
Champagne Vinaigrette, 124
Champagne vinegar
Champagne Vinaigrette, 124
Kalamata Oil Vinaigrette, 125
Cheese. *See* Blue cheese; Goat cheese; Manchego cheese; Mozzarella cheese; Parmesan cheese; Ricotta
Cherry tomatoes. *See also* Roma tomatoes; Tomatoes
Arugula with Strawberries and Vanilla Champagne Vinaigrette, 104, *105*
Green and Yellow Bean Salad with Heirloom Tomatoes, Olive Tapenade, and Grapefruit Vinaigrette, *108*, 109
Roasted Cherry Tomatoes and Broccoli, *72-73*, 74
Roasted Tomatoes, 176
Watermelon, Cucumber and Tomato Skewers with Vanilla-Honey Gastrique, 76, *77*
Chicken
Asian Chicken Salad, *106*, 107
BBQ Chicken and Pesto Pizza, 188
Grilled Chicken Kebabs with Garlic Flatbread, Tzatziki Sauce, and Greek Salad, *182*, 183-185
Herb Chicken with Heirloom Tomato Provençal Zucchini Noodles, and Calaypso Beans, *172-173*, 174-175
Chicken stock
Green Curry Paste, 147
Kale and Veggie Soup, 92, *93*
Parmesan Polenta, 145
Towers of Classic Meatballs with Marinara Sauce and Parmesan Polenta, 56-57
Chili-Lime Vinaigrette, 107, 125
Chili paste, 179
Chilled Avocado Soup with Roasted Corn Salsa, *79*, 80
Chimichurri Sauce, 176
Chocolate
Chocolate Ice Cream, 270
Chocolate Mousse with Salted Almonds, *266*, 267
Chocolate Peanut Butter Cookies, 258, *259*
Chocolate Torte, *256*, 257
Macadamia Chocolate Muffins, 241
Cipollini Onions, 198
Citrus Vinaigrette, 116
Almond Coleslaw, 112
Coconut
Coconut Almond Protein Bars, 218, *219*
Coconut Cilantro Rice, 147
Coconut Macaroon, 246
Coconut Pistachio Muffins, 243
Coconut Vanilla Bean Ice Cream, 270
Coconut cream: Lemon Squares with Whipped Coconut Cream, *250*, 251
Coconut milk
Carrot Coconut Soup, 86, *87*
Coconut Vanilla Bean Ice cream, 270
Green Smoothie, 202
Lemon Blueberry Muffins, 242
Lobster Curry, 148
Pineapple Coconut Smoothie, 202
Pumpkin Coconut Pie with Whipped Coconut Cream, *262*, 263
Coconut oil: Lemon Squares with Whipped Coconut Cream, *250*, 251
Coconut yogurt
Lemon Blueberry Muffins, 242
Macadamia Chocolate Muffins, 241
Cooke, Curtis, *21*
Cooking, Philosophy of, 20-23
Corn
Roasted Corn Salsa, 80
Skillet Zucchini and Corn, 167
Cornish Game Hens with Grilled Zucchini, Roasted Tomatoes and Chimichurri, 176, *177*
Cranberries: Coconut Almond Protein Bars, 218, *219*
Cream cheese: Vanilla Cheesecake with Berny Compote, 253
Crispy Tortillas, 155
Cucumbers
Bloody Mary Gazpacho, 84, *85*
Caviar Salmon Cucumber Crudités, *60*, 60-61, *61*
Cirpollini Cucumber Salsa, 84
Kale Salad with Persian Cucumbers, Salted Pepitas, and Whole Grain Mustard Vinaigrette, 110, *111*
Watermelon Cucumber Tomato Skewers, 76, *77*
Curry Oil, 98

D

Desserts
Cal-a-Vie Carrot Cake with Lemon Curd, 248, *249*
Chocolate Ice Cream, 270
Chocolate Mousse with Salted Almonds, *266,* 267
Chocolate Peanut Butter Cookies, 258, *259*
Chocolate Torte, *256,* 257
Coconut Macaroon, 246
Coconut Vanilla Bean Ice Cream, 270
Green Tea Ice Cream, 271
Lemon Squares with Whipped Coconut Cream, *250,* 251
Melon Sorbet, 271
Meyer Lemon Sorbet, 272
Peach Blueberry Cobbler, 260, *261*
Peanut Butter Ice Cream, 272
Pistachio Ice Cream, 273
Pumpkin Coconut Pie with Whipped Coconut Cream, *262,* 263
Strawberry Rhubarb Streusel, 264, *265*
Strawberry Sorbet, 271
Vanilla Cheesecake with Berry Compote, 252, 253
Vanilla Ice Cream, 273
Vanilla Panna Cotta with Citrus Gelée, 254, *255*
Dirty dozen, 276
Duck Breast with Spaghetti Squash, Olive, Golden-Raisin Relish and Spiced Yogurt, *178,* 179-181

E

Eggplant: Baba Ganoush, 64, *64-65*
Eggs
Broccoli Frittata with Broccoli Balsamic Salad, *221,* 222-223
Eggs Benedict Towers, *224,* 225-226
hard-boiled
Caviar Salmon Cucumber Crudités, *60,* 60-61, *61*
Huevos Rancheros, *228-229,* 230
Pancakes with Blueberry Compote, 232, *233*
Waffles with Strawberry Sauce and Maple Syrup, 234, *235*
English peas: Sautéed Peas, 142
Entrees
BBQ Chicken and Pesto Pizza, 188
Beef Tenderloin with Red Wine Demi-Glace Mashed Sweet Potatoes and Green Beans, 132-133
Bison Lasagna Rolls with Basil Pesto and Toasted Garlic, *134,* 135-136
Cal-a-Vie Pizza Three Ways, 186, *187*
Cornish Game Hens with Grilled Zucchini, Roasted Tomatoes and Chimichurri, 176, *177*
Duck Breast with Spaghetti Squash, Olive Golden-Raisin Relish and Spiced Yogurt, *178,* 179-181
Garlic and Mushroom Pizza, 189
Grilled Chicken Kebabs with Garlic Flatbread, Tzatziki Sauce, and Greek Salad, *182,* 183-185
Herb Chicken with Heirloom Tomato Provençal Zucchini Noodles, and Calaypso Beans, *172-173,* 174-175
Herb Shrimp with Puttanesca Sauce, Parmesan Polenta, and Swiss Chard, *144,* 145
King Salmon with Honey Sesame Glaze, Soba Noodles, and Green Beans, *158,* 159-160
Lemon-Garlic Shrimp with Sautéed Asparagus, 163, *163*
Lobster Curry with Baby Carrots, Beech Mushrooms, Snap Peas, and Coconut Cilantro Rice, 147-148
Loup de Mer with Thai Chili Glaze Vinaigrette and Roasted Broccoli, 164, *165*
Marinara and Turkey Sausage Pizza, 189
Pork Tenderloin with Honey Mustard, Parsnip Mash and Savoy Cabbage, 128
Roasted Lamb Loin Chops with Beluga Lentil Ragu and King Trumpet Mushrooms, *138,* 139-140
Roasted Ora King Salmon with Romesco Sauce, Skillet Zucchini and Corn, *166,* 167
Roasted Rack of Lamb with Sautéed Peas and Piperade Sauce, 142, *143*
Sea Bass Veracruz with Wild Rice and Broccolini, *169,* 170
Seared Branzino with Chanterelle Mushroom Puree and Roasted Brussels Sprouts, *150-151,* 152
Shrimp Taco Bowl, *154,* 155-156
Turkey Burgers on Homemade Wheat Buns with Sweet Potato Fries and Almond Coleslaw, 190, *191,* 192
Espelette aioli: Poached Shrimp with Persimmon Salsa and Aioli in Endive Boats, 58, *59*

F

Farm to table philosophy, 20
Fennel, Carrot, Apple, and Bibb Lettuce Salad with Green Goddess Dressing, 102, *103*
Fish and seafood
Herb Shrimp with Puttanesca Sauce, Parmesan Polenta, and Swiss Chard, *144,* 145
King Salmon with Honey Sesame Glaze, Soba Noodles, and Green Beans, *158,* 159-160
Lemon-Garlic Shrimp with Sautéed Asparagus, 163, *163*
Lobster Curry with Baby Carrots, Beech Mushrooms, Snap Peas, and Coconut Cilantro Rice, 147-148
Loup de Mer with Thai Chili Glaze Vinaigrette and Roasted Broccoli, 164, *165*
mercury in, 280
Roasted Ora King Salmon with Romesco Sauce, Skillet Zucchini and Corn, *166,* 167
Sea Bass Veracruz with Wild Rice and Broccolini, *169,* 170
Seared Branzino with Chanterelle Mushroom Puree and Roasted Brussels Sprouts, *150-151,* 152
Shrimp Taco Bowl, *154,* 155-156
Flatbread
Garlic Flatbread, 183
Grilled Garlic Flatbread, 185
Tomato Broccoli Flatbread, *72-73,* 74
Flour. *See* Almond flour; Arrowhead Mills® Flour; Gluten free flour; High gluten fiber; Whole wheat pastry flour

G

Garbanzo beans
Cal-a-Vie Traditional Hummus, 206
Greek Salad, 184
Red Pepper Hummus, 207
Garden Pumpkin Soup with Goat Cheese Crema and Salted Pepitas, 88, *89*
Garlic and Mushroom Pizza, 189
Garlic Flatbread
Grilled Chicken Kebabs with Garlic Flatbread, Tzatziki Sauce, and Greek Salad, *182,* 183-185
Gastriques
Maple Gastrique, 113
Vanilla-Honey Gastrique, 76, *77*
Gazpacho, Bloody Mary, 84, *85*
Glazes, Honey Sesame, 160
Gluten free flour
Apple Spice Muffins, 240
Cal-a-Vie Carrot Cake with Lemon Curd, 248, *248-249*
Carrot Apple Muffins, 241
Chocolate Peanut Butter Cookies, 258, *259*
Chocolate Torte, *256,* 257
Coconut Pistachio Muffins, 243
Lemon Blueberry Muffins, 242
Lemon Poppyseed Muffins, 242
Macadamia Chocolate Muffins, 241
Pancakes with Blueberry Compote, 232, *233*
Strawberry Lemon Muffins, 243
Welcome Banana Muffins, *238,* 239
Zucchini Muffins, 240
Gluten free pizza crusts
Tomato Broccoli Flatbread, *72-73,* 74
Goat cheese
Arugula with Strawberries and Vanilla Champagne Vinaigrette, 104, *105*
Goat Cheese Crema, 88
Peach Salad with Spinach, Toasted Pecans, and White Balsamic Vinaigrette, *112,* 113
Roasted Beet Salad with Toasted Hazelnuts and Citrus Vinaigrett, 116, *117*
Golden Lentil Soup, *90,* 91

Golden raisins
Balsamic Broccoli Salad, 222
Olive Golden-Raisin Relish, 179
Olive-, Relish, 179
Grapefruit Vinaigrette, 124
Grapes, Spiced Poached Pear with Mixed Greens, and Hazelnuts, *118,* 119
Greek Salad, 184
Greek yogurt
Lemon Poppyseed Muffins, 242
Strawberry Lemon Muffins, 243
Green beans
Beef Tenderloin with Red Wine Demi-Glace, Mashed Sweet Potatoes, and Green Beans, 132, *133*
Green and Yellow Bean Salad with Heirloom Tomatoes, Olive Tapenade and Grapefruit Vinaigrette, *108,* 109
Green and Yellow Bean Salad with Heirloom Tomatoes, Olive Tapenade, and Grapefruit Vinaigrette, *108,* 109
King Salmon with Honey Sesame Glaze, Soba Noodles, and Green Beans, *158-159,* 159-160
Green bell pepper: Bloody Mary Gazpacho, 84, *85*
Green Curry Paste, 147
Green Goddess Dressing, 102
Green onions: Asian Chicken Salad, *106,* 107
Green Tea Ice Cream, 271
Grilled Chicken Kebabs with Garlic Flatbread, Tzatziki Sauce, and Greek Salad, *182,* 183-185
Grilled Garlic Flatbread, 185
Grilled Peaches, 113
Ground beef: Towers of Classic Meatballs with Marinara Sauce and Parmesan Polenta, 56-57

H

Haricot verts. *See* Green beans
Havens, John, 2, *4,* 5, 9, 12
Havens, Terri, 2, *4,* 5, 12
Hazelnuts
Roasted Beet Salad with Toasted Hazelnuts and Citrus Vinaigrette, 116, *117*
Spiced Poached Pear with Mixed Greens, Grapes, and Hazelnuts, *118,* 119
Heirloom Tomato Provençal, 174
Herb Chicken with Heirloom Tomato Provençal Zucchini Noodles, and Calaypso Beans, *172-173,* 174-175
Herb Mayonnaise, 192
Herb Ricotta, 136
Herb Shrimp with Puttanesca Sauce, Parmesan Polenta, and Swiss Chard, *144,* 145
High gluten flour
Cal-a-Vie Pizza Three Ways, 186, *187*
Grilled Chicken Kebabs with Garlic Flatbread, Tzatziki Sauce, and Greek Salad, *182,* 183-185
Turkey Burgers on Homemade Wheat Buns with Sweet Potato Fries and Almond Coleslaw, 190, *191,* 192
Honey mustard, 128
Honey Sesame Glaze, 160
Hot Salsa, 216
Huevos Rancheros, *228-229,* 230

J

Jalapeño
Chili-Lime Vinaigrette, 107
Golden Lentil Soup, *90,* 91
Jalapeño Vinaigrette, 125
Pico de Gallo, 155
Roasted Corn Salsa, 80

K

Kalamata Olive Vinaigrette, 125
Kale
Green Smoothie, 202
Kale and Veggie Soup, 92, *93*
Kale Salad with Persian Cucumbers, Salted Pepitas, and Whole Grain Mustard Vinaigrette, 110, *111*
Kebabs
Grilled Chicken Kebabs with Garlic Flatbread, Tzatziki Sauce, and Greek Salad, *182,* 183-185
Watermelon Cucumber Tomato Skewers, 76, *77*
King Salmon with Honey Sesame Glaze, Soba Noodles, and Green Beans, *158,* 159-160
King Trumpet Mushrooms, 140

L

Lamb
Roasted Lamb Loin Chops with Beluga Lentil Ragu and King Trumpet Mushrooms, *138,* 139-140
Roasted Rack of Lamb with Sautéed Peas and Piperade Sauce, 142, *143*
Lemon
Lemon Blueberry Muffins, 242
Lemon-Garlic Shrimp with Sautéed Asparagus, 163, *163*
Lemon-Lime Vinaigrette, 155
Lemon Poppyseed Muffins, 242
Lemon Squares with Whipped Coconut Cream, *250,* 251
Lemongrass: Carrot Coconut Soup, 86, *87*
Lentils
Golden Lentil Soup, *90,* 91
Roasted Lamb Loin Chops with Beluga Lentil Ragu and King Trumpet Mushrooms, *138,* 139
Lettuce. *See also* Arugula; Mixed greens
Fennel, Carrot, Apple, and Bibb Lettuce Salad with Green Goddess Dressing, 102, *103*
Shrimp Taco Bowl, *154,* 155-156
Lime
Asian Chicken Salad, *106,* 107
Bloody Mary Gazpacho, 84
Chile-Lime Vinaigrette, 125
Jalapeño Vinaigette, 125
Lobster Curry with Baby Carrots, Beech Mushrooms, Snap Peas, and Coconut Cilantro Rice, *146,* 147
Loup de Mer with Thai Chili Glaze Vinaigrette and Roasted Broccoli, 164, *165*
Roasted Corn Salsa, 80
Shrimp Taco Bowl, *154,* 155
Lime salt, 84
Limes: Green Curry Paste, 147
Lobster Curry with Baby Carrots, Beech Mushrooms, Snap Peas, and Coconut Cilantro Rice, 147-148
Loup de Mer with Thai Chili Glaze Vinaigrette and Roasted Broccoli, 164, *165*

M

Macadamia Chocolate Muffins, 241
Manchego cheese: Kale Salad with Persian Cucumbers, Salted Pepitas, and Whole Grain Mustard Vinaigrette, 110, *111*
Maple gastrique, 113
Marinara and Turkey Sausage Pizza, 189
Marinara Sauce
Bison Lasagna Rolls with Basil Pesto and Toasted Garlic, *134,* 135
Marinara and Turkey Sausage Pizza, 189
Towers of Classic Meatballs with Marinara Sauce and Parmesan Polenta, 56-57
Marinated Olives, 212
Massages, 9
Mayonnaise, herb, 192
Medium Salsa, 216
Melon Sorbet, 271
Mercury in fish, 280
Meyer Lemon Sorbet, 272
Milk. *See also* Almond milk; Buttermilk; Coconut milk; Soy milk
Waffles with Strawberry Sauce and Maple Syrup, 234, *235*
Mixed greens
Roasted Beet Salad with Toasted Hazelnuts and Citrus Vinaigrette, 116, *117*
Spiced Poached Pear with Mixed Greens, Grapes, and Hazelnuts, *118,* 119
Mozzarella cheese: BBQ Chicken and Pesto Pizza, 188

Muffins
Apple Spice Muffins, 240
Carrot Apple Muffins, 241
Coconut Pistachio Muffins, 243
Lemon Blueberry Muffins, 242
Lemon Poppyseed Muffins, 242
Macadamia Chocolate Muffins, 241
Strawberry Lemon Muffins, 243
Welcome Banana Muffins, *238,* 239
Zucchini Muffins, 240
Mushrooms
Cashew-Stuffed Mushrooms, *66,* 67
Chanterelle Mushroom Puree, 152
Garlic and Mushroom Pizza, 189
Lobster Curry with Baby Carrots, Beech Mushrooms, Snap Peas, and Coconut Cilantro Rice, *146,* 147
Roasted Lamb Loin Chops with Beluga Lentil Ragu and King Trumpet Mushrooms, *138,* 139
Mustard, honey, 128

N

Nutritionist yeast: Cashew Cream, 67
Nuts. *See* Almonds; Cashews; Pecans; Pine nuts; Pistachios; Walnuts

O

Oats
Steel-Cut Oatmeal with Fruit Compote, 236, *237*
Strawberry Rhubarb Streusel, 264, *265*
Olives
Green and Yellow Bean Salad with Heirloom Tomatoes, Olive Tapenade, and Grapefruit Vinaigrette, *108,* 109
Kalamata Oil Vinaigrette, 125
Olive Golden-Raisin Relish, 179
Olive Tapenade, 63
Veracruz Sauce, 170
Onions. *See also* Green onions; Pearl onions; Red onions
Beef Tenderloin with Red Wine Demi, Mashed Sweet Potatoes, and Green Beans, *130-131,* 132-133
Bison Lasagna Rolls with Basil Pesto and Toasted Garlic, *134,* 135
Cipollini Onions, 198
Golden Lentil Soup, *90,* 91
Orange Vinaigrette, 115, 125

P

Pancakes with Blueberry Compote, *231,* 232, *333*
Parmesan cheese
BBQ Chicken and Pesto Pizza, 188
Broccoli Soup with Parmesan Crisps, *82,* 83
Green and Yellow Bean Salad with Heirloom Tomatoes, Olive Tapenade, and Grapefruit Vinaigrette, *108,* 109
Parmesan Polenta, 145
Parsnips
Parsnip-Apple Soup, 94, *95*
Parsnip Mash, 128, 198
Pork Tenderloin with Honey Mustard, Parsnip Mash, and Savoy Cabbage, 128, *129*
Roasted Roots, 196
Pasta: Bison Lasagna Rolls with Basil Pesto and Toasted Garlic, 136
Peaches
Peach Blueberry Cobbler, 260, *261*
Peach Salad with Spinach, Toasted Pecans, and White Balsamic Vinaigrette, *112,* 113
Peanuts
Peanut Butter Ice Cream, 272
Peanut Chili Vinaigrette, 71
Roasted Brussels Sprouts with Peanut Chili Vinaigrette, 71
Pearl onions: Carrot Sunchoke Hash, 197
Pears
Petite Arugula Salad with Pears and Candied Walnuts, *114,* 115
Spiced Poached Pear with Mixed Greens, Grapes, and Hazelnuts, *118,* 119
Peas. *See* Black-eyed peas; Snap peas
Pecans, Peach Salad with Spinach, Toasted, and White Balsamic Vinaigrette, *112,* 113
Pepitas, Salted, 88, 110
Peppercorn: Poached Bosc Pears, 119
Pepperoncinis: Grilled Chicken Kebabs with Garlic Flatbread, Tzatziki Sauce and Greek Salad, *182,* 183-185, *179*
Peppers. *See* Arbol chili peppers; Bell peppers; Jalapeño, Arbol chili peppers; Thai chile peppers
Pesto
Basil Pesto, 135, 174
Jalapeño Pesto, 188
Petite Arugula Salad with Pears and Candied Walnuts, *114,* 115
Pickled Shallots, 104
Pico de Gallo, 155
Pine nuts
Basil Pesto, 174
Olive Golden-Raisin Relish, 179
Piperada Sauce, 142
Pistachios
Coconut Pistachio Muffins, 243
Pistachio Ice Cream, 273
Pizza
BBQ Chicken and Pesto Pizza, 188
Cal-a-Vie Pizza Three Ways, 186, *187*
Garlic and Mushroom Pizza, 189
Marinara and Turkey Sausage Pizza, 189
Pizza crusts: Roasted Cherry Tomatoes and Broccoli, *72-73,* 74
Pizza Dough, 186
Poached Globe Artichoke Hearts, 63
Poached Shrimp with Persimmon Salsa, 58, *59*
Polenta
Parmesan Polenta, 145
Towers of Classic Meatballs with Marinara Sauce and Parmesan Polenta, 56-57
Porcini Stock, 139
Pork Tenderloin with Honey Mustard, Parsnip Mash, and Savoy Cabbage, 128
Poultry. *See* Chicken; Cornish game hens; Duck; Turkey
Protein powder
Blackberry Lemon Smoothie, 202
Coconut Almond Protein Bars, 218, *219*
Green Tea Mango Smoothie, 203
Peach Maple Smoothie, 203
Pineapple Coconut Smoothie, 202
Pumpkin
Garden Pumpkin Soup with Goat Cheese Crema and Salted Pepitas, 88, *89*
Pumpkin Coconut Pie with Whipped Coconut Cream, *262,* 263
Puttanesca Sauce, 145

R

Raisins. *See* Golden raisins
Red bell peppers
Grilled Chicken Kebabs with Garlic Flatbread, Tzatziki Sauce, and Greek Salad, *182,* 183-185
Piperada Saucer, 142
Roasted Red Bell Pepper, 63
Romesco Sauce, 167
Red onions
Greek Salad, 184
Grilled Chicken Kebabs with Garlic Flatbread, Tzatziki Sauce, and Greek Salad, *182,* 183-185
Grilled Chicken Kebabs with Garlic Flatbread, Tzatziki Sauce, and Greek Salad, *182,* 183-185
Sautéed Red Onions, 192
Red Pepper Hummus, 207
Red wine
Beef Tenderloin with Red Wine Demi-Glace, Mashed Sweet Potatoes, and Green Beans, *130-131,* 132-133
Beluga Lentil Ragu, 139
Marinara Sauce, 56, 135, 189
Red Wine Demi-Glace, 133
Red Wine Honey Sauce, 140

Roasted Lamb Loin Chops with Beluga Lentil Ragu and King Trumpet Mushrooms, *138,* 139
Spiced Poached Pear with Mixed Greens, Grapes, and Hazelnuts, *118,* 119
Relish, Olive-Golden Raisin, 179
Revitalizer, 213
Rice
Coconut Cilantro Rice, 147
Sea Bass Veracruz with Wild Rice and Broccoli, *169,* 170
Spanish, 156
Wild, 170
Ricotta
Herb Ricotta, 136
Roasted Cherry Tomatoes and Broccoli, *72-73, 74*
Strawberry Lemon Muffins, 243
Roasted Beet Salad with Toasted Hazelnuts and Citrus Vinaigrette, 116, *117*
Roasted Brussels Sprouts with Peanut Chili Vinaigrette, *70,* 71
Roasted Cauliflower Soup with Curry Oil, *96-97,* 98
Roasted Corn Salsa, 80
Roasted Lamb Loin Chops with Beluga Lentil Ragu and King Trumpet Mushrooms, *138,* 139-140
Roasted Ora King Salmon with Romesco Sauce, Skillet Zucchini and Corn, *166,* 167
Roasted Rack of Lamb with Sautéed Peas and Piperade Sauce, 142, *143*
Roasted Roots, 196
Roasted Tomatoes, 176
Roma tomatoes. *See also* Cherry tomatoes; Tomatoes
Persimmon Salsa, 58
Piperada Sauce, 142
Romesco Sauce, 167

S

Salad dressings. *See also* Vinaigrettes
Green Goddess Dressing, 102
Salads
Arugula with Strawberries and Vanilla Champagne Vinaigrette, 104, *105*
Asian Chicken Salad, *106,* 107
Fennel, Carrot, Apple, and Bibb Lettuce Salad with Green Goddess Dressage, 102, *103*
Greek Salad, 184
Green and Yellow Bean Salad with Heirloom Tomatoes, Olive Tapenade and Grapefruit Vinaigrette, *108,* 109
Kale Salad with Persian Cucumbers, Salted Pepitas, and Whole Grain Mustard Vinaigrette, 110, *111*
Peace Salad with Spinach, Toasted Pecans, and White Balsamic Vinaigrette, *112,* 113
Petite Arugula Salad with Pears and Candied Walnuts, *114,* 115
Roasted Beet Salad with Toasted Hazelnuts and Citrus Vinaigrette, 116, *117*
Spiced Poached Pear with Mixed Greens, Grapes, and Hazelnuts, *118,* 119
Texas Caviar, 120, *120-121*
Salmon
Caviar Salmon Cucumber Crudités, *60,* 60-61, *61*
King Salmon with Honey Sesame Glaze, Soba Noodles, and Green Beans, *158, 158-159,* 159-160
Roasted Ora King Salmon with Romesco Sauce, Skillet Zucchini and Corn, *166,* 167
Salsa
Cirpollini Cucumber Salsa, 84
Poached Shrimp with Persimmon Salsa and Aioli in Endive Boats, 58, *59*
Roasted Corn Salsa, 80
Roasted Tomatillos Salsa, 214
Salso Verde, 152
Seared Branzino with Chanterelle Mushroom Puree and Roasted Brussels Sprouts, 152, *153*
Salted Pepitas, 88, 110
Sauces
BBQ Sauce, 188
Bolognese sauce, 135
Chimichurri Sauce, 176
Heirloom Tomato Provençal, 174
Bison Lasagna Rolls with Basil Pesto and Toasted Garlic, *134,* 135
Marinara and Turkey Sausage Pizza, 189
Towers of Classic Meatballs with Marinara Sauce and Parmesan Polenta, 56-57
Piperada Saucee, 142
Puttanesca Sauce, 145
Red Wine Honey Sauce, 140
Romesco Sauce, 167
Sweet and Sour Sauce, 159
Tzatsiki Sauce, 184
Veracruz Sauce, 170
Sautéed Peas, 142
Seafood. *See* Fish and seafood
Seared Branzino with Chanterelle Mushroom Puree and Roasted Brussels Sprouts, *150-151,* 152
Shallots: Arugula with Strawberries and Vanilla Champagne Vinaigrette, 104, *105*
Sherry vinegar: Peach Salad with Spinach, Toasted Pecans, and White Balsamic Vinegar, *112,* 113
Shrimp
buying, 163
Herb Shrimp with Puttanesca Sauce, Parmesan Polenta, and Swiss Chard, *144,* 145
Lemon-Garlic Shrimp with Sautéed Asparagus, 163, *163*
Poached Shrimp with Persimmon Salsa and Aioli in Endive Boats, 58, *59*
Shrimp Taco Bowl, *154,* 155-156
Sides
Carrot Sunchoke Hash, 197
Cherry Root Mash, 196
Parsnip Mash and Cipollini Onions, 198
Roasted Roots, 196
Spaghetti Squash, 199
Swiss Chard, 199
Slaw: Almond Coleslaw, 192
Smoothies
Banana Almond Smoothie, 203
Blackberry Lemon Smoothie, 202
Green Smoothie, 202
Green Tea Mango Smoothie, 203
Peach Maple Smooths, 203
Pineapple Coconut Smoothie, 202
Strawberry Banana Smoothie, 203
Snacks
Baked Pita Chips, 207
Barbecue Spiced Snack Nuts and Marinated Olives, *210,* 211
Cal-a-Vie Popcorn, *208,* 209
Cal-a-Vie Traditional Hummus, 206
Carrot Hummus, 206
Coconut Almond Protein Bars, 218, *219*
Hot Salsa, 216
Marinated Olives, 212
Medium Salsa, 216
Red Pepper Hummus, 207
Revitalizer, 213
Snap peas
Blanched Carrots and Peas, 148
Sautéed Peas, 142
Soba noodles, 160
Soups
Bloody Mary Gazpacho, 84, *85*
Broccoli Soup with Parmesan Crisps, *82,* 83
Carrot Coconut Soup, 86, *86-87*
Chilled Avocado Soup with Roasted Corn Salsa, *79,* 80
Garden Pumpkin Soup with Goat Cheese Crema and Salted Pepitas, 88, *89*
Golden Lentil Soup, *90,* 91
Kale and Veggie Soup, 92, *93*
Parsnip-Apple Soup, 94, *95*
Roasted Cauliflower Soup with Curry Oil, *96-97,* 98
Sour cream: Lemon Blueberry Muffins, 242
Soy milk
Apple Spice Muffins, 240
Green Tea Ice Cream, 271
Green Tea Mango Smoothie, 203
Pancakes with Blueberry Compote, 232, *233*

Peanut Butter Ice Cream, 272
Pistachio Ice Cream, 273
Vanilla Ice Cream, 273
Zucchini Muffins, 240
Spaghetti Squash, 180, 199
Spanish Rice, 156
Spiced Poached Pear with Mixed Greens, Grapes, and Hazelnuts, *118,* 119
Spiced Yogurt, 179
Spinach
Blackberry Lemon Smoothie, 202
Peach Salad with, Toasted Pecans, and White Balsamic Vinaigrette, *112,* 113
Sautéed Spinach, 225
Squash. *See* Butternut squash; Spaghetti squash
Star anise pods: Poached Bosc Pears, 119
Steel-Cut Oatmeal with Fruit Compote, 236, *237*
Stock. *See* Beef stock; Beef stock, Chicken stock; Chicken stock; Porcine stock; Veal stock; Vegetable stock
Strawberries
Arugula with Strawberries and Vanilla Champagne Vinaigrette, 104, *105*
Strawberry Lemon Muffins, 243
Strawberry Rhubarb Streusel, 264, *265*
Strawberry Sorbet, 271
Sunchoke, Carrot, Hash, 197
Sweet and Sour Sauce
King Salmon with Honey Sesame Glaze, Soba Noodles, and Green Beans, *158-159,* 159-160
Sweet potatoes
Beef Tenderloin with Red Wine Demi-Glace, Mashed Sweet Potatoes, and Green Beans, 132, *133*
Roasted Roots, 196
Roasted Sweet Potato Hash, 225
Sweet Potato Fries, 192
Swiss Chard, 145, 199

T

Tamari sauce: King Salmon with Honey Sesame Glaze, Soba Noodles, and Green Beans, *158,* 159
Tasari sauce: Asian Chicken Salad, *106,* 107
Texas Caviar, 120, *120-121*
Thai chili peppers: Loup de Mer with Thai Chili Glaze Vinaigrette and Roasted Broccoli, 164, *165*
Thai Chili Glaze Vinaigrette, 164
Tomatillos, Roasted, Salsa, 214
Tomatoes. *See also* Cherry tomatoes; Roma tomatoes
Bloody Mary Gazpacho, 84, *85*
Chilled Avocado Soup with Roasted Corn Salsa, 80
Heirloom Tomato Provençal, 174
Marinara and Turkey Sausage Pizza, 189
Marinara Sauce, 135
Pico de Gallo, 155
Roasted Corn Salsa, 80
Romesco Sauce, 167
Texas Caviar, 120, *121*
Towers of Classic Meatballs with Marinara Sauce and Parmesan Polenta, 56-57
Veracruz Sauce, 170
Tom, May, 24
Tortillas, Crispy, 155
Towers of Classic Meatballs with Marinara Sauce and Parmesan Polenta, 56-57
Turkey
Marinara and, Sausage Pizza, 189
Turkey Burgers on Homemade Wheat Buns with Sweet Potato Fries and Almond Coleslaw, 190, *191,* 192
Tzatsiki Sauce: Grilled Chicken Kebabs with Garlic Flatbread, Tzatziki Sauce, and Greek Salad, 184

U

Unbleached white flour
Cal-a-Vie Pizza Three Ways, 186, *187*
Turkey Burgers on Homemade Wheat Buns with Sweet Potato Fries and Almond Coleslaw, 190, *191,* 192

V

Vanilla Champagne Vinaigrette, 104
Vanilla Cheesecake with Berry Compote, 252, 253
Vanilla-Honey Gastrique, 76, *77*
Vanilla Ice Cream, 273
Vanilla Panna Cotta with Citrus Gelée, 254, *255*
Veal stock: Red Wine Demi-Glace, 133
Vegetable stock
Carrot Coconut Soup, 86, *87*
Garden Pumpkin Soup with Goat Cheese Crema and Salted Pepitas, 88, *89*
Golden Lentil Soup, *90,* 91
Parsnip-Apple Soup, 94, *95*
Roasted Cauliflower Soup with Curry Oil, *96-97,* 98
Wild Rice, 170
Veracruz Sauce, 170
Vinaigrettes. *See also* Salad dressings
Banyuls Vinaigrette, 119
Champagne Vinaigrette, 124
Chili-Lime Vinaigrette, 107, 125
Citrus Vinaigrette, 116
Grapefruit Vinaigrette, *108,* 109, 124
Jalapeño Vinaigrette, 125
Kalamata Olive Vinaigrette, 125
Lemon-Lime Vinaigrette, 155
Orange Vinaigrette, 115, 125
Peanut Chili Vinaigrette, 71
Red Wine Vinaigrette, 184
Thai Chili Glaze Vinaigrette, 164
Vanilla Champagne Vinaigrette, 104
White Balsamic Vinaigrette, 124
Whole Grain Mustard Vinaigrette, 110

W

Waffles with Strawberry Sauce and Maple Syrup, 234, *235*
Walnuts, Candied, 115
Watermelon, Cucumber, and Tomato Skewers with Vanilla-Honey Gastrique, 78, *79*
Welcome Banana Muffins, *238,* 239
Whole Grain Mustard Vinaigrette, 110
Whole wheat pastry flour
Cal-a-Vie Pizza Three Ways, 186, *187*
Grilled Chicken Kebabs with Garlic Flatbread, Tzatziki Sauce, and Greek Salad, *182,* 183-185
Strawberry Rhubarb Streusel, 264, *265*
Turkey Burgers on Homemade Wheat Buns with Sweet Potato Fries and Almond Coleslaw, 190, *191,* 192
Wild rice, 170
Wine, 37, 38, *38, 39, 40, 41, 42. See also* Red wine tasting of, 161
Wonton, Baked, Strips, 107
Worful, Gina, 24

Y

Yams. *See* Sweet potatoes
Yeast. *See* Nutritionist yeast
Yellow bell peppers
Grilled Chicken Kebabs with Garlic Flatbread, Tzatziki Sauce, and Greek Salad, *182,* 183-185
Texas Caviar, 120, *121*
Yellow wax beans: Green and Yellow Bean Salad with Heirloom Tomatoes, Olive Tapenade, and Grapefruit Vinaigrette, *108,* 109
Yogurt. *See* Coconut yogurt; Greek yogurt
Spiced Yogurt, 179

Z

Zucchini
Skillet Zucchini and Corn, 167
Zucchini Muffins, 240
Zucchini Noodles, 14
Zumba, 28

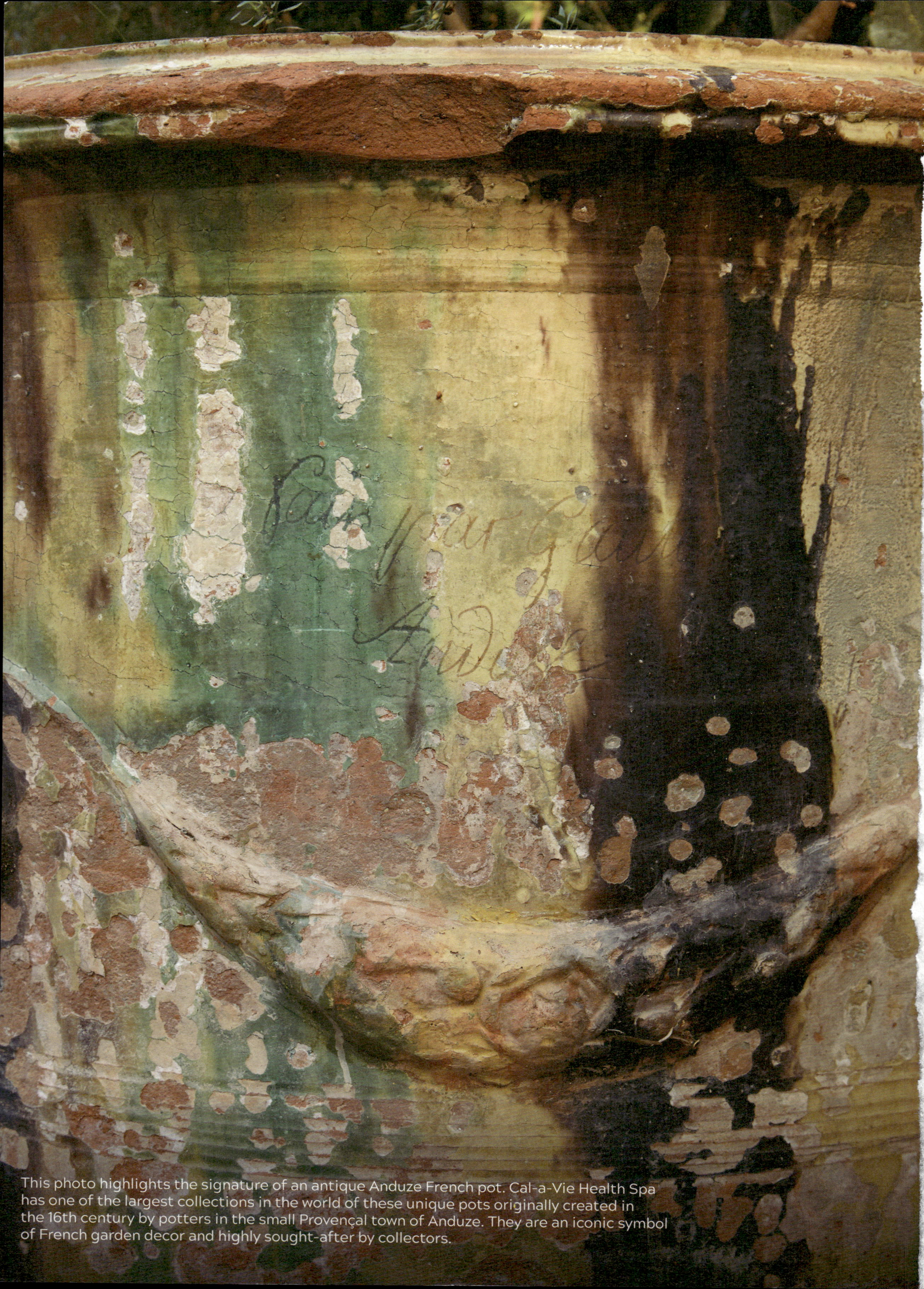

This photo highlights the signature of an antique Anduze French pot. Cal-a-Vie Health Spa has one of the largest collections in the world of these unique pots originally created in the 16th century by potters in the small Provençal town of Anduze. They are an iconic symbol of French garden decor and highly sought-after by collectors.

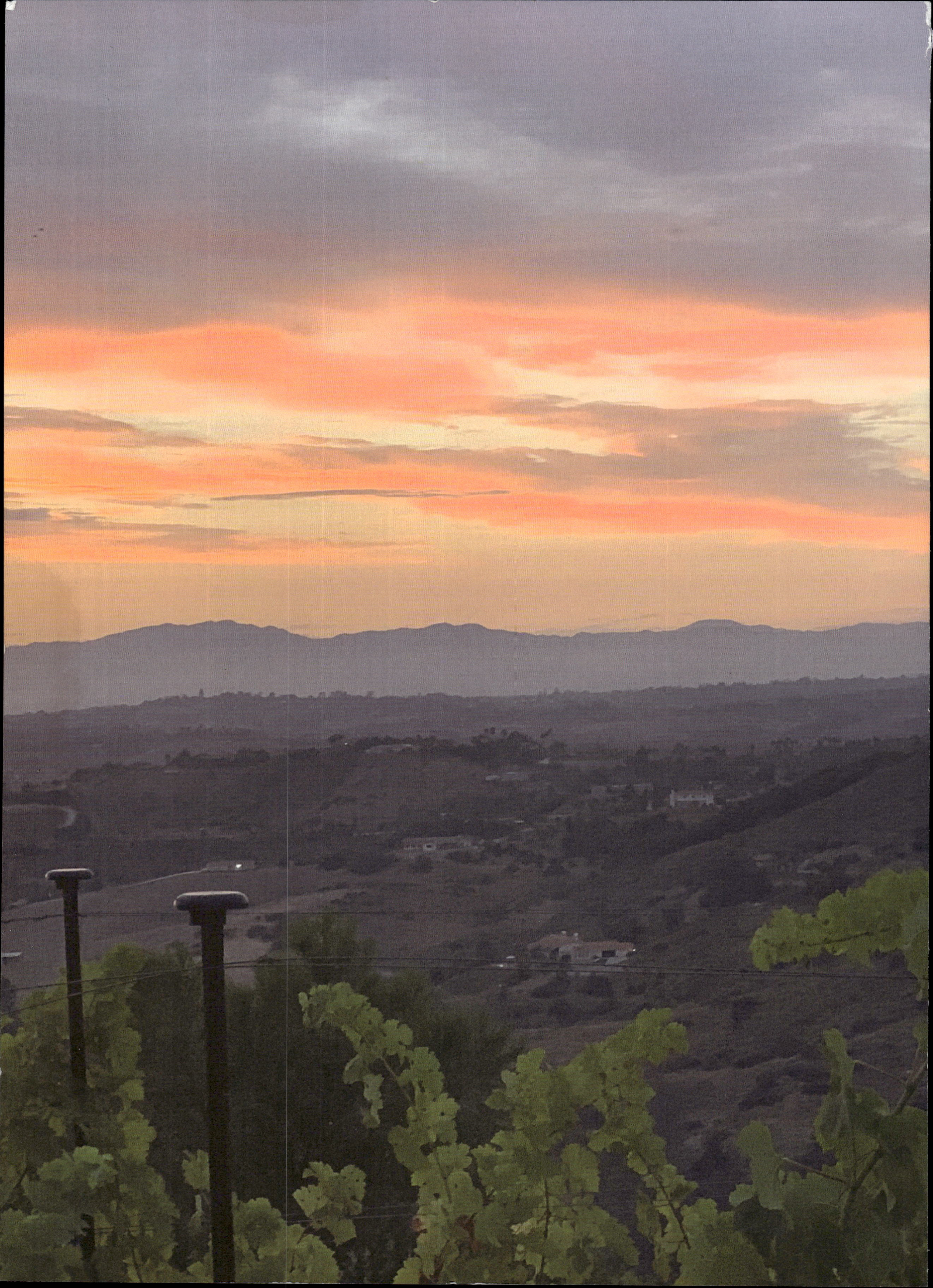